Emergency Medicine Pearls

Jill M. Baren, MD, FACEP, FAAP
Assistant Professor
Departments of Emergency Medicine and Pediatrics
University of Pennsylvania School of Medicine
Attending Physician
Division of Emergency Medicine
The Children's Hospital of Philadelphia
    and
Department of Emergency Medicine
Hospital of the University of Pennsylvania
Philadelphia, Pennsylvania

Elizabeth R. Alpern, MD, MSCE
Assistant Professor
Department of Pediatrics
University of Pennsylvania School of Medicine
    and
Attending Physician
Division of Emergency Medicine
The Children's Hospital of Philadelphia
Philadelphia, Pennsylvania

HANLEY & BELFUS
An Affiliate of Elsevier

HANLEY & BELFUS, INC.
An Affiliate of Elsevier

The Curtis Center
Independence Square West
Philadelphia, Pennsylvania 19106

Note to the reader: Although the techniques, ideas, and information in this book have been carefully reviewed for correctness, neither the authors nor the publisher can accept any legal responsibility for any errors or omissions that may be made. Neither the authors nor the publisher makes any guarantee, expressed or implied,with respect to the material contained herein.

Library of Congress Control Number: 2003107384

EMERGENCY MEDICINE PEARLS   ISBN 1-56053-575-X

Last digit is the print number: 9 8 7 6 5 4 3 2 1

CONTENTS

CONTRIBUTORS

Stephanie B. Abbuhl, MD
Medical Director and Associate Professor, Department of Emergency Medicine, University of Pennsylvania School of Medicine, Philadelphia, Pennsylvania

Evaline A. Alessandrini, MD, MSCE
Assistant Professor, Departments of Pediatrics, Emergency Medicine, and Epidemiology, University of Pennsylvania School of Medicine, Philadelphia; Attending Physician, Division of Emergency Medicine, The Children's Hospital of Philadelphia, Philadelphia, Pennsylvania

Elizabeth R. Alpern, MD, MSCE
Assistant Professor, Department of Pediatrics, University of Pennsylvania School of Medicine, Philadelphia; Attending Physician, Division of Emergency Medicine, The Children's Hospital of Philadelphia, Philadelphia, Pennsylvania

Charlene H. An, MD
Resident, Department of Emergency Medicine, Hospital of the University of Pennsylvania, Philadelphia, Pennsylvania

Paul A. Andrulonis, MD
Attending Physician, Department of Emergency Medicine, Pennsylvania Hospital, Philadelphia; Clinical Assistant Professor, Department of Emergency Medicine, University of Pennsylvania School of Medicine, Philadelphia, Pennsylvania

Roger Allen Band, MD
Resident, Department of Emergency Medicine, Hospital of the University of Pennsylvania, Philadelphia, Pennsylvania

Jill M. Baren, MD
Assistant Professor, Departments of Emergency Medicine and Pediatrics, University of Pennsylvania School of Medicine, Philadelphia; Attending Physician, Department of Pediatrics, Division of Emergency Medicine, The Children's Hospital of Philadelphia, and Department of Emergency Medicine, Hospital of the University of Pennsylvania, Philadelphia, Pennsylvania

Louis M. Bell, MD
Chief, Division of General Pediatrics, The Children's Hospital of Philadelphia, Philadelphia; Professor, Department of Pediatrics, University of Pennsylvania School of Medicine, Philadelphia, Pennsylvania

Hillary R. Bogner, MD, MSCE
Assistant Professor, Department of Family Practice and Community Medicine, University of Pennsylvania School of Medicine, Philadelphia; Attending Physician, Hospital of the University of Pennsylvania and Presbyterian Hospital, Philadelphia, Pennsylvania

Linda L. Brown, MD
Fellow, Division of Emergency Medicine, The Children's Hospital of Philadelphia, Philadelphia; Instructor, Department of Pediatrics, University of Pennsylvania School of Medicine, Philadelphia, Pennsylvania

Elizabeth A. Bushra, MD
Assistant Clinical Professor, Department of Emergency Medicine, University of Pennsylvania School of Medicine, Philadelphia, Pennsylvania

Joseph S. Bushra, MD
Assistant Professor, Department of Emergency Medicine, Temple University School of Medicine, Philadelphia, Pennsylvania

Diane P. Calello, MD
Fellow, Department of Pediatrics, Division of Emergency Medicine, The Children's Hospital of Philadelphia, Philadelphia, Pennsylvania

Brendan G. Carr, MD, MA
Resident, Department of Emergency Medicine, Hospital of the University of Pennsylvania, Philadelphia, Pennsylvania

Esther H. Chen, MD
Instructor, Department of Emergency Medicine, University of Pennsylvania School of Medicine, Philadelphia, Pennsylvania

Robert Louis Cloutier, MD
Assistant Professor, Department of Emergency Medicine, Oregon Health and Science University, Portland; Adjunct Assistant Professor, Department of Pediatrics, Doernbecher Children's Hospital, Portland, Oregon

Lauren P. Daly, MD
Instructor, Department of Pediatrics, University of Pennsylvania School of Medicine, Philadelphia; Fellow, Division of Emergency Medicine, The Children's Hospital of Philadelphia, Philadelphia, Pennsylvania

Elizabeth M. Datner, MD
Assistant Professor, Department of Emergency Medicine, Hospital of the University of Pennsylvania, Philadelphia, Pennsylvania

Reza J. Daugherty, MD
Fellow, Division of Emergency Medicine, The Children's Hospital of Philadelphia, Philadelphia, Pennsylvania

Anthony J. Dean, MD
Assistant Professor, Department of Emergency Medicine, University of Pennsylvania School of Medicine, Philadelphia; Attending Physician, Department of Emergency Medicine, University of Pennsylvania Medical Center, Philadelphia, Pennsylvania

Francis Jerome DeRoos, MD
Program Director and Assistant Professor, Department of Emergency Medicine, Division of Clinical Toxicology, Hospital of the University of Pennsylvania, Philadelphia, Pennsylvania

Edward T. Dickinson, MD
Assistant Professor and Director of EMS Field Operations, Department of Emergency Medicine, Hospital of the University of Pennsylvania, Philadelphia, Pennsylvania

Aaron Donoghue, MD
Fellow, Department of Critical Care Medicine, Division of Emergency Medicine, The Children's Hospital of Philadelphia, Philadelphia, Pennsylvania

Ugo A. Ezenkwele, MD, MPH
Clinical Instructor, Department of Emergency Medicine, New York University/Bellevue Hospital Center, New York, New York

Worth W. Everett, MD
Clinical Instructor, Department of Emergency Medicine, University of Pennsylvania School of Medicine, Philadelphia, Pennsylvania

M. Bradley Falk, MD
Resident, Department of Emergency Medicine, Hospital of the University of Pennsylvania, Philadelphia, Pennsylvania

Joel A. Fein, MD
Associate Professor, Department of Pediatrics, University of Pennsylvania School of Medicine, Philadelphia; Attending Physician, Division of Emergency Medicine, The Children's Hospital of Philadelphia, Philadelphia, Pennsylvania

Eron Friedlaender, MD
Instructor, Department of Pediatrics, University of Pennsylvania School of Medicine, Philadelphia; Attending Physician, Division of Emergency Medicine, The Children's Hospital of Philadelphia, Philadelphia, Pennsylvania

Howard A. Greller, MD
Fellow, Medical Toxicology, Division of Emergency Medicine, Bellevue/New York University Medical Center, New York, New York

Kevin Hardy, MD
Assistant Professor, Department of Emergency Medicine, University of Pennsylvania School of Medicine, Philadelphia, Pennsylvania

Judd E. Hollander, MD
Professor, Department of Emergency Medicine, and Clinical Research Director, University of Pennsylvania School of Medicine, Philadelphia, Pennsylvania

Marilyn V. Howarth, MD
Assistant Professor, Department of Emergency Medicine, Division of Occupational Medicine, University of Pennsylvania School of Medicine, Philadelphia; Director, Occupational and Environmental Consultation Services, Hospital of the University of Pennsylvania, Philadelphia, Pennsylvania

Vivian Hwang, MD
Fellow and Clinical Instructor in Pediatrics, Division of Emergency Medicine, The Children's Hospital of Philadelphia, Philadelphia; Attending Physician, Department of Emergency Medicine, Hospital of the University of Pennsylvania, Philadelphia, Pennsylvania

Paul Ishimine, MD
Assistant Professor, Departments of Pediatrics and Medicine, University of California School of Medicine, San Diego; Attending Physician, Department of Emergency Medicine, Children's Hospital and Health Center, and UCSD Medical Center, San Diego, California

Cynthia Jacobstein, MD
Assistant Professor, Department of Pediatrics, University of Pennsylvania School of Medicine, Philadelphia; Attending Physician, Department of Pediatrics, Division of Emergency Medicine, The Children's Hospital of Philadelphia, Philadelphia, Pennsylvania

Russell J. Karten, MD
Clinical Assistant Professor, Department of Emergency Medicine, University of Pennsylvania School of Medicine, Philadelphia, Pennsylvania

Allyson A. Kreshak, MD
Resident, Department of Emergency Medicine, Hospital of the University of Pennsylvania, Philadelphia, Pennsylvania

Paul Y. Ko, MD
Resident, Department of Emergency Medicine, Hospital of the University of Pennsylvania, Philadelphia, Pennsylvania

Steven Larsen, MD
Associate Professor, Department of Emergency Medicine, University of Pennsylvania School of Medicine, Philadelphia, Pennsylvania

Jane M. Lavelle, MD
Associate Director, Department of Pediatrics, Division of Emergency Medicine, The Children's Hospital of Philadelphia, Philadelphia; Associate Professor, Department of Pediatrics, University of Pennsylvania School of Medicine, Philadelphia, Pennsylvania

Thomas Joseph Lydon, MD, PhD
Resident, Department of Emergency Medicine, Hospital of the University of Pennsylvania, Philadelphia, Pennsylvania

Rex Mathew, MD
Resident, Department of Emergency Medicine, Hospital of the University of Pennsylvania, Philadelphia, Pennsylvania

C. Crawford Mechem, MD
Associate Professor, Department of Emergency Medicine, University of Pennsylvania School of Medicine, Philadelphia; Director, Emergency Medical Services, Philadelphia Fire Department, Philadelphia, Pennsylvania

Sumeru G. Mehta, MD, MPH
Resident, Department of Emergency Medicine, Hospital of the University of Pennsylvania, Philadelphia, Pennsylvania

Zachary F. Meisel, MD, MPH
Chief Resident, Department of Emergency Medicine, Hospital of the University of Pennsylvania, Philadelphia, Pennsylvania

Angela M. Mills, MD
Resident and Lecturer, Department of Emergency Medicine, University of Pennsylvania School of Medicine, Philadelphia, Pennsylvania

Cynthia J. Mollen, MD, MSCE
Assistant Professor, Department of Pediatrics, University of Pennsylvania School of Medicine, Philadelphia; Attending Physician, Division of Emergency Medicine, The Children's Hospital of Philadelphia, Philadelphia, Pennsylvania

Frances M. Nadel, MD
Assistant Professor, Department of Pediatrics, Division of Emergency Medicine, University of Pennsylvania School of Medicine, Philadelphia; Attending Physician, The Children's Hospital of Philadelphia, Philadelphia, Pennsylvania

Karen O'Connell, MD
Fellow, Department of Emergency Medicine, The Children's Hospital of Philadelphia, Philadelphia; Clinical Instructor, University of Pennsylvania School of Medicine, Philadelphia, Pennsylvania

Kevin C. Osterhoudt, MD
Assistant Professor, Department of Pediatrics, University of Pennsylvania School of Medicine, Philadelphia; Attending Physician, Department of Pediatrics, Division of Emergency Medicine, The Children's Hospital of Philadelphia, Philadelphia; Associate Medical Director, The Poison Control Center, Philadelphia, Pennsylvania

Chirag Patel, MD
Resident, Department of Emergency Medicine, Hospital of the University of Pennsylvania, Philadelphia, Pennsylvania

Y. Veronica Pei, MD, MEd
Resident, Department of Emergency Medicine, University of Pennsylvania Medical Center, Philadelphia, Pennsylvania

Charles V. Pollack, Jr, MD, MA
Chair, Department of Emergency Medicine, Pennsylvania Hospital, Philadelphia; Associate Professor, Department of Emergency Medicine, University of Pennsylvania School of Medicine, Philadelphia, Pennsylvania

Stefanie Porges, MD
Assistant Clinical Professor, Department of Emergency Medicine, University of Pennsylvania School of Medicine, Philadelphia, Pennsylvania

Jill C. Posner, MD
Assistant Professor, Department of Pediatrics, University of Pennsylvania School of Medicine, Philadelphia; Attending Physician, Division of Emergency Medicine, The Children's Hospital of Philadelphia, Philadelphia, Pennsylvania

John Pryor, MD
Assistant Professor, Department of Surgery, University of Pennsylvania School of Medicine, Philadelphia, Pennsylvania

Amy L. Puchalski, MD
Fellow, Department of Pediatrics, Division of Emergency Medicine, The Children's Hospital of Philadelphia; Instructor, Department of Pediatrics, University of Pennsylvania School of Medicine, Philadelphia, Pennsylvania

Anthony W. Rekito, MD
Resident, Department of Emergency Medicine, University of Pennsylvania Health System, Philadelphia, Pennsylvania

Iris M. Reyes, MD, FACEP
Assistant Professor, Department of Emergency Medicine, University of Pennsylvania School of Medicine, Philadelphia; Associate Medical Director, Department of Emergency Medicine, Hospital of the University of Pennsylvania, Philadelphia, Pennsylvania

Bruce D. Rubin, MD
Clinical Instructor, Department of Emergency Medicine, Hospital of the University of Pennsylvania, Philadelphia, Pennsylvania

Richard J. Scarfone, MD
Assistant Professor, Department of Pediatrics, University of Pennsylvania School of Medicine, Philadelphia; Attending Physician, Division of Emergency Medicine, The Children's Hospital of Philadelphia, Philadelphia, Pennsylvania

Sandra Schwab, MD
Resident, Department of Pediatrics, The Children's Hospital of Philadelphia, Philadelphia, Pennsylvania

Todd C. Severson, MD
Resident, Department of Emergency Medicine, Hospital of the University of Pennsylvania, Philadelphia, Pennsylvania

Purvi D. Shah, MD
Resident, Department of Emergency Medicine, Hospital of the University of Pennsylvania, Philadelphia, Pennsylvania

Kathy N. Shaw, MD, MSCE
Professor, Department of Pediatrics, University of Pennsylvania School of Medicine, Philadelphia; Chief, Division of Emergency Medicine, The Children's Hospital of Philadelphia, Philadelphia, Pennsylvania

Suzanne Moore Shepherd, MD, DTM&H
Associate Professor, Department of Emergency Medicine, Hospital of the University of Pennsylvania, and Director of Education and Research, PENN Travel Medicine, Philadelphia, Pennsylvania

William H. Shoff, MD, DTM&H
Associate Professor, Department of Emergency Medicine, University of Pennsylvania Health System, and Director, PENN Travel Medicine, Philadelphia, Pennsylvania

Allison R. Silver, MD
Clinical Assistant Professor, Department of Emergency Medicine, University of Pennsylvania School of Medicine, Philadelphia; Attending Physician, University of Pennsylvania Health System, Philadelphia, Pennsylvania

Philip R. Spandorfer, MD
Assistant Professor, Department of Pediatrics, Division of Emergency Medicine, University of Pennsylvania School of Medicine, Philadelphia; Attending Physician, Division of Emergency Medicine, The Children's Hospital of Philadelphia, Philadelphia, Pennsylvania

Nancy N. Sun, MD
Chief Resident, Department of Emergency Medicine, Hospital of the University of Pennsylvania, Philadelphia, Pennsylvania

Kevin M. Takakuwa, MD
Resident, Department of Emergency Medicine, Hospital of the University of Pennsylvania, Philadelphia, Pennsylvania

George A. Woodward, MD, MBA
Associate Professor, Department of Pediatrics, Division of Emergency Medicine, University of Pennsylvania School of Medicine, Philadelphia; Medical Director, Transport Services, The Children's Hospital of Philadelphia, Philadelphia, Pennsylvania

Joseph J. Zorc, MD
Assistant Professor, Departments of Pediatrics and Emergency Medicine, University of Pennsylvania School of Medicine, Philadelphia; Attending Physician, The Children's Hospital of Philadelphia, Philadelphia, Pennsylvania

PREFACE

Emergency Medicine Pearls is the result of a collaboration between Emergency Medicine Physicians at the University of Pennsylvania and its affiliated hospitals: The Hospital of the University of Pennsylvania, The Children's Hospital of Philadelphia, Presbyterian Medical Center, and Pennsylvania Hospital. Each author has been a resident, fellow, attending physician, or faculty member in our collective organization at some point in time, and thus has experienced and benefited from the remarkable teaching and learning that takes place in our institutions. We are proud to produce a book that reflects the collegial nature of our daily practice and scholarly activity.

Patients requiring the services of emergency medicine bring us many surprises as well as predictable problems. Our approach to problem solving addresses the dual need to recognize common illnesses and injuries while always being prepared to face the unexpected. This book reflects such an approach and we hope is representative of the challenges inherent in the care of emergency patients.

We are especially appreciative of the contributions from our residents and fellows and the time and effort on the part of the many faculty participants. They stimulate all of us to do our best as teachers. Our emergency medicine and pediatric emergency medicine mentors have made invaluable contributions to our knowledge, and this effort is a small way to perpetuate their dedication and wisdom.

Jill M. Baren, MD
Elizabeth R. Alpern, MD
EDITORS

ACKNOWLEDGMENT

We gratefully acknowledge the assistance of Jacqueline Mahon who knew exactly how to keep us on track and provided excellent technical expertise for the project.

We also thank the patients who have allowed us to cultivate the "pearls" of emergency medicine, for without them and their trust in our care, this book could never have been written.

Dedication

To my parents for their love and encouragement, which allowed me to learn and achieve.
To my husband for his love, support, and understanding, which allow me to succeed.
To my children for their love and acceptance, which allow me to be happy.
To a special friend, who inspires me to live and work with passion. ~ JMB

To my husband for his patience, insight, and love; all of which give me strength and peace.
To my family for their love and support, as well as for teaching me that the quest for knowledge and wisdom mark the path. ~ ERA

Roger A. Band, MD
Worth Everett, MD

PATIENT 1

A 54-year-old man with a distended, tender abdomen

A 55-year-old man with a history of alcoholic liver disease and hepatitis C presents for evaluation of progressive abdominal distention, dyspnea, abdominal pain, and fever. He denies any other symptoms. He admits to occasional noncompliance with his medications, which include lactulose, spironolactone, and furosemide.

Physical Examination: Temperature 38.5°C; pulse 110; respirations 22; blood pressure 133/52. General: appears uncomfortable. Skin: warm, no diaphoresis, multiple spider angiomas. HEENT: icteric sclera, dry mucous membranes. Cardiac: regular tachycardia without murmurs or gallops. Chest: shallow breaths, decreased to auscultation bilaterally. Abdomen: distended, protuberent abdomen with caput medusae, distant but present bowel sounds, moderate diffuse tenderness, fluid wave present (see figure). Extremities: bilateral lower extremity edema to the knee without cyanosis, 2+ symmetric radial and femoral pulses. Digital rectal examination: normal. Neurologic: awake, alert, no asterixis.

Laboratory Findings: CBC: WBC 11,900/μl, hemoglobin 12.7 g/dL, platelets 528,000/μl. Blood chemistries: normal. Coagulation profile: prothrombin time 13.9, INR 1.4. LFTs: elevated total bilirubin of 3.0 mg/dL. Chest x-ray: poor inspiratory effort, bibasilar atelectasis. Ascites fluid analysis: WBC 820/μl (42% PMNs), RBC 544/μl. Ultrasound: see figure.

Questions: This patient with known cirrhosis and abdominal pain is at risk for what potentially fatal disease? What diagnostic procedure is essential in this setting? What are the key management issues regarding this patient?

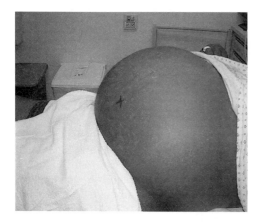 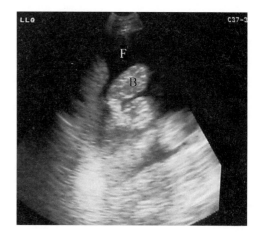

Diagnosis and Treatment: Spontaneous bacterial peritonitis (SBP). Following diagnostic paracentesis, early and aggressive broad-spectrum antibiotic coverage should be initiated. All patients should be hospitalized for intravenous antibiotics while blood and ascites fluid cultures are monitored to identify the causitive organism(s).

Discussion: SBP is a condition defined by infection of ascites fluid in the absence of other identifiable infectious sources within the peritoneum or adjacent tissues. The mortality rate of a single episode of SBP has been estimated at 20–40%, even with aggressive therapy. Among cirrhotic patients with ascites, the incidence of SBP is 10–35%. Estimated 1-year survival rates after a first episode of SBP are 30–50%. The high mortality rate of this disease reflects the fact that it is a condition that can easily be overlooked, particularly when it occurs in the setting of other serious conditions such as gastrointestinal bleeding, hepatorenal syndrome, and hepatic failure.

Although the exact mechanisms are still speculative, the pathogenesis of SBP is a multifactorial process that includes translocation of native bowel flora, a compromised hepatic reticuloendothelial system, and an impaired ability for both microbial compliment activation and opsonization in the ascites fluid. Translocation is further facilitated by portal hypertension with subsequent bowel wall edema and microbial overgrowth from slowed intestinal motility. Gram-negative enteric organisms are the most common isolates, with *Escherichia coli* and *Klebsiella pneumoniae* being the most prevalent. However, owing to the increased frequency of abdominal instrumentation and expanded use of antibiotic prophylaxis, gram-positive (*Streptococcus pneumoniae*) and multiple-drug-resistant organisms have emerged over the last 15 years.

SBP is an entity most commonly seen in patients with advanced liver disease. Patients typically complain of abdominal pain, either acute or insidious in onset, associated with signs of peritoneal irritation, fever, chills, hemodynamic instability, or all of the above. The presenting symptoms can also be subtle, thus requiring clinicians to be vigilant in maintaining a high index of suspicion for the disease. In an estimated 10% of SBP cases, the patients are asymptomatic. Although patients with cirrhosis are predisposed to develop SBP, the diagnosis should be considered in any patient with ascites (e.g., secondary to congestive heart failure, nephrotic syndrome, mixed connective tissue disease).

Examining the ascites fluid is essential to diagnosing SBP. A diagnostic paracentesis should be performed in the following instances: all cases of new-onset ascites, patients with ascites and symptoms suggestive of SBP, and patients with known liver disease with a sudden change in mental status. A paracentesis can also relieve pain by reducing pressure on the abdominal wall. Although most patients with ascites have various degrees of liver impairment, clinicians should not delay a diagnostic paracentesis while waiting for coagulation profile results. Rates of coagulopathy-associated paracentsis complications are less than 1%.

Ascites fluid should be sent for culture and blood cell count. Injection of 10 ml of ascites fluid into each standard blood culture bottle increases culture yield by 90%. Early diagnosis of SBP relies on the initial findings, with an emphasis on the polymorphonuclear (PMN) component of the cell count. In general, a PMN count of greater than 250 cells/μl is considered highly suggestive for SPB and the level at which empiric therapy for SBP should be started. A PMN count of greater than 500 cells/μl is the best overall predictor of SBP. Assessing other components of the ascites fluid (protein, glucose, pH, etc.) in the emergency department setting adds little to decisions regarding therapeutic choices. Secondary SBP should be considered in patients with cultures that are positive for more than one organism or who fail to respond to standard antimicrobal therapy. Abdominal surgery, recent abdominal instrumentation, or a perforated viscus are common precedents of secondary SBP.

Management of SBP involves early diagnosis and intravenous antibiotics. Antibiotic selection should be broad enough to cover gram-negative and gram-positive organisms. Cefotaxime is the most extensively studied agent, but a combination of penicillin and a sulfa drug or clavulanic acid, or a fluoroquinolone have similar efficacy. Initial treatment should be administered intravenously. Nephrotoxic medications such as aminoglycosides are not considered appropriate choices to treat SBP. Recent studies have suggested that albumin infusion may decrease the incidence of renal failure and improve mortality in the setting of SBP, although this remains unproven in any large-scale trials.

The present patient had an obvious protuberant abdomen. Bedside ultrasonography was used to identify and mark a pocket of ascites fluid (see *F* in figure; *B* = bowel). Ultrasonography is a valuable asset to identify small or loculated fluid collections and to avoid unnecessary complications such as bowel perforation. The patient was started on a course of intravenous cefotaxime with improvement in his symptoms. He remained stable through-out his stay in the emergency department and in the hospital. Ascites fluid cultures grew *Escherichia* *coli*. The patient was discharged home 5 days later and scheduled for a transjugular intrahepatic portosystemic shunt (TIPS) procedure as an outpatient.

Clinical Pearls

1. The diagnosis of SBP should be considered in patients with new-onset ascites; in patients with known ascites with abdominal pain, fever, chills, or hypotension; and in patients with known liver failure and changes in mental status.

2. The mortality rate of a single episode of SBP is between 20 and 40%.

3. Ascites fluid analysis and culture are essential to establishing the diagnosis, but treatment is based on preliminary cell count results in the emergency department.

REFERENCES

1. Navasa FJ, Gomez J, Colmenero J, Vila J, Arroyo V, Rodes J: Bacterial infections in cirrhosis: Epidemiological changes with invasive procedures and norfloxacin prophylaxis. Hepatology 35:140–148, 2002.
2. Mowat C, Stanley AJ: Review article: Spontaneous bacterial peritonitis—diagnosis, treatment and prevention. Aliment Pharmacol Ther 15:1851–1859, 2001.
3. Sort P, Navasa M, Arroyo V, et al: Effect of intravenous albumin on renal impairment and mortality in patients with cirrhosis and spontaneous bacterial peritonitis. N Engl J Med 341:403–409, 1999.
4. Dupeyron C, Campillo B, Mangeney N, et al: Changes in nature and antibiotic resistance of bacteria causing peritonitis in cirrhotic patients over a 20 year period. J Clin Pathol 51:614–616, 1998.
5. Garcia-Tsao G: Spontaneous bacterial peritonitis. Gastroenterol Clin North Am 21:257–275, 1992.
6. Runyon BA, Canawati HN, Akriviadis EA: Optimisation of ascitic fluid culture technique. Gastroenterology 95:1351–1355, 1988.

PATIENT 2

A 26-month-old boy with fever and decreased activity

A previously healthy 26-month-old boy is brought to the emergency department by his mother and father. They state that he has had a tactile fever for 1½ days with decreased activity and oral intake over the past 12–18 hours. He has had rhinorrhea and has been crying more often than usual. He has not had any vomiting, diarrhea, or cough. There are sick contacts at his home and day-care site. His parents have been treating his fever with acetaminophen, but he has not had any other prescribed or over-the-counter medications. His urine output is slightly less than normal for him. He has not had any rashes noted.

Physical Examination: Vital signs: temperature 38.4°C rectally; pulse 218; respiratory rate 42; blood pressure 95/53. General: well-nourished and developed child lying quietly in the bed. HEENT: eyes open spontaneously, PERRL (pupils equal, round, reactive to light), crusted nasal discharge, dry lips and tacky mucous membranes, pearly tympanic membranes bilaterally. Chest: clear to auscultation. Cardiac: regularly tachycardiac. Abdomen: bowel sounds present, soft, nontender, nondistended abdomen, liver palpable 2 cm below right costal margin. Extremities: warm, 3-second capillary refill.

Laboratory/Radiographic Findings: Hemoglobin 12.3 g/dl, WBC 9200/μl, platelets 245,000/μl. Electrolytes within normal limits. Electrocardiogram: see figure. Chest x-ray: no infiltrates, normal heart size.

Question: What is the most likely diagnosis?

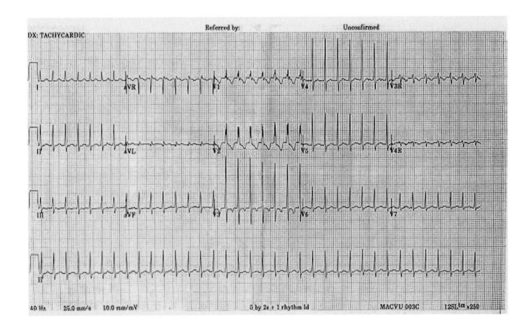

Diagnosis: Supraventricular tachycardia

Discussion: Supraventricular tachycardias (SVT) are the most frequent form of pediatric arrhythmias, with an incidence of 0.1–0.4%. More than 60% of initial presentations of SVT occur in infants within the first year of life and an additional 20% in children 1–5 years of age. Although most children with SVT have a structurally normal heart, up to one quarter may have associated congenital anomalies. Fever, infections, and drug exposures (antihistamines, caffeine, phenothiazines) are associated with SVT.

There are two mechanisms, reentrant circuits and automatic tachycardias, that cause SVT in children. Reentrant circuits account for the vast majority of cases (>80%). In these cases, an accessory pathway conducts electrical current between the atrium and ventricles. In sinus rhythm, if the conduction is from the atrium to the ventricle, a pre-excited area of ventricle may be represented by a delta wave on ECG. This is typical of Wolff-Parkinson-White syndrome. If the accessory pathway conducts from the ventricle to the atrium, this may not be detected on ECG.

During tachycardias, the electrical impulse may be conducted antegrade through the AV node and retrograde through the accessory pathway (orthodromic) or antegrade through the accessory pathway and retrograde through the AV node (antedromic). Orthodromic conduction is more common. Although rare, if atrial flutter or fibrillation is present, reentrant pathways may allow for ventricular fibrillation, resulting in syncope or sudden death.

The other main mechanism for pediatric SVT is enhanced automaticity from abnormal foci. These resultant tachycardias are named by the area of ectopic foci, as atrial ectopic or junctional ectopic tachycardia.

SVT episodes in preverbal children are especially difficult to detect and may go on for a prolonged period of time prior to medical attention. The nonspecific symptoms of lethargy or irritability may be mistaken for sepsis, toxic ingestion, or respiratory distress. Cardiovascular decompensation may occur if the dysrhythmia is sustained over a prolonged period of time. A high index of suspicion must be maintained to correctly recognize SVT in the young child. If vital signs are appropriately checked during the physical examination, the cause of the symptoms will become evident. SVT is defined by a heart rate >180 beats/min in children and >220 beats/min in infants. Dehydration, fever, or crying may momentarily raise a child's heart rate into the above ranges, but sinus tachycardia as associated with these states will be more variable than true SVT and will decrease as the child quiets or the fever is treated with an antipyretic. A full 12-lead ECG should be obtained if SVT is considered. P-waves are usually not discernable or, if present, have an abnormal axis. The QRS complex is most often narrow.

Treatment of SVT depends on the clinical status of the patient. If the child has a stable cardiovascular state, vagal maneuvers or an ice bag applied to the face may be attempted to break the SVT. Ice to the face, coughing, or other Valsalva maneuvers will slow atrioventricular (AV) node conduction and may terminate the arrhythmia. Rapid intravenous push of adenosine (0.1 mg/kg/dose) followed by rapid saline flush is the drug of first choice for terminating SVT. Administration results in transient AV node block. The successful cardioversion rate of SVT in pediatric patients with adenosine is >70%. If the initial administration is not successful, the dose may doubled and repeated up to 0.3 mg/kg or the adult dose of 6–12 mg. Side effects of flushing, vomiting, dyspnea, or bradycardia may be associated with its administration.

If the child is hemodynamically unstable, synchronized cardioversion with 0.5–1 J/kg is indicated. Once the arrhythmia has resolved, very young children are started on digitalis to prevent recurrence. Verapamil should be avoided in young children, as it is associated with hypotension, cardiovascular collapse, and even death.

In the present patient, as an intravenous catheter was being inserted, the child spontaneously converted from a heart rate of 215 to 145. He began crying loudly and became increasing active in the few minutes following the intravenous catheter placement. Cardiology was consulted and the patient was admitted to the hospital for further evaluation.

Clinical Pearls

1. SVT may be brought on by sympathomimetics in over-the-counter cough/cold preparations, fever, or infection.

2. In young children, SVT may be associated with vague, nonspecific symptoms.

3. Adenosine is the drug of first choice for children with hemodynamically stable SVT that does not respond to vagal maneuvers.

4. Cardioversion at 0.5–1 J/kg is indicated in cases of imminent or existing cardiovascular collapse.

REFERENCES

1. Bauersfeld R, Pfammatter JP, Jeaggi E: Treatment of supraventricular tachycardia in the new millenium: Drugs or radiofrequency catheter ablation? Eur J Pediatr 160:1–9, 2001.
2. Gewitz MH, Vetter VL: Cardiac emergencies. In Fleisher GR, Ludwig S (eds): Textbook of Pediatric Emergency Medicine, 4th ed. Philadelphia, Lippincott Williams & Wilkins, 2000, pp 676–681.
3. Ethridge SP, Judd VE: Supraventricular tachycardia in infancy: Evaluation, management, and follow-up. Arch Pediatr Adolesc Med 153:267–271, 1999.
4. Losek JD, Endom E, Dietrich A, et al: Adenosine and pediatric supraventricular tachycardia in the emergency department: Multicenter study and review. Ann Emerg Med 33:185–191, 1999.
5. Chameides L, Hazinski MF (eds): Pediatric Advanced Life Support. Dallas, American Heart Association, 1997.

PATIENT 3

A 29-year-old woman with left shoulder pain

A 29-year-old woman with a past medical history significant for anemia and recent elective abortion presents to the emergency department complaining of left shoulder pain. She has a 1-week history of fever, chills, myalgias, and malaise. Ibuprofen has provided pain relief. Over the last 4 days, she noted left shoulder stiffness that rapidly progressed to severe pain and immobility. Her primary care physician diagnosed a viral illness. The patient also reports mild diarrhea and nasal congestion but denies other symptoms. She has never used intravenous drugs.

Physical Examination: Temperature 39°C; pulse 130; respirations 20; blood pressure 112/66. HEENT: no nasal discharge, no erythema of the throat, no tonsillar enlargement. Neck: supple, no lymphadenopathy. Heart: regular tachycardia, no murmurs, rubs, or gallops. Lungs: normal. Abdomen: normal. Extremities: left shoulder—diffuse tenderness and decreased range of motion; no erythema, warmth, or swelling; pulses normal; all other joints normal. Skin: no rashes or petechiae. Genitalia: scant brown vaginal discharge, otherwise normal. Rectal: normal. Neurologic: normal.

Laboratory Findings: CBC: WBC 8300/μl (88% neutrophils, 9% lymphocytes), Hgb 8.9 g/dl, Hct 26.6; normal platelets. Blood chemistries: normal. Urinalysis: normal. Left shoulder synovial fluid: WBC 56,000/μL (98% neutrophils, 1% lymphocytes), RBC 22,000/μL. Gram stain: rare gram-positive cocci. Blood and synovial fluid cultures: pending. Cervical cultures: pending. Left shoulder radiograph: normal.

Questions: What is the most likely cause for this patient's symptoms? What therapy should be initiated immediately?

Diagnosis and Treatment: Septic arthritis. Initial therapy should include immediate intravenous antibiotics and orthopedic consultation.

Discussion: Septic arthritis is an orthopedic emergency requiring prompt treatment. The most common causative agent in an adult is *Staphylococcus aureus,* but *Streptococcus* species, *Neisseria gonorrhoeae,* and *Haemophilus* species are also prevalent. Infectious arthritis may result from hematogenous spread, adjacent soft tissue or bony infection, direct inoculation, or postoperative contamination. In the present case, the causative agent was group B beta-hemolytic *Streptococcus (S. agalactiae),* most likely spread hematogenously during her elective abortion.

Septic arthritis usually affects one joint, but gonococcal arthritis is often polyarticular in nature. The most commonly affected joints, in decreasing order of involvement, are the knee, hip, shoulder, ankle, wrist, and elbow. Typical clinical findings include fever, tenderness, decreased range of motion, effusion, erythema, and warmth. Rheumatologic conditions such as gout may mimic septic arthritis, and synovial fluid analysis may be similar as well. Patients at risk for septic arthritis include the immunocompromised, those with chronic disease, intravenous drug users, those with previous rheumatologic disease, and patients with prosthetic joints.

Evaluation of a patient with suspected septic arthritis should include a careful history and physical examination. Special attention should be paid to behaviors or recent procedures that may place the patient at risk. Routine laboratory tests—CBC and blood chemistries—should be obtained, and arthrocentesis should be performed. A synovial fluid WBC count greater than 50,000/μl strongly suggests septic arthritis (see table). A Gram stain and culture of joint fluid (including gonococcal culture), blood cultures, and a radiograph of the affected joint should be obtained. Ultrasonography, MRI, and serologic markers for rheumatoid conditions are additional tests that may be helpful. Empiric antibiotic therapy should cover *Staphylococcus* and *Streptococcus* species (nafcillin or vancomycin) and *Neisseria gonorrhoeae* if clinically indicated (ceftriaxone). Prompt orthopedic consultation should be obtained, as many patients will require open drainage in the operating room.

The present patient was treated with intravenous antibiotics, and blood and synovial cultures grew group B *Streptococcus.* The patient underwent three additional arthrocenteses and ultimately required arthroscopic surgery. Incision and drainage were successfully performed; biopsies of the adjacent cartilage also grew *Streptococcus.* The patient received 4 weeks of intravenous penicillin G with good clinical results.

Synovial Fluid Analysis

	NORMAL	NONINFLAMMATORY	INFLAMMATORY	SEPTIC
Gross Appearance	Clear	Clear	Turbid	Turbid
WBC/μl	<200	<2000	2000–50,000	>50,000
%PMNs	<25	<25	>50	>75
Glucose (% serum)	>95	>95	75–100	<50
Culture	Negative	Negative	Negative	Usually positive
Examples	N/A	Degenerative joint disease, trauma	Gout, pseudogout, rheumatoid arthritis, Lyme disease	*Staphylococcus, Streptococcus, Gonococcus*

Clinical Pearls

1. Delays in diagnosis and treatment of septic arthritis may lead to permanent joint damage, osteomyelitis, sepsis, or death.

2. Early in the course of the illness, plain radiographs are likely to be normal.

3. Arthrocentesis with Gram stain and culture should be performed in any patient with clinical suspicion for septic arthritis. A joint fluid WBC count of $>50,000/\mu l$ makes the diagnosis likely.

4. Immediately begin intravenous antibiotics for suspected septic arthritis and obtain orthopedic consultation.

5. Maintain high clinical suspicion for septic arthritis in the elderly, patients with recent surgery, penetrating trauma, intravenous drug use, immunocompromised hosts, or those with underlying medical or rheumatologic conditions.

REFERENCES

1. Munoz G: Septic Arthritis (on-line). eMedicine. Orthopedic Surgery. Accessed 2003 at http://www.emedicine.com.
2. Brusch JL: Septic Arthritis (on-line). eMedicine. Medicine, Ob/Gyn, Psychiatry, and Surgery. Accessed 2002 at http://www.emedicine.com.
3. Onadeko O, Parsh B, Scott J, Wilson D: Index of suspicion. Case 3. Diagnosis: Septic arthritis. Pediatr Rev 21:67,70–71, 2000.
4. McAllister DR, Parker RD, Cooper AE, et al: Outcomes of postoperative septic arthritis after anterior cruciate ligament reconstruction. Am J Sports Med 27:562–570, 1999.
5. Donatto, KC: Orthopedic management of septic arthritis. Rheum Dis Clin North Am 24:275–286, 1998.
6. Hakim-Elahi E, Tovell HM, Burnhill MS: Complications of first-trimester abortion: A report of 170,000 cases. Obstet Gynecol 76:129–135, 1990.

PATIENT 4

A 3-month-old infant with excessive crying

The parents of a previously healthy 3-month-old boy bring him to the emergency department for excessive crying. They state that he was acting normally until he awoke from an afternoon nap. Since then, he has been crying inconsolably. He has not had fever, cough, rhinorrhea, vomiting, or diarrhea. There is no history of trauma and he has not been given any medications.

Physical Examination: Vital signs: temperature 37.2°C rectally; pulse 190; respiratory rate 44; blood pressure 96/50. General: Well-nourished infant, crying inconsolably. HEENT: Anterior fontanel open and flat, no scalp abrasions or contusions, PERRL, TMs pearly bilaterally, mild clear nasal discharge, mucous membranes moist, no oral lesions. Chest: clear to auscultation. Cardiac: tachycardia, regular rhythm. Abdomen: nondistended, bowel sounds present, soft, nontender, no organomegaly. Genitourinary: normal Tanner stage 1 genitalia, circumsized, testes descended with normal lie, normal cremasteric reflexes bilaterally, no inguinal hernia. Extremities: edema and erythema of the third finger with blanching of the skin adjacent to the proximal interphalangeal joint (see figure).

Question: What are the diagnostic considerations?

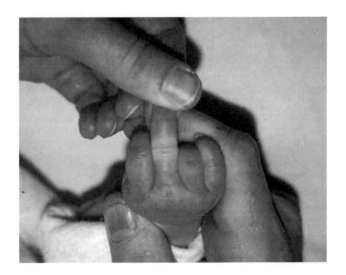

Diagnosis: Strangulated digit due to hair-thread tourniquet

Discussion: An infant cries to express his needs and emotions such as hunger, fatigue, discomfort (e.g., cold, dirty diaper), pain, and the desire to be held. By a few months of age, most parents will be able to discern differences in their infant's cry and can respond accordingly. However, excessive, inconsolable crying can be frightening for even the most experienced parent and may prompt a visit to the emergency department. An organized approach to the evaluation of the crying infant is important to identify the occasional physical cause and to provide guidance to unnerved families.

A careful history and physical examination will exclude most serious conditions. The history should ascertain the onset of the crying and thoroughly review all systems to identify systemic symptoms. Irritability associated with feeding may be a symptom of gastroesophageal reflux or cardiac ischemia (a rare cause of excessive crying due to anomalous origin of left coronary artery from pulmonary artery [ALCAPA]). A history of recent immunizations, trauma, or medications should be sought. For the physical examination, the baby should be completely undressed, including the diaper. The thorough examination should include attention to the vital signs, as fever may indicate infection, tachycardia may suggest arrhythmia, and hyperpnea may be a sign of acidosis. The child's head should be inspected for signs of trauma and for fullness of the fontanel, suggesting meningitis or increased intracranial pressure. The eyes should be examined with flourescein dye to evaluate for corneal abrasion, even in infants without conjunctival injection or tearing, and the lids should be everted to evaluate for foreign body. Fundoscopy should be attempted to assess for retinal hemorrhages, a sign of child abuse. Otoscopy might reveal otitis media or hemotypanum. The mouth and oropharynx must be carefully inspected to look for stomatitis or erupting teeth. The cardiac examination should assess for signs of congestive heart failure or arrythmia. Abdominal and rectal examinations should be performed to look for signs of intussusception or anal fissure. The genitals must be inspected carefully for testicular torsion, incarcerated hernia, or strangulation of the penis or clitoris by hair or thread. Careful palpation of the extremities and joints to identify focal areas of tenderness (occult fracture) or limitation of mobility (septic arthritis) is important. Each digit should be inspected carefully for strangulation by hair or thread.

Many patients will have normal physical examinations. Screening laboratory tests can be limited to urinalysis and urine culture. If the diagnosis remains unclear, a period of observation is warranted. One study (Poole, 1991) concluded that infants who cease crying either before or during the initial evaluation are unlikely to have serious disease, whereas infants who continue to cry excessively are more likely have a serious condition.

Colic, or periodic episodes of excessive crying, usually begins in the second to third week of life. The attacks occur more commonly in the late afternoon or evening and may last for several hours. Commonly, the crying progresses to a piercing scream, and the infant draws his legs up and develops abdominal distension and flatus, thereby leading the parent to believe that the infant is experiencing abdominal pain. There is no cure for colic, and the diagnosis is made only when the crying episodes are repeated and stereotypical, and other causes of crying are excluded.

The condition known as "hair-tourniquet syndrome," "hair thread tourniquet," "hair wrapping," and "toe tourniquet" occurs most commonly in infants and consists of strangulation of the affected area by a hair or synthetic fiber. Toes are afflicted most commonly, but hair tourniquet syndrome may involve the fingers, penis, or clitoris. It is postulated that repeated flexion and extension of digits or movement of the hips in the presence of hair or clothing fibers results in an encircling of the fibers with subsequent constriction of venous blood and lymphatic flow. Left untreated, the constriction may result in gangrene, amputation, and permanent damage.

Removal of the hair or fibers will reverse the constriction. In the present patient, the physician cut the hair by isolating it from the underlying skin by sliding a fine forceps beneath the strands and then cutting through them with a scalpel onto the probe. Alternatively, depilatory agents could have been used. This method is not recommended if the underlying skin is eroded and will be ineffective in removing thread or synthetic fibers.

Clinical Pearls

1. Excessive crying may represent normal infant communication or indicate a serious condition.

2. A thorough history and physical examination will reveal the diagnosis in most cases.

3. The physical examination should include careful inspection of the digits and penis or clitoris to evaluate for strangulation due to an encircling hair or thread.

4. Hair thread tourniquets are a relatively common, reversible cause of excessive crying in infants.

REFERENCES

1. Pawel BB, Henretig FM: Crying and colic in early infancy. In Fleisher GR, Ludwig S (eds): Textbook of Pediatric Emergency Medicine, 4th ed. Philadelphia, Lippincott Williams & Wilkins, 2000, pp 193–195, 1499, 1871–1872.
2. Loiselle J, Cook RT: Hair tourniquet removal. In Henretig FM, King C (eds): Textbook of Pediatric Emergency Procedures. Baltimore, Williams & Wilkins, 1997, pp 1183–1187.
3. Conners G: Index of suspicion. Pediatr Rev 18:283–286, 1997.
4. Poole SR: The infant with acute, unexplained, excessive crying. Pediatrics 88:450–455, 1991.
5. Barton DJ, Sloan GM, Nichter LS, Reinisch JF: Experience and reason—Briefly recorded: Hair-thread tourniquet syndrome. Pediatrics 82:925–928, 1988.

Esther H. Chen, MD
Judd E. Hollander, MD

PATIENT 5

A 65-year-old woman with chest pain

A 65-year-old woman with a history of insulin-dependent diabetes mellitus, hypertension, chronic renal failure, and transient ischemic attacks presents with chest pain beginning 1 hour prior to ED arrival. She has accompanying shortness of breath and diaphoresis. In the ambulance, she was noted to be bradycardic and hypotensive.

Physical Examination: Temperature 35.5°C; pulse 74; respirations 14; blood pressure 94/32. Skin: cool, moist extremities. HEENT: normal. Chest: shallow breathing, diminished breath sounds at bases bilaterally. Cardiac: distant heart sounds, regular rate and rhythm without murmurs. Abdomen: normal. Rectal hemoccult negative. Extremities: 1+ pitting edema, 2+ peripheral pulses. Neuromuscular: alert, normal.

Laboratory Findings: CBC: normal. Blood chemistries: normal except BUN 90, creatinine 6.9, glucose 248. ECG (see figure): bradycardia with an ectopic atrial focus, normal axis, incomplete right bundle-branch block, 1-mm ST elevation lead III, aVF, 1-mm ST depression in lead I, aVL. Chest radiograph: cardiomegaly, otherwise normal.

Questions: What is the appropriate treatment for this patient? What questions need to be answered prior to treatment? The patient developed acute left arm weakness after treatment. What is the immediate next step?

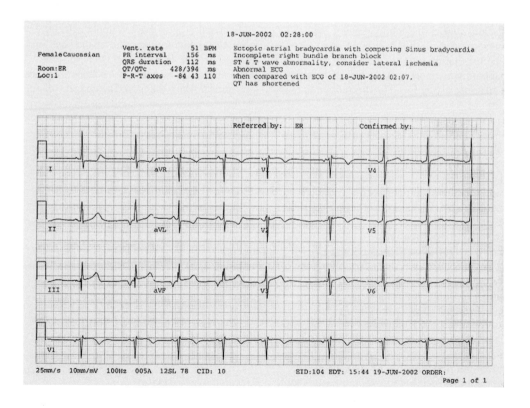

Diagnosis and Treatment: Acute inferior wall myocardial infarction. Therapy includes fibrinolytic therapy (FT) in addition to aspirin, heparin, and consideration of nitroglycerin and beta-blocking agents. The patient developed neurologic symptoms after FT. The differential diagnosis of acute neurologic events after FT includes intracranial hemorrhage bleed (which can be diagnosed with computed tomography of the head) and aortic dissection (which can be diagnosed with computed tomography of the chest or esophageal echocardiography).

Discussion: The differential diagnosis of acute chest pain is broad, although acute coronary syndromes (ACS) are the most common serious cause of chest pain. Clinical features such as character or location of pain are generally unhelpful in conclusively ruling out ACS. Recent guidelines for prompt treatment of acute myocardial infarction (AMI) with fibrinolytics has established significant time pressure to determine when fibrinolysis is indicated. Although the risk-benefit analysis of treating AMI patients with FT clearly falls on the beneficial side, there are downsides to the use of these agents. One must be careful to avoid giving fibrinolytic agents to patients who do not have AMIs, specifically to patients who have serious conditions that may be exacerbated by FT, such as aortic dissection, pericarditis, or pericardial effusion/tamponade (see table below).

The frequency of ACS as the cause of acute chest pain is approximately 80-fold greater than aortic dissection. Approximately 4% of patients with acute aortic dissection present with ECG findings suggestive of AMI, most commonly in dissections that involve the coronary arteries. Of all patients who meet criteria for FT, about 3% have an aortic dissection. The mortality rate in patients with aortic dissection who are inadvertently treated with FT approaches 100%.

Using a chest radiograph to rule out aortic dissection prior to therapy may not be helpful, because a widened mediastinum, a classic sign of aortic dissection, is not uniformly present. Withholding therapy that reduces mortality in patients at high risk for AMI is not appropriate. Therefore, in patients with acute chest pain and ECG abnormalities, fibrinolysis is still indicated, despite the fact that a small percentage of these patients will ultimately have a non-ACS diagnosis and potentially complicated clinical course. Clinicians should be aware of conditions that may have ST segment elevation in the absence of ischemia (see table next page).

The present patient was initially diagnosed with an acute inferior wall myocardial infarction, and received fibrinolysis on the basis of the ECG. With therapy, her ST segments returned to baseline, and her symptoms improved, although her blood pressure remained low. Approximately 40 minutes later, in the cardiac care unit, the patient developed sudden and progressive left upper extremity weakness. Computed tomography of the head was performed, which showed no acute hemorrhage. Subsequently, a transesophageal echocardiogram was performed, which diagnosed acute aortic dissection.

Contraindications to Fibrinolytic Therapy

Absolute Contraindications
    Previous hemorrhagic stroke at any time
    Bland strokes of CVA in past year
    Known intracranial neoplasm
    Active internal bleeding (excluding menses)
    Suspected aortic dissection
Relative Contraindications
    Severe uncontrolled blood pressure (>180/100 mm Hg)
    History of prior CVA of known intracranial pathology
    Current use of anticoagulants with INR >2–3
    Known bleeding diathesis
    Recent trauma (past 2 weeks)
    Prolonged CPR >10 minutes
    Major surgery <3 weeks
    Noncompressible vascular punctures
    Recent internal bleeding (2–4 weeks)
    Prior allergic reaction to streptokinase (should not receive streptokinase)
    Pregnancy
    Active peptic ulcer disease
    History of chronic severe hypertension

Early repolarization
Left ventricular hypertrophy
Pericarditis
Myocarditis
Left ventricular aneurysms
Idiopathic hypertrophic subaortic stenosis
Hypothermia
Paced rhythms
Left bundle branch block

Clinical Pearls

1. There are no definite clinical features that accurately distinguish ACS from aortic dissection.

2. Although ECG abnormalities in the setting of acute chest pain usually suggest ACS, the rare diagnosis of aortic dissection should be considered.

3. Patients who meet criteria for fibrinolysis should be promptly treated to reduce morbidity and mortality from AMI. Therapy should not be withheld to obtain results from time-consuming tests to rule out other diagnoses unless there is a high suspicion of a serious condition that can be worsened by rapid administration of FT.

REFERENCES

1. Kodolitsch Y, Schwartz AG, Nienaber CA: Clinical prediction of acute aortic dissection. Arch Intern Med 160:2977–2982, 2000.
2. Armstrong WF, Bach DS, Carey LM, et al: Clinical and echocardiographic findings in patients with suspected acute aortic dissection. Am Heart J 136:1051–1060, 1998.
3. Khoury NE, Borzak S, Gokli A, et al: "Inadvertent" thrombolytic administration in patients without myocardial infarction: Clinical features and outcome. Ann Emerg Med 28:289–293, 1996.
4. Hirata K, Kyushima M, Asato H: Electrocardiographic abnormalities in patients with acute aortic dissection. Am J Cardiol 76:1207–1212, 1995.

Linda Brown, MD
Richard Scarfone, MD

PATIENT 6

A 13-month-old boy with sleepiness and poor feeding

A 13-month-old boy is evaluated in the emergency department because of excessive somnolence and decreased feeding. He has been sleeping more than usual and has been difficult to arouse for 1 day. He has not played with his toys and has not wanted to eat or drink for the past 7 hours. He has not had a fever, and there is no history of head injury, known ingestion, or seizure. He does not take medication, and he vomited once in the ED waiting room.

Physical Examination: Temperature 36.8°C; pulse 128; respirations 32; blood pressure 82/50. General: lethargic, floppy child; mucous membranes are slightly dry and capillary refill is 2 seconds. Chest: clear. Cardiac: tachycardia without murmur. Abdomen (see figure): active bowel sounds, soft, distended, diffusely tender without masses. Neurologic: nonfocal with cranial nerves intact.

Laboratory Findings: Hematocrit 36%, WBC count 19,700/μl, platelets 342,000/μl. Electrolytes within normal limits. Abdominal x-ray: paucity of air in distal colon, multiple dilated loops of bowel, and air/fluid levels (see figure).

ED Course: One hour after ED arrival, the patient passed a large, bloody stool.

Question: What is the most likely diagnosis?

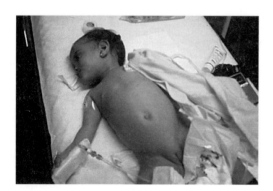 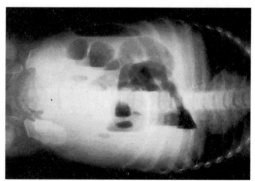

Diagnosis: Intussusception

Discussion: Intussusception is the most common abdominal surgical emergency in children <2 years old. Approximately two thirds of patients presenting with this diagnosis are <1 year old, with a peak incidence between 5 and 9 months. It is more common in boys by a 2:1 ratio. It occurs when a segment of intestine envelops a more proximal segment, resulting in obstruction. Most commonly, the point of obstruction is at the ileocolic junction (80%), and it is postulated that hypertrophied Peyer's patches, inflamed after a viral illness, may precipitate this event. In children older than 2 years, however, there is often a more specific lead point identified, such as a Meckel's diverticulum, polyp, or tumor.

Clinical manifestations are highly variable but often include crampy abdominal pain, vomiting, and irritability. The parents may report witnessing spasms of pain, associated with the child drawing the legs upward, followed by periods of lethargy. Lethargy alone may also be the chief symptom, with some infants presenting in a "shock-like" state. The cause for this profound change in mental status is not entirely clear but may be due, in part, to endogenous cytokine release from the entrapped bowel. The presence of "currant-jelly" stools is a classic, but late, finding in intussusception and may be present in 50–85% of confirmed cases. This finding is believed to be secondary to compression of the mesenteric veins by the obstructed segment of bowel. With worsening obstruction, the mesenteric arteries may also be compressed and may potentially lead to ischemia or perforation. However, the absence of these grossly bloody and mucus-laden stools does not rule out the diagnosis, since up to 25% of children present with heme-negative stools. Overall, the presence of colicky abdominal pain, vomiting, rectal bleeding, right upper quadrant mass, and male sex have been identified as clinical predictors of intussusception.

Physical examination of the child often reveals a distended, tender abdomen, and, in some cases, a sausage-shaped structure may be palpated in the right upper quadrant. Laboratory study findings are usually normal. The utility of plain abdominal radiographs in the diagnosis of intussusception has often been debated. Several large studies have found that approximately 40–60% of patients with confirmed intussusception have a soft tissue mass on their abdominal plain radiographs, 25–50% have findings consistent with bowel obstruction, and up to 25% have normal study findings. The plain radiograph may also reveal evidence of bowel perforation, which would be a contraindication for radiographic reduction. Since the sensitivity of plain radiographs is less than 100%, the diagnosis is not excluded if radiographs are normal.

Sonography has been found to be both sensitive and specific for the diagnosis of intussusception, with false-negative rates approaching 0% in some reports. However, patients with positive ultrasonograms will need to proceed directly to fluoroscopy, where an air or barium contrast enema can be both diagnostic and therapeutic. Success rates of 55–70% have been reported after hydrostatic barium reduction and 70–90% for pneumatic reduction. Recurrence rates after enema reduction have been reported in the range of 1–5%. Surgical intervention may be required when enemas are unsuccessful or cannot be performed because of perforation.

In the present patient, the profound lethargy with no obvious explanation and the patient's emesis and abnormal plain radiographs led to the suspicion of intussusception as a possible diagnosis. The patient's intussusception was successfully reduced with hydrostatic barium enema.

Clinical Pearls

1. Lethargy may be the only presenting symptom in an infant with intussusception.
2. A history of episodic and severe crying or lethargy, even in the presence of a well-appearing child, may be enough to pursue the diagnosis.
3. The absence of heme-positive, or "currant-jelly," stools does not rule out intussusception.
4. Normal plain abdominal radiographs may be seen in patients with intussusception.
5. Most cases of intussusception can be radiologically reduced without surgery.

REFERENCES

1. Kupperman N, O'Dea T, Pinckney L, Hoecker C: Predictors of intussusception in young children. Arch Pediatr Adolesc Med 154:250–255, 2000.
2. Parashar UD, Holman RC, Cummings KC, et al: Trends in intussusception-associated hospitalizations and deaths among US infants. Pediatrics 106:1413–1421, 2000.
3. Schaufer L, Mahboubi S: Abdominal emergencies. In Fleischer GR, Ludwig S (eds): Textbook of Pediatric Emergency Medicine, 4th ed. Philadelphia, Lippincott, Williams & Wilkins 2000, pp 1513–1538.
4. Birkhahn R, Fiorini M, Gaeta TJ: Painless intussusception and altered mental status. Am J Emerg Med 17:345–347, 1999.
5. Harrington L, Connolly B, Hu X, et al: Ultrasonographic and clinical predictors of intussusception. J Pediatr 132:836–839, 1998.
6. Yamamoto LG, Morita SY, Boychuk RB, et al: Stool appearance in intussusception: Assessing the value of the term "currant jelly." Am J Emerg Med 15:293–298, 1997.
7. Lee JM, Kim H, Byun JY, et al: Intussusception: Characteristic radiolucencies on the abdominal radiographs. Pediatr Radiol 24:293–295, 1994.
8. Smith DS, Bonadio WA, Losek JC, et al: The role of abdominal x-rays in the diagnosis and management of intussusception. Pediatr Emerg Care 8:325–327, 1992.

Elizabeth M. Datner, MD

PATIENT 7

A 22-year-old gravid woman with abdominal pain after a motor vehicle collision

A 22-year-old woman is brought to the emergency department after a motor vehicle collision. She is reporting abdominal cramping and is known to be 28 weeks pregnant. She is lying supine on a backboard with a cervical collar in place (see figure).

Physical Examination: Temperature 37°C; pulse 118; respirations 28; blood pressure 95/62. Skin: cool and clammy. HEENT: normal. Chest: rapid respirations, clear to auscultation anteriorly. Cardiac: regular tachycardia without murmurs, gallops, or rubs. Abdomen: slightly protuberant lower abdomen, tenderness to palpation of uterine fundus, fundal height 32 cm, otherwise soft without guarding or rebound. No fetal movement is palpable. Extremities: no injuries noted. Neurologic: slightly agitated but following commands, awake, alert, and oriented to person, place, and time. Rectal: no blood. Vagina: scant gross blood.

Laboratory Findings: CBC: normal. Blood chemistries: normal, Urinalysis: normal, positive urine HCG. Radiographs: cervical: normal, chest: normal, pelvis: normal with 28-week fetus. Emergency bedside sonogram: 28-week fetus with fetal heart rate 40 bpm.

Question: What are the emergency physician's priorities in caring for the pregnant trauma victim?

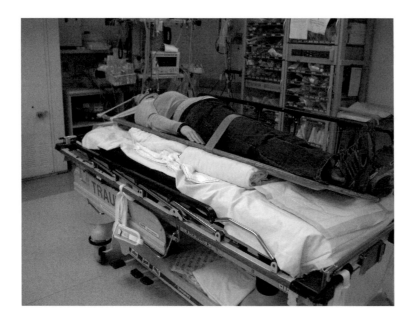

Diagnosis and Treatment: This relatively minor trauma resulted in placental abruption and fetal distress. Immediate interventions should involve hemodynamic support of the mother, immediate and ongoing cardiotocographic monitoring of the fetus, and emergency cesarean section if maternal mortality occurs or fetal distress is identified. The emergency physician must provide hemodynamic support for the mother as a top priority and as part of the primary trauma assessment and must act to identify potential life-threats to the fetus.

Discussion: Injury is common in pregnancy, occurring in as many as 6–7% of pregnant patients and accounting for significant trauma and morbidity for both mother and fetus. Trauma is the number one cause of maternal death. Maternal trauma, however, accounts for a greater number of fetal deaths than maternal deaths, since fetal death can result from direct fetal injury, maternal shock, and placental abruption.

Fetal fatality typically occurs as a result of cranial injury in cases of blunt trauma or direct injury in cases of penetrating trauma. Maternal shock results in fetal death secondary to decreased uterine perfusion. The uteroplacental mass is a passive, low-resistance vascular system. As such, uterine hypoperfusion precedes maternal shock. Early evaluation of fetal heart tones can identify fetal distress and act as an early indicator of maternal instability. Placental abruption is the premature separation of the placenta from the uterine wall that occurs as the result of a shearing force. Placental abruption secondary to trauma, due to either direct force to the abdomen or deceleration, can result in fetal death and can be easily missed. It is the most common cause of fetal death secondary to maternal trauma because it can occur in the setting of minor trauma. Fetal deaths occur in 20–30% of cases of placental abruption. Maternal complications of abruption include hypovolemia and resultant hypotension.

A suspicion of the diagnosis of placental abruption is based on the history and physical examination, including fetal heart rate determination and cardiotocographic monitoring. Findings suggestive of placental abruption include vaginal bleeding, uterine cramping or contractions, maternal hypovolemia, expanding uterine size, and fetal heart rate abnormalities. Placental abruption can occur in a delayed fashion but usually occurs within the first 48 hours after trauma. Approximately 25% of placental abruptions are concurrent with the trauma and may be detected on the initial trauma evaluation. Cases of delayed abruption can be detected with ongoing monitoring.

Pregnant trauma patients should be managed as nonpregnant trauma patients with the addition of early evaluation of the fetus and early hemodynamic support of the mother. The mother should always be given oxygen and fluids and turned or tilted onto her left side to avoid aortocaval compression by the gravid uterus. Pregnant patients develop hypoxia quickly, have decreased buffering capacity, and are at increased risk for aspiration and other factors that complicate airway management. They should be intubated early when airway management appears necessary. All standard tests and radiographs should be performed on the pregnant trauma patient. Abdominal and pelvic computed tomography is the only radiographic study that provides enough radiation to the fetus to complicate organogenesis (9–60 days). All advanced cardiac and advanced trauma life support drugs should be used in caring for the pregnant trauma patient; however, gestational exposure to amiodarone carries a potential risk. Amiodarone is a category D drug that has demonstrated risk to the fetus of causing hypo-or hyperthyroidism. Its use may be warranted in life-threatening situations.

In the present case, the diagnosis of fetal distress was made with the initial evaluation of fetal heart tones that demonstrated bradycardia. The fetus was delivered by emergency cesarean section in the trauma bay and was resuscitated and admitted to the neonatal intensive care unit. The mother was not found to have any additional injuries, and placental abruption was confirmed during cesarean section as the cause of fetal distress.

Clinical Pearls

1. Pregnant patients beyond 16 weeks gestation should be placed in a left lateral decubitus position or tilted to the left side and maintained in that position to prevent aortocaval compression.

2. Trauma protocols are the same for pregnant patients as for nonpregnant patients with the addition of including the fetus in the initial evaluation, providing support of maternal physiology (oxygen, fluids, displacing the uterus), and considering emergency cesarean section.

3. Emergency physicians should know how to perform emergency cesarean sections in cases of impending or actual maternal cardiac arrest.

4. Placental abruption should be sought and ruled out even in cases of minor trauma.

5. Maternal trauma may be an initial episode of domestic abuse; thus, all injured pregnant patients should be carefully evaluated for domestic abuse and home safety.

REFERENCES

1. Horon IL, Cheng D: Enhanced surveillance for pregnancy-associated mortality—Maryland, 1993–1998. JAMA 285:1455–1459, 2001.
2. Magee LA, Downar E, Sermer M, et al: Pregnancy outcome after gestational exposure to amiodarone in Canada. Am J Obstet Gynecol 172:1307–1311, 1995.

Joel Fein, MD

PATIENT 8

A 4-year-old girl with painless vaginal bleeding for 1 day

A 4-year-old girl is brought to the emergency department after her parents noted blood spots in her underwear that evening. She denies injury or itching in her perineum but does report that it burns when she urinates. She attends preschool classes at a local facility but denies that anyone is touching her "privates." She does not report vaginal or anal pain, vomiting, abdominal pain, diarrhea, or urinary frequency or hesitancy.

Physical Examination: Vital signs: normal for age. Abdomen: nontender, good bowel sounds, no masses palpated. Vaginal examination: doughnut shaped red-purple mass with central indentation (see figure). No blood present in the vaginal introitus. Tanner I with regard to breast and pubic hair.

Questions: What is the most likely diagnosis? What are other possible diagnoses to consider in a prepubertal girl with vaginal bleeding? What is the appropriate initial management?

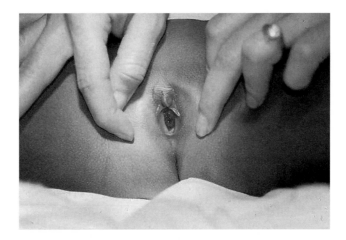

Diagnosis: Urethral prolapse

Discussion: This girl has bleeding due to local irritation of the urethral mucosa, which has prolapsed through its meatus. The physical examination in girls with urethral prolapse reveals a swollen, well-defined, dark red, doughnut-shaped tissue in the vaginal introitus. The urethral lumen often can be visualized in the center of this mass. Urethral prolapse is a common cause of vaginal bleeding in African-American girls between the ages of 3 and 10 years. Reported causes include poor adherence between smooth muscle layers in association with episodic increases in intra-abdominal pressure, such as associated with constipation or severe coughing.

Other possible causes of vaginal bleeding in prepubertal girls include vaginal foreign body, vaginitis, trauma, sexual abuse, condyloma acuminatum, precocious puberty, hemangioma, and benign and malignant tumors. Other causes of a mass that can be seen protruding through the urethra are prolapsed ureterocele or bladder and urethral or bladder polyp.

If the mucosa appears healthy and not necrotic, the child with urethral prolapse can be treated expectantly with sitz-baths four times each day and topical estrogen cream applied to the urethral area twice each day. Many cases resolve within a few weeks and do not recur. Surgical resection of redundant mucosa may be required if there is necrotic tissue or symptoms do not resolve within a few weeks. The estrogen cream serves the added benefit of preventing labial adhesions that occur due to inflammation and bleeding.

The present patient was treated with sitz-baths and estrogen cream with complete resolution of the urethral prolapse.

Clinical Pearls

1. Urethral prolapse is a relatively common cause of prepubertal vaginal bleeding in African-American girls.

2. Many cases of urethral prolapse resolve spontaneously, without surgical intervention.

3. Applying estrogen cream to the urethral area and labia minora of girls with urethral prolapse can be curative and also prevents labial adhesions.

REFERENCES
1. Valerie E, Gilchrist BF, Frischer J, et al: Diagnosis and treatment of urethral prolapse in children. Urology 54:1082–1084, 1999.
2. Flanagan J, Cram J: Index of suspicion. Case 3. Urethral prolapse. Pediatr Rev 20:137, 139–140, 1998.
3. Shetty AK, Coffman K, Harmon E: Urethral prolapse. J Pediatr 133:552, 1998.
4. Anveden-Hertzberg L, Gauderer MW, Elder JS: Urethral prolapse: An often misdiagnosed cause of urogenital bleeding in girls. Pediatr Emerg Care 11:212–214, 1995.

Joseph Bushra, MD

PATIENT 9

A 38-year-old woman with generalized weakness

A 38-year-old woman with a history of gastritis presents to the emergency department with progressive weakness over 3 weeks. Her symptoms began with tingling in her feet and progressed to bilateral leg weakness. She is no longer able to get out of bed and lately has started dropping objects out of her hands. She was recently seen in the emergency department and treated for dehydration. She is now unable to raise her arms above her head to brush her hair. She has had no recent illness and has no other symptoms.

Physical Examination: Temperature 37.3°C, pulse 130, respirations 20, blood pressure 116/62, pulse oximetry 92% on room air. Skin: no lesions. HEENT: dry mucous membranes, otherwise normal. Neck: normal. Lungs: clear to auscultation bilaterally, respirations shallow. Heart: tachycardia without murmurs or gallops. Abdomen: normal. Back: nontender, no palpable deformity. Extremities: no atrophy or fasciculations, no edema. Neurologic: Awake, alert, and oriented, cranial nerves intact, muscle strength 3/5 in bilateral upper extremities and 2/5 in bilateral lower extremities, sensation intact, deep tendon reflexes absent at Achilles, patella, biceps, and triceps, unable to perform cerebellar or gait testing due to weakness.

Laboratory Findings: CBC: normal. Blood chemistries: normal. Creatine phosphokinase: 93. ABG: pH 7.41, PCO_2 33, PO_2 104 on room air. CSF studies: RBC 0, WBC 0, CSF glucose 72 (normal 50–80), CSF protein 61 (normal 15–45). Forced vital capacity (FVC) 800 ml (normal 5000 ml), negative inspiratory force (NIF) 5 cm H_2O (normal 90 cm H_2O).

Questions: What is the most likely cause of this patient's weakness? What procedure may be immediately necessary? What is the most effective treatment for her condition?

Diagnosis and Treatment: Guillain-Barré syndrome. The present patient required intubation for respiratory failure. Treatment was initiated with intravenous immunoglobulin (IVIg) in the intensive care unit.

Discussion: Guillain-Barré syndrome (GBS) is the most common cause of acute generalized paralysis in the developed world. In its early stages, patients report distal paresthesias and mild weakness, and the diagnosis is often missed initially, as in the present case. The weakness worsens and ascends proximally and can extend to the respiratory muscles, causing respiratory failure. The pathophysiology is that of a demyelinating polyneuropathy, but the exact cause remains unclear. A large number of cases occur after a viral illness, and a smaller but significant number of cases occur after infection with *Campylobacter jejuni*. It is thought that these infectious agents and the human myelin sheath have some structural similarity, and that the immune response against the former may be responsible for the destruction of the latter (molecular mimicry). The resulting failure of nerve conduction causes profound muscle weakness.

The diagnosis of GBS is a clinical one. Patients usually complain of paresthesias preceding muscle weakness. The most common findings on examination are symmetric muscle weakness and diminished or absent deep tendon reflexes. Many patients display autonomic instability, like the present patient, with tachycardia and mild hypotension. GBS may also affect the cranial nerves. A rare variant of GBS is called Miller-Fisher syndrome and is characterized by ataxia, ophthalmoplegia, and areflexia. The usual course of GBS is advancing weakness over 1 to 3 weeks, followed by a plateau phase and then slow resolution. Mild cases may not affect the patient's ability to walk, whereas severe cases may require mechanical ventilation for years. A small number of patients may relapse after recovery.

The differential diagnosis of GBS is broad (see table). Emergency department management of patients suspected of having GBS should include ruling out these potential diagnoses, performing confirmatory studies, and careful monitoring of respiratory parameters. The most important confirmatory study that should be performed in the ED is a lumbar puncture. Classically, patients with GBS manifest *albuminocytologic dissociation,* that is, an elevation of CSF protein without CSF pleocytosis. This finding may not be present early in the disease, so its absence does not rule out the diagnosis. It is also essential to measure FVC and NIF in the emergency department. If FVC is less than 1000 ml and NIF is less than 20 cm H_2O, the need for mechanical ventilation should be anticipated. Electromyelography on an inpatient can confirm the demyelinating nature of the disease.

The treatment of GBS involves plasmapheresis and/or IVIg. A recent study of patients with severe GBS showed no difference in outcome among patients receiving either of these treatments or both in combination. Selection of the appropriate treatment depends on availability and patient-specific factors and should be made in consultation with a neurologist.

Differential Diagnosis of Guillain-Barré Syndrome

	REFLEXES	CSF PLEOCYTOSIS	PARESTHESIAS	SENSORY LOSS	ALBUMINOCYTOLOGIC DISSOCIATION
Spinal cord compression	Variable	Variable	Yes	Yes	No
Transverse myelitis	Increased	Yes	Yes	Yes	No
Myasthenia gravis	Decreased or normal	No	No	No	No
Multiple sclerosis	Variable	No	Yes	Yes	No
GBS	Decreased or absent	No	Yes	No	Yes

Clinical Pearls

1. The diagnosis of Guillain-Barré syndrome is made clinically, but paresthesias, weakness, and areflexia are the classic findings.

2. Emergency department measurement of respiratory parameters is essential to anticipate respiratory complications.

3. CSF findings are often normal, but lumbar puncture is necessary to rule out other causes of ascending weakness and paralysis.

REFERENCES

1. Bushra JS: Miller-Fisher syndrome: An uncommon acute neuropathy. J Emerg Med 18:427–430, 2000.
2. Hughes RAC, and the Plasma Exchange/Sandoglobulin Guillain-Barré Syndrome Trial Group: Randomised trial of plasma exchange, intravenous immunoglobulin, and combined treatments in Guillain-Barré syndrome. Lancet 349:225–230, 1997.
3. Rees JH, Soudain SE, Gregson NA, Hughes RAC: *Campylobacter jejuni* infection and Guillain-Barré Syndrome. N Engl J Med 333:1374–1379, 1995.
4. Ropper AH: The Guillian-Barré syndrome. N Engl J Med 326:1130–1136, 1992.
5. Singer JI, Back K: Postural guarding and hypertension as initial manifestations of Guillain-Barré syndrome. Am J Emerg Med 7:177–179, 1989.
6. Fisher M: An unusual variant of acute idiopathic polyneuritis (syndrome of ophthalmoplegia, ataxia, and areflexia). N Engl J Med 255:57–65, 1956.

Cynthia J. Mollen, MD, MSCE

PATIENT 10

A 6-day-old girl with eye discharge

A 6-day-old girl presents to the emergency department with her mother, who reports that the baby has had a 1-day history of eye discharge. The baby had been doing well at home until the day prior to her visit, when crusted eye discharge was noted upon awakening in the morning. The patient's mother also reports that the patient's eye is red. The baby has not had fever, rhinorrhea, cough, vomiting, or diarrhea. She has been eating well, with good urine output and normal activity. She was born at 39 weeks by normal spontaneous vaginal delivery and was discharged at 48 hours of life. The patient's mother had received appropriate prenatal care; she reports a history of both *Neisseria gonorrhoeae* and *Chlamydia trachomatis* infection in the past, for which she received treatment. She had rupture of membranes 6 hours before delivery and did not receive peripartum antibiotics.

Physical Examination: Vital signs: temperature 36.4°C rectally; pulse 140; respiratory rate 42; blood pressure 84/47. General: well-appearing infant girl in no acute distress. HEENT (*see* figure): flat anterior fontanel; left eye with palpebral conjunctival injection and thick, yellowish discharge; right eye with minimal palpebral conjunctival injection and no discharge; no nasal discharge; no oral lesions. Chest: clear to auscultation. Cardiac: RRR without murmur. Abdomen: soft, nontender, nondistended; no masses; no hepatosplenomegaly; normoactive bowel sounds. Genitourinary: normal Tanner 1 female. Extremities: normal. Skin: no lesions or rash. Neurologic: strong suck and grasp; symmetric Moro reflex; normal tone.

Laboratory Findings: Gram stain of eye discharge: moderate WBCs; no organisms seen.

Questions: What is the patient's most likely diagnosis? What other laboratory tests should be ordered? What is the treatment?

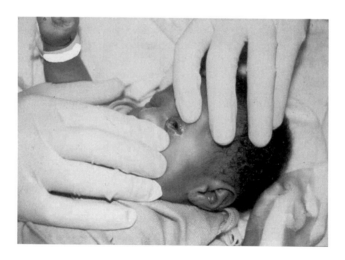

Diagnosis: With no organisms seen on Gram stain, chlamydial conjunctivitis is the most likely diagnosis. Eye discharge should be sent for bacterial culture, and conjunctival scraping should be sent for *C. trachomatis* culture. Topical erythromycin ointment would be effective for chlamydial conjunctivitis; however, oral erythromycin therapy is necessary to eradicate nasopharyngeal carriage of *C. trachomatis* to prevent subsequent pneumonia.

Discussion: Neonatal conjunctivitis is defined as conjunctivitis occurring in the first 4 weeks of life. Chemical irritation or infection with *C. trachomatis, N. gonorrhoeae,* other bacteria, or herpes simplex virus can cause conjunctivitis in this age group. The epidemiology of neonatal conjunctivitis has changed dramatically over the last 100 years owing to the introduction of neonatal ocular prophylaxis. Gonococcal disease, once an important cause of blindness in infants, is now relatively uncommon in industrialized countries. *C. trachomatis* is now the most common identifiable infectious cause of neonatal conjunctivitis in the United States. Clinically, there is much overlap of the various types of conjunctivitis, making definitive diagnosis on the basis of history and physical examination findings alone quite difficult.

Conjunctivitis that occurs in the first 24 hours of life is almost always chemical, unless the mother has a history of prolonged rupture of membranes. Silver nitrate, used in the delivery room as ocular prophylaxis, is the most common culprit, although antibiotic ointments can cause irritation as well. Povidone-iodine solution has been studied for prophylaxis, because of its low cost and wide availability, especially in developing countries, and has been found to be effective and less toxic. Chemical conjunctivitis resolves spontaneously in 3 to 4 days.

Gonococcal conjunctivitis is the most serious form of neonatal conjunctivitis. Infection can rapidly lead to corneal involvement and subsequent globe rupture. In addition, bacteremia and meningitis can occur in untreated patients. Fortunately, with mandated neonatal ocular prophylaxis, the incidence of this infection has dropped dramatically. However, the failure rate of antimicrobial prophylaxis is about 1%; in addition, infants born in nonhospital settings may not receive prophylaxis. Therefore, it is important to consider infection with *N. gonorrhoeae* in every infant with purulent conjunctivitis.

Most infants with gonococcal conjunctivitis present between 2 and 5 days of life, although the incubation period can be longer; in addition, symptoms can appear sooner if the mother had prolonged rupture of membranes. The infection is generally hyperacute, with thick, purulent discharge. A sample of the discharge should be sent for Gram stain and culture. Diagnosis is usually made by identifying gram-negative intracellular diplococci on Gram stain, which are present in about 95% of cases. All patients with gonococcal conjunctivitis should be hospitalized and treated with hourly saline eye irrigation until the discharge disappears. Blood, CSF, and urine cultures should be sent to the laboratory for all ill-appearing or febrile infants. In patients with nondisseminated infection, a single dose of ceftriaxone or cefotaxime is sufficient treatment; ceftriaxone should be avoided in patients with hyperbilirubinemia because it can displace bilirubin from albumin binding sites. Patients with disseminated disease should be treated for 7 to 14 days. Treatment for presumed concomitant *C. trachomatis* infection should be initiated as well.

Conjunctivitis due to *C. trachomatis* can manifest with a range of severity, from a mild hyperemia with minimal mucoid discharge to severe hyperemia with copious purulent discharge, chemosis, and pseudomembrane formation. Generally, this infection appears between 5 and 14 days of life. Given that the prevalence of *C. trachomatis* infection among pregnant women varies from 2% to 37% (with most estimates ranging between 6% and 12%) and that approximately 50% of infants born vaginally to infected mothers will acquire the organism, *Chlamydia* is a common cause of neonatal conjunctivitis. Cases have also been reported in some infants delivered by cesarean section with intact membranes. The risk of conjunctivitis is 25%–50% in infants who have acquired the organism, and neonatal ocular prophylaxis does not prevent infection.

Definitive diagnosis of *Chlamydia* conjunctivitis is made by culture; culture specimens must contain epithelial cells and be obtained using a wireshafted Dacron-tipped swab and the appropriate media. Cotton- and calcium alginate–tipped swabs and wooden-shafted swabs can be toxic to the organism. Rapid nucleic acid detection techniques have not been well tested on conjunctival specimens and in general should not be used in this setting. Infants with *Chlamydia* conjunctivitis should be treated with oral erythromycin for 14 days; topical treatment alone will not eradicate the organism from the nasopharynx, which is necessary to reduce the risk of subsequent pneumonia. Of note, an association between oral erythromycin and infantile hypertrophic pyloric stenosis has been reported in infants younger than 6 weeks of age. Because the link is not confirmed, and alternative therapies for *C. trachomatis* are not well studied, the American Academy of Pediatrics still recommends the use of erythromycin in these patients. Parents should be informed of the signs and symptoms of pyloric stenosis and instructed to contact their physician if symptoms develop.

Bacteria other than *N. gonorrhoeae* can also cause neonatal conjunctivitis. In general, infection is thought to occur after exposure to maternal vaginal flora; therefore, bacterial conjunctivitis is rare in a neonate born by cesarean section without rupture of membranes. The most common pathogenic organisms in this setting are *Streptococcus pneumoniae* and *Haemophilus influenzae;* multiple studies have found that these organisms are present in <1% of infants without conjunctivitis. The role of *Staphylococcus aureus* in neonatal conjunctivitis is controversial. *S. aureus* has been isolated from as many as 45% of infants with conjunctivitis but is also commonly cultured from neonates without conjunctivitis. One theory is that *S. aureus* thrives in the wet environment created

by the infection, rather than causing the infection itself. Other *Neisseria* species, other *Streptococcus* species, various gram-negative enteric rods, and, rarely, *Pseudomonas* species have also been implicated in neonatal conjunctivitis. It can be difficult to distinguish clinically conjunctivitis caused by these bacteria from conjunctivitis due to *C. trachomatis* and *N. gonorrhoeae,* although most other bacterial infections have longer incubation periods and less severe symptoms. The Gram stain, as discussed, is crucial in making an initial distinction between the various types of conjunctivitis. Bacterial culture samples should be sent to the laboratory as well to confirm the diagnosis. If bacterial conjunctivitis is suspected, empiric topical treatment should be initiated; treatment should continue for 7 days.

The present patient was treated with oral erythromycin for 14 days. Her conjunctival scraping culture confirmed the diagnosis of *C. trachomatis* conjunctivitis; her bacterial culture was negative. She did well.

Neonatal Conjunctivitis

TYPE	DISTINGUISHING FEATURES	TREATMENT
Chemical	Occurs in first 24 hours of life; most likely diagnosis in first 24 hours unless there was prolonged rupture of membranes	None
Chlamydial	Usually occurs at 6 to 14 days of age (but variable); spectrum of physical findings, from mild conjunctival injection to severe conjunctival injection with profuse purulent discharge.	PO erythromycin 50 mg/kg per day in divided in four doses for 14 days
Gonococcal	Usually occurs at 2 to 5 days of age (but variable); hyperacute; hyperpurulent. Gram stain with gram-negative, intracellular diplococci	• Nondisseminated infection: Ceftriaxone 25 to 50 mg/kg IV or IM, max 125 mg, ×1 dose *or* Cefotaxime 100 mg/kg IV or IM ×1 dose • Disseminated infection: Ceftriaxone as above *or* Cefotaxime 50 mg/kg IV or IM divided BID (arthritis/septicemia, treat for 7 days; meningitis, treat for 14 days)
Other bacterial infection	Varying degrees of conjunctival injection and discharge; difficult to distinguish clinically from other forms. Gram stain with many WBCs, +organisms	Topical antibiotics, e.g., erythromycin ointment or bacitracin/polymixin B ointment, four times a day for 7 days

Table continues

TYPE	DISTINGUISHING FEATURES	TREATMENT
Herpes simplex virus	Generally occurs in association with infection at other sites, such as skin, or with disseminated disease. Careful physical examination for vesicles is crucial.	Full sepsis work-up IV acyclovir 60 mg/kg per day divided in three doses for 14 to 21 days (depending on site of infection)

Clinical Pearls

1. All neonates with conjunctivitis should have a sample of the eye discharge sent to the laboratory for Gram stain during the ED visit to rule out gonococcal infection.

2. Gonococcal conjunctivitis is a medical emergency, because infection can spread to the cornea and lead to globe rupture, even after antibiotic treatment.

3. Prophylactic eye ointment applied at birth does not prevent chlamydial conjunctivitis.

REFERENCES

1. Isenberg SJ, Apt L, Campeas D: Ocular applications of povidone-iodine. Dermatology 204(suppl 1): 92–95, 2002.
2. Dunn PM: Dr. Carl Crede and the prevention of ophthalmia neonatorum. Arch Dis Child 83:F158–F159, 2000.
3. American Academy of Pediatrics: Chlamydial infections. In: Pickering LK (ed): 2000 Red Book: Report of the Committee on Infectious Diseases, 25th ed. Elk Grove Village, IL: American Academy of Pediatrics, 2000, pp 208–212.
4. American Academy of Pediatrics: Gonococcal Infections. In: Pickering LK (ed): 2000 Red Book: Report of the Committee on Infectious Diseases, 25th ed. Elk Grove Village, IL: American Academy of Pediatrics, 2000, 254–260.
5. Gigliotti F: Acute conjunctivitis. Pediatr Rev 16:203–207, 1995.
6. Isenberg SJ, Apt L, Wood M: A controlled trial of povidone-iodine as prophylaxis against ophthalmia neonatorum. N Engl J Med 332:562–566, 1995.
7. Hammerschlag MR: Neonatal conjunctivitis. Pediatr Ann 22:346–351, 1993.
8. Ohara MA: Ophthalmia neonatorum. Pediatr Clin North Am 40:715–725, 1993.

Esther H. Chen, MD
Judd E. Hollander, MD

PATIENT 11

A 77-year-old-woman with unresponsiveness

A 77-year-old woman with a history of severe hypertension, myocardial infarction, renal insufficiency (baseline creatine 2.5), and renal artery stenosis was recently admitted to the hospital with severe uncontrolled hypertension. Her blood pressure was ultimately controlled on clonidine 0.3 mg BID, verapamil 120 mg TID, hydrochlorthiazide 50 mg BID, vasotec 20 mg BID, and minoxodil 5 mg BID (added during the admission). The patient was discharged after 1 week in the hospital with an average blood pressure of 150/90. She was seen daily by a home health nurse. Four days after discharge, she developed lightheadedness that was worse in the late afternoon hours and progressed over the next several days. On presentation to the ED, the patient was noted to be unresponsive. Her family reported no other past medical history.

Physical Examination: Blood pressure 210/110, pulse 110, respiratory rate 20. HEENT: no papilledema. Neck: supple, no jugular vein distention. Chest: clear. Cardiac: RRR, grade II/VI systolic murmur (old). Abdomen: normal bowel sounds, nontender, no organomegaly. Rectal: hemoccult negative. Neuromuscular: withdraws to pain, nonfocal.

Questions: What immediate diagnostic test and therapy should be initiated in this patient? What are the most likely causes of this patient's signs and symptoms?

Diagnosis and Clinical Course: Medication-induced hypoglycemia. This patient immediately received intravenous dextrose, naloxone (Narcan), and thiamine. She became more responsive and gradually returned to normal. Her fingerstick glucose level was found to be 20 mg/dl. No one in the patient's house was diabetic. The physicians caring for the patient examined her medications. The new prescription for minoxidil actually contained Micronase (glyburide) tablets. These two medications were stored adjacent to each other on the pharmacy shelf. The patient's hypoglycemia was caused by a medication error in which her antihypertensive medication was substituted with an oral hypoglycemic medication, thus explaining her worsening hypertension and symptomatic hypoglycemia.

Discussion: Unexpected and recurrent hypoglycemia in a nondiabetic patient requires that several possibilities be considered, including various medical conditions (see table) and pharmacologic agents. Drug-induced hypoglycemia caused by inadvertent poisoning is sometimes due to a simple error in medication ordering, dispensing, or administration process. Prescription medications as well as commonly abused substances, such as alcohol, opioids, and cocaine, cause hypoglycemia either primarily or as a side effect (see table).

The National Coordinating Council for Medication Error Reporting and Prevention (NCCMERP) defines a medication error as any preventable event that may cause or lead to inappropriate medication use or patient harm while the medication is in the control of the health care professional, patient, or consumer. A recent review of the Adverse Event Reporting System (AERS) over a 6-year period showed that of 469 of 5366 (8.7%) cases of medication error resulted in death. Errors originating in ambulatory pharmacies caused approximately 4.7% of these deaths, with more than 15% due to inadvertent substitution of one product for another.

Further confusion may be caused by similar-sounding drug names, similar-appearing packages, or difficult to read labels, compounded by poor handwriting on prescriptions. In-hospital medication errors can cause significant morbidity and mortality. The Institute for Safe Medication Practices (ISMP) publishes a report of serious drug-related complications, of which approximately 25% are due to labeling and packaging issues. It estimates that only 1 to 2% of events are actually reported. Medication errors should always be considered as part of the differential diagnosis of a patient with sudden, unexplained altered mental status.

Medical Conditions that Cause Hypoglycemia[1,3]

Addison's disease
Panhypopituitarism
Carcinomas (insulinoma, extrapancreatic tumors)
Reactive hypoglycemia
Cirrhosis/liver failure
Chronic renal insufficiency
Acquired immunodeficiency syndrome
Autoimmune disorders (systemic lupus erythematosus,
  Graves' disease)
Septicemia
Shock
Wasting syndrome/malnutrition

Medications that Cause Hypoglycemia[3]

Beta-blockers
Disopyramide
Hypoglycemic agents
Pentamidine
Quinine and its derivatives
Salicylates
Streptozocin
Sulfonamides
Valproic acid
Insulin

Clinical Pearls

1. Acute hypoglycemia should be considered immediately in any patient with altered mental status.

2. Pharmacologic agents other than oral hypoglycemic agents and insulin may cause recurrent, profound hypoglycemia.

3. Medications errors that originate in ambulatory pharmacies may be due to poor handwriting on prescriptions, similar-sounding drug names, or similar-appearing packages.

REFERENCES

1. Bates DW: Unexpected hypoglycemia in a critically ill patient. Ann Intern Med 137:E110–117, 2002.
2. Marks V, Teale JD: Drug-induced hypoglycemia. Endocrinol Metab Clin North Am 28:555–577, 1999.
3. Bosse GM: Antidiabetic and hypoglycemic agents. In Goldfrank LR, Flomenbaum NE (eds): Goldfrank's Toxicologic Emergencies, 7th ed. New York, McGraw-Hill, 2002, pp. 593–605.
4. Phillips J, Beam S, Brinker A, et al: Retrospective analysis of mortalities associated with medication errors. Am J Health Syst Pharm 58:1835–1841, 2001.
5. Kenagy JW, Stein GC: Naming, labeling, and packaging of pharmaceuticals. Am J Health Syst Pharm 58:2033–2041, 2001.

Jill C. Posner, MD

PATIENT 12

An 11-year-old boy with fever, myalgias, and rash

An 11-year-old, previously healthy boy presents to the emergency department with fevers and progressively worsening rash. Ten days prior, he first developed "flu-like" symptoms, including low-grade fever (to 37.8°C) and myalgias. A few days later, a 3 cm erythematous macular skin lesion appeared on his left torso. In the following days, the lesion enlarged and developed central clearing. In addition, he began to experience bilateral knee and ankle pain without swelling of the joints. The symptoms persisted and 3 days ago several additional skin lesions developed on his back, legs, and face, similar in appearance to the first. He reports having intermittent headache and neck stiffness although denies these symptoms at the present time. He is an avid outdoor sports enthusiast and recently returned from a fishing trip in the Pennsylvania mountains.

Physical Examination: Vital signs: temperature 36.8°C orally; pulse 115, respiratory rate 16, blood pressure 106/68. General: well appearing. HEENT: normal. Neck: no meningismus, no Kernig's or Brudzinski's signs. Chest: clear to auscultation. Cardiac: regular rate and rhythm without murmurs, rubs, or gallops. Abdomen: normal. Extremities: No edema or erythema, full range of motion at all joints. Neurologic: alert and oriented, cranial nerves intact, strength and sensation normal, normal deep tendon and Babinski reflexes, normal gait. Skin: eight target lesions varying in diameter from 4 to 8 cm located on the left jaw angle, both cheeks (see figure), left upper torso (see figure), left abdomen, left back, right thigh, and right leg.

Laboratory Findings: CBC: normal. Blood chemistries: normal. Liver function tests: normal. CSF analysis: WBCs 20/hpf (4% segmented neutrophils, 15% monocytes, 64% lymphocytes, 1% eosinophils, 15% atypical lymphocytes), RBCs 0/hpf, glucose 48 mg/dl, protein 34 mg/dl. CSF gram stain: few WBC, no bacteria. Electrocardiogram: normal.

Question: What is the diagnosis?

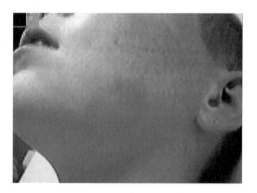 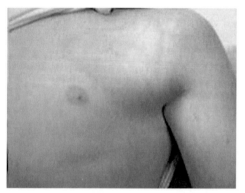

Diagnosis: Early disseminated Lyme disease

Discussion: Lyme disease, caused by infection with the spirochete *Borrelia burgdorferi,* is transmitted to humans via the blood meal of an infected *Ixode*s tick. Although it occurs throughout the world, Lyme disease in the United States occurs primarily in three geographic regions. More than 90% of the 16,000 cases reported annually to the Centers for Disease Control and Prevention originate in the Northeastern and mid-Atlantic states, with the remainder mostly reported in the Midwest (Wisconsin and Minnesota) and northern California and Oregon. A tick may become infected at any stage of its life cycle; however, the nymphal tick, emerging in the spring, is responsible for most human transmission.

The clinical manifestations of Lyme disease are divided into three phases: early localized, early disseminated, and late disease. A distinct rash, erythema migrans (EM), characterizes early localized disease appearing at the site of the tick bite 7 to 10 days later. It begins as an erythematous macule or papule and expands for days to weeks to form a large, annular lesion that is at least 5 cm in diameter. It can vary in shape and the degree of central clearing. The lesion may be uniformly erythematous, may look like a target, or occasionally may have a vesicular or necrotic center. The rash itself is generally asymptomatic, but there may be associated "flu-like" systemic symptoms such as fever, malaise, myalgia, headache, regional lymphadenopathy, or arthralgia. The differential diagnosis of the EM rash includes erythema multiforme, contact dermatitis, urticaria, nummular eczema, granuloma annulare, tinea corporis, and other insect bites.

The most common manifestation of early disseminated Lyme disease is multiple EM. Secondary lesions, resulting from spirochetemia and dermal dissemination, appear 3 to 5 weeks after the tick bite. These lesions are usually similar in appearance to the primary lesion, although they may be smaller in size. Systemic symptoms are common. Other manifestations of early disseminated disease include central nervous system and cardiac dysfunction. About 15% of untreated patients in the United States develop dissemination to the central nervous system resulting in meningitis, cranial nerve palsies (most commonly of the facial nerve), cerebellar ataxia, and motor or sensory radiculoneuropathies. Cardiac involvement is rare, affecting about 5% of untreated patients, most commonly in the form of atrioventricular block.

Late Lyme disease, which occurs weeks to months after the initial tick bite, is most commonly manifested by mono- or oligoarticular arthritis. Sixty percent of untreated patients develop arthritis in the large joints, most commonly the knee. The affected joint may become warm, swollen, and painful, although generally not to the degree of a "septic" joint. Despite adequate antibiotic therapy, about 10% of patients have persistent or recurrent joint inflammation. Encephalitis, encephalopathy (mild, subtle cognitive dysfunction), and polyneuropathy are also rare manifestations of late Lyme disease.

Nearly 90% of patients with Lyme disease develop the primary EM rash. Patients with EM may be diagnosed clinically, as serodiagnostic test results are often negative in early disease. For others, the diagnosis of Lyme disease can be difficult. Commercially available serologic kits can be rather insensitive, and testing should be performed at an experienced reference laboratory. A "two-step process" for the detection of serum antibody response to *B. burgdorferi* is generally recommended. The enzyme immunoassay (EIA) is performed first, followed by the Western immunoblot test to corroborate positive or equivocal EIA results. A negative EIA result requires no further immunoblot testing. The immunoglobin IgM specific antibody titer usually peaks between 3 and 6 weeks after infection, IgG titers usually rise more slowly and peak weeks to months later, and both titers may persist for many years despite cure. Because the sensitivity of a diagnostic test is dependent on the disease prevalence, caution should be taken in using Lyme serologic tests for screening purposes for patients with chronic, nonspecific symptoms. In these instances, false-positive findings are common. The polymerase chain reaction assay has been used investigationally for decades and is now available for reference laboratory use. In most clinical settings, its use is limited by its low sensitivity, and it should be used as only as an adjunct in the evaluation for Lyme disease.

The treatment of Lyme disease depends on the stage of the disease and organ system(s) involved (see table). For patients who are allergic to penicillin, cefuroxime axetil and erythromycin are alternative drugs.

Currently, controversy abounds regarding the utility of prophylactic antibiotic treatment following a tick bite and the cost-effectiveness of the Lyme disease vaccine. The American Academy of Pediatrics Committee on Infectious Diseases, in at least two published documents, have come out strongly against the routine use of antimicrobial agents to prevent Lyme disease, even after a

DISEASE CATEGORY	DRUG(S) AND DOSE
Early localized disease	
≥ 8 years old	Doxycycline, oral regimen, 100 mg BID for 14–21 days
All ages	Amoxicillin, oral regimen, 25–50 mg/kg per day divided into two doses (max, 2 g/d) for 14–21 days
Early disseminated and late disease	
Multiple EM	Same oral regimen as for early disease but for 21 days
Isolated facial palsy	Same oral regimen as for early disease but for 21–28 days (corticosteriods should not be given)
Arthritis	Same oral regimen as for early disease but for 28 days
Persistent/recurrent arthritis	Ceftriaxone, 75–100 mg/kg, IV or IM, once daily (max, 2 g/d) for 14–21 days; or penicillin, 300,000 U/kg per day IV given in divided doses every 4 hours (maximum, 20 million U/d) for 14–21 days
Carditis	Ceftriaxone or penicillin: see persistent or recurrent arthritis
Meningitis or encephalitis	Ceftriaxone or penicillin: see persistent or recurrent arthritis

From the Committee on Infectious Diseases: Red Book: Report of the Committee on Infectious Diseases, 25th ed. Lyme Disease—CD-Rom 2002. Elk Grove, IL, American Academy of Pediatrics; with permission.

known deer tick bite in an endemic area. The Academy recommendations concerning the vaccine are specific: consider administration of the vaccine for persons 15 years of age or older whose activities in a high-risk area result in frequent or prolonged exposure to ticks. Routine vaccination is not recommended for those who have minimal or no exposure to infected ticks, even if living in high- or moderate-risk areas.

Most effective at reducing the risk of developing Lyme disease is the adoption of personal protective measures, including the avoidance of high-risk, heavily wooded areas, wearing protective clothing such as hats, long-sleeved shirts, and long pants, and applying insect repellent with *n,n,*-diethylmetatoluamide (DEET) (<30%). Daily tick checks should be routine in families with high tick exposure.

In the present patient, the history of headache and neck stiffness is an important indicator that dissemination to the central nervous system may have occurred. The physical examination provided no evidence of meningitis, yet cerebrospinal fluid (CSF) analysis led to the diagnosis of Lyme meningitis and a markedly different treatment regimen than if the patient had been diagnosed with multiple EM alone. Intravenous ceftriaxone was administered in the ED and the patient was admitted to the general ward. The CSF culture for bacteria was negative, as expected. The CSF Lyme polymerase chain reaction assay finding was also negative, not unexpected given the low sensitivity of this test. However, the serum immunotests were markedly positive based on the Centers for Disease Control and Prevention criteria. During the hospitalization, the patient underwent placement of a peripheral intravenous central catheter, and arrangements for home care nursing were made to facilitate his completing the 30-day course of therapy as an outpatient. Importantly, preventive measures were reviewed with the patient and the family upon hospital discharge.

Clinical Pearls

1. Prompt recognition and treatment of Lyme disease in its early stages can reduce morbidity.

2. Erythema migrans is a distinct, diagnostic rash seen in the majority of patients with Lyme disease.

3. Serologic studies for unclear cases should be ordered with discretion and interpreted with caution, based on the individual patient's pretest probability of disease and the disease prevalence.

4. Prevention education should emphasize measures to avoid tick bites.

REFERENCES

1. Bunikis J, Barbour AG: Laboratory testing for suspected Lyme disease. Med Clin North Am 86:311–340, 2002.
2. Mollen CJ, Bell LM: Tick-borne illnesses in the United States. Pediatr Case Rev 1:14–25, 2002.
3. Steere AC: Lyme disease. N Engl J Med 345:115–123, 2001.
4. Committee on Infectious Diseases: Red Book: Report of the Committee on Infectious Diseases, 25th ed. Lyme Disease—CD-Rom 2002. Elk Grove, IL, American Academy of Pediatrics.
5. Shapiro ED, Gerber MA: Lyme disease. Clin Infect Dis 31:533–542, 2000.
6. Committee on Infectious Diseases: Prevention of Lyme disease. Pediatrics 105:142–147, 2000.
7. Preim S, et al: An optimized PCR leads to rapid and highly sensitive detection of *Borrelia burgdorferi* in patients with Lyme borreliosis. J Clin Microbiol 35:685–690, 1997.
8. Nocton JJ, et al: Detection of *Borrelia burgdorferi* DNA by polymerase chain reaction in cerebrospinal fluid in Lyme neuroborreliosis. J Infect Dis 174:623–627, 1996.

Paul A. Andrulonis, MD

PATIENT 13

A 68-year-old woman with upper back pain

A 68-year-old woman presents to the emergency department with an upper back injury after straining to lift a sewing machine. The pain is described as throbbing. She denies any other symptoms.

Physical Examination: Temperature 36.3°C, pulse 67, respiratory rate 18, blood pressure 214/102, pulse oximetry 98% on room air. Skin: normal. HEENT: normal. Cardiac: regular rate and rhythm without murmurs or rubs. Chest: breath sounds equal and clear. Back: bilateral paraspinal muscle tenderness to palpation in region of vertebrae T_5 to T_{10}. Abdomen: normal. Neurologic: normal.

Laboratory Findings: WBC 8400/μl, Hgb 12.9 g/dl, CPK 119 ng/ml, CPK-MB 1.1 ng/ml, troponin < 0.2 u/l. ECG: normal sinus rhythm, left ventricular hypertrophy with repolarization changes, QRS axis 39. No previous ECG available. Chest radiograph: (see figure) aortic uncoiling, no pulmonary disease.

Questions: How would you treat this patient? Is any further work-up indicated?

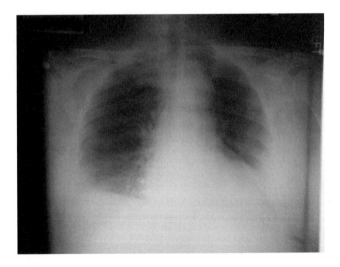

Diagnosis and Treatment: Blood pressure was rechecked—the right upper extremity blood pressure was 148/115, and the left was 180/116. Computed tomography (CT) of the chest with contrast revealed an aortic dissection distal to the left subclavian artery extending to the aortic bifurcation. The patient was admitted to a monitored bed, treated medically, and discharged from the hospital 11 days later.

Discussion: Aortic dissection occurs when blood flows from the aortic intimal lining into the aortic media, creating a false lumen. The initial insult most commonly is an intimal tear. Less frequently, dissection results from hemorrhage of the vaso vasorum into the media with expansion of the hematoma through the intima into the aortic lumen. Two variants of dissection are aortic intramural hematoma (hematoma without an intimal flap) and penetrating atherosclerotic aortic ulcer, which may lead to hematoma and aneurysm formation.

Aortic dissection predominates among men with chronic hypertension in the sixth to seventh decade of life. Other predisposing factors include cocaine use, pregnancy, Marfan's syndrome, Turner's syndrome, connective tissue disease, vasculitis, coarctation of the aorta, and congenital heart disease. The risk of dissection associated with atherosclerotic changes has not been well defined.

Two anatomic classification systems are used to describe aortic dissection. In the Stanford system, type A dissection involves the ascending aorta with or without extension into the descending aorta; type B involves only the descending aorta. In the DeBakey system, type I dissection involves both the ascending and the descending aorta, type II only involves the ascending aorta, and type III is confined to the descending aorta. Dissections are considered acute if symptoms last less than 2 weeks and chronic if present for more than 2 weeks.

Pain is the most common presenting symptom of aortic dissection and occurs in 90 to 95% of patients. The location of pain may be in the chest, back or abdomen. One third of patients initially have abdominal pain, frequently in the epigastrum. Classic chest and back pain is also seen in about one third of patients. Painless dissection is reported in up to 10% of cases. Other signs and symptoms of dissection include absent pulses, hypotension, acute aortic regurgitation murmur, cardiac tamponade, hemothorax, peripheral neuropathy, Horner's syndrome, acute stroke, spinal cord ischemia, and mesenteric ischemia. Ortner's syndrome (hoarseness from compression of the left recurrent laryngeal nerve) caused by the dissection is an uncommon presentation.

Death from acute aortic dissection usually results from aortic rupture, acute aortic valve regurgitation, cardiac tamponade or hypotension and multi-organ failure. Mortality rates increase 1 to 3% each hour following the onset of dissection. It is estimated that 21% of patients die prior to reaching the hospital; in-hospital mortality rates are approximately 30% and 10% for proximal and distal dissections, respectively.

The electrocardiogram often shows nonspecific abnormalities. Evidence of acute myocardial infarction may be present if the dissection has propagated into the coronary arteries. Chest radiograph offers poor sensitivity in detecting a dissection. Sixteen percent of patients have a normal chest x-ray, 23% show a tortuous aorta, and less than 50% show a widened mediastinum. CT, transesophageal echocardiogram (TEE) and magnetic resonance imaging (MRI) are far superior for diagnostic evaluation. CT offers a sensitivity of 94% but is rarely able to detect an intimal flap or the presence of aortic regurgitation. TEE is becoming the diagnostic modality of choice. Sensitivity approaches 98% and it allows for evaluation of the intimal flap location, aortic regurgitation, and coronary vessel involvement. TEE also offers the advantage of being a rapid bedside procedure. MRI has the highest sensitivity but is often considered impractical for acutely ill patients because of the prolonged time for the study outside of the emergency department. Recent studies have begun to explore the use of a blood assay that detects heavy chain smooth muscle myosin as a marker for dissection. Initial reports of 91% sensitivity and 98% specificity for the presence of aortic dissection are encouraging.

The goal of therapy is to reduce pulsatile blood flow, which limits propagation of the dissection. Medical treatment alone is indicated for patients with uncomplicated distal dissections, and there is no advantage to surgical treatment in terms of survival rate. Intravenous beta-blockers are first-line therapy targeting heart rate of less than 60. The preferred initial agents are labetalol 20 mg IV every 10 minutes for a maximum of 300 mg or an esmolol infusion given as a bolus of 500 μg/kg followed by 50 to 150 μg/kg/min. Sodium nitroprusside 0.3 to 0.5 μg/kg/min is added to assist in blood pressure reduction. Blood pressure should be lowered as much as the patient is able to tolerate.

Proximal dissections have a much higher incidence of life-threatening complications and therefore require prompt surgical intervention. Surgery reduces the mortality rate from greater than 50%

to less than 36% but may be contraindicated in certain patients (e.g., acute stroke patients). Descending dissections that are rapidly expanding, produce intractable pain, or impair blood flow to extremities or vital organs also require surgical treatment. The goal of surgery is to obliterate the intimal flap, thereby obstructing blood flow into the media. Fifty percent of surgical patients have a persistent dissection, and 15% require a second operation for dissection within their lifetime.

Clinical Pearls

1. Up to 40% of patients with aortic dissection may be initially misdiagnosed, and up to 35% are diagnosed postmortem.

2. Dissections occur two to three times more frequently than abdominal aortic aneurysmal rupture. Consider the diagnosis in all patients with chest pain, back pain, or epigastric pain.

3. Reproducible muscular pain or other atypical symptoms do not exclude significant pathology such as dissection.

REFERENCES

1. Khan IA, Nair CK: Clinical, diagnostic and management perspectives of aortic dissection. Chest 122:311–328, 2002.
2. Manning WJ: Clinical manifestations and diagnosis of aortic dissection. UpToDate 2002. www.uptodate.com.
3. Manning WJ: Management of aortic dissection. UpToDate 2002. www.uptodate.com.
4. Sullivan PR, Wolfson AB, Leckey RD, Burke JL: Diagnosis of acute thoracic aortic dissection in the emergency department. Am J Emerg Med 18:46–50, 2000.
5. Khan IA, Wattanasauwan N, Ansari AW: Painless aortic dissection as hoarseness of voice—Cardiovocal syndrome: Ortner's syndrome. Am J Emerg Med 17:361–363, 1999.

Elizabeth R. Alpern, MD, MSCE

PATIENT 14

A 12-year-old girl with abdominal pain and inability to urinate

A previously healthy 12-year-old girl was referred from an outside emergency department for evaluation of possible appendicitis. The patient reports lower abdominal pain over 4 days and inability to urinate for 24 hours. She states that she is hungry but unable to eat secondary to the abdominal pain. She has had recent urinary frequency and dysuria followed by the inability to void despite the ongoing sensation of urinary urgency. She has been afebrile and has not vomited. She had a bowel movement this morning which she describes as hard in nature. She has not started menstruating yet and denies any sexual activity or vaginal discharge. She has had intermittent abdominal pains in the last few months, but none so severe that she sought medical attention. She has not taken any medications and is accompanied by her mother and older sister to the ED.

Physical Examination: Vital signs: Temperature 37.6°C orally; pulse 108; respiratory rate 18; blood pressure 115/70. General: Well-nourished and well-developed adolescent girl in moderate discomfort. Chest: clear to auscultation. Cardiac: RRR without murmur. Abdomen: distended lower abdomen, tenderness to suprapubic area with palpable midline mass, no hepatosplenomegaly, no rebound. Rectal examination: brown, hard stool, guaiac test negative. Torso: no costovertebral angle tenderness. Genitourinary: Tanner 3 breast development, Tanner 3 pubic hair, and external female genitalia with bluish bulging membrane at vaginal introitus (see figure).

Laboratory Findings: Urine βHCG: negative; Urinalysis: pH 7.0, specific gravity 1.010, negative for leukocytes, nitrites, ketones, glucose, protein; electrolytes, BUN, and Cr within normal limits.

ED Course/Radiographic Findings: A Foley catheter is placed and 700 ml of urine obtained. On re-examination, the patient's abdomen is less distended but still with a fullness to the suprapubic area. Ultrasonography is performed, which notes a homogeneous avascular mass within the expected region of the lumen of vagina and uterus and normal kidney structure.

Question: What is the most likely diagnosis?

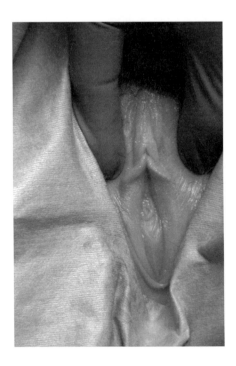

Diagnosis: Imperforate hymen with hematocolpos

Discussion: Evaluation of the adolescent female with abdominal pain is fraught with difficulties and, at the very least, must include consideration of gastrointestinal, genitourinary, and psychological etiologies. A complete physical examination, including rectal, external genitalia, and pelvic examination, is indicated. The diagnosis of imperforate hymen with hematocolpos and urinary retention was immediately evident upon examination of the external genitalia in this case. A bluish intralabial membrane was identified bulging with retained menstrual blood. Historical finding consistent with this diagnosis include primary amenorrhea despite advancing Tanner stage breast and pubic hair development and cyclic (monthly) abdominal pain.

The hymen divides the vagina from the urogenital sinus. It is embryologically derived from the epithelium of the urogenital sinus. An imperforate hymen is the result of a failure of degeneration of the central epithelial cells and occurs in approximately 0.1% of full-term girl births. Although it is usually not associated with other congenital anomalies, transverse vaginal septum, vaginal atresia, and dysplastic kidneys have been reported in conjunction with a finding of imperforate hymen.

An imperforate hymen may be clinically evident at any age with close examination. However, complications are most notable in the newborn and adolescent age ranges. Hydrocolpos, accumulation of mucus or blood in the vagina stimulated from circulating maternal hormones, is usually diagnosed in the neonatal period. In the pubertal patient, hematocolpos is the accumulation of menstrual blood in the vagina due to an imperforate hymen. Hematometra (blood retained in the uterus) or hematosalpinx (blood in the fallopian tube) have been described when hematocolpos goes unrecognized. Urinary retention and constipation may result from compression of the urethra or rectum by the distended vagina. Infection, with retained blood as the culture medium, must also be considered.

Diagnosis is determined by inspection. Ultrasonography will confirm the diagnosis and may identify any associated urogenital anomalies. Surgical repair will allow for excision of redundant hymenal tissue and evacuation of old menstrual blood. Infection is a risk, but when hematocolpos is the only complication of imperforate hymen, the prognosis is excellent.

In the present patient, surgical consultation was obtained and she was taken to the operating room for definitive treatment.

Clinical Pearls

1. Cyclic abdominal pain in an adolescent girl with primary amenorrhea may indicate an imperforate hymen with hematocolpos.

2. Hematocolpos, hematometra, and hematosalpinx are complications of imperforate hymen in the menarchal adolescent girl.

3. Ultrasonography can may be used to diagnose associated urogenital anomalies.

4. Surgical hymenotomy is definitive treatment for imperforate hymen and its complications.

REFERENCES
1. Bogen DL, Gehris RP, Bellinger MF: Imperforate hymen with hydrocolpos. Arch Pediatr Adolesc Med 154:959–960, 2000.
2. Bakos O, Berglund L: Imperforate hymen and ruptured hematosalpinx: Case report with a review of the literature. J Adolesc Health 24:226–228, 1999.
3. Schneider K, Hong J, Fong J, Sanders CG: Hematocolpos as an easily overlooked diagnosis. Curr Opin Pediatri 11:249–252, 1999.

Brendan Carr, MD, MA
Elizabeth M. Datner, MD

PATIENT 15

A 28-year-old man with a hand laceration after an assault

A 28-year-old man presents to the emergency department with a 6-cm laceration to the dorsum of his nondominant left hand. He reports that his injury occurred 30 minutes prior to arrival when his ex-girlfriend "sliced him" with a steak knife during an argument. He is accompanied by a police officer who explains that she is going to take him to police headquarters to file for a restraining order against the assailant once medical treatment is complete.

Physical Examination: Temperature 36.7°C, pulse 85, respiratory rate 16, blood pressure 118/74. General: No distress, left hand wrapped in a kitchen towel soaked with blood. Skin: warm and dry, no other visible injuries. Extremities: left hand with 6-cm laceration over dorsum with no tendon involvement, no foreign body, no active bleeding. The wound is gaping but the edges are not jagged and can be easily approximated. Neurologic: full extension of all digits on left hand at all joints, sensation is intact to light touch and pinprick distal to the wound.

Laboratory Findings: No laboratory tests are performed.

Questions: What important public health issue is illustrated by this case? What is the role of the emergency physician in such cases?

Diagnosis: Domestic violence (DV). DV is the perpetration and maintenance of power and control that one adult (or adolescent) yields over an intimate partner. The term is meant to include past and present intimate partners and is applicable to homosexual and heterosexual relationships. The power and control within the relationship are maintained through physical assaults, physical threats, sexual assault, coercion, social isolation, financial dependence, threats to harm loved ones, and mental and emotional abuse.

Discussion: The United States Department of Justice collects data on violent crimes in the form of the National Crime Victimization Survey (NCVS). In 1998, victims reported that approximately 1 million violent crimes were committed by current or former intimate partners. Approximately 85% of intimate partner crimes were committed against women.

The ED is a likely place for intimate partner violence (IPV) to be detected. It remains difficult to estimate the number of victims of IPV that are seen in emergency departments annually because the relationship of the assailant is often not known. A 1981 study investigating DV victims in the ED found that 22% of adults had been victims of DV. Another study found that about half of women who were victims of DV-related homicides had been seen in an ED within the preceding 2 years. Additional work on the role of screening for DV in trauma patients demonstrated a rise in incidence from about 5% to 30% when patients were screened during their ED visit.

In the last several decades, there has been an increase in the awareness of DV and its impact on health. The AMA states that "physicians should routinely inquire about physical, sexual, and psychological abuse as part of the medical history." Despite these efforts, screening for DV is not a routine part of health care in the United States, even though screening for less prevalent diseases is commonplace. A methodology called "RADAR" is now taught in medical schools around the country. RADAR reminds clinicians to (**R**) routinely screen female patients, (**A**) ask direct questions, (**D**) document findings, (**A**) assess patient safety, and (**R**) review options and referrals.

Interest on the part of the physician alone may have a significant impact on how a DV victim perceives his or her abuse. Clinicians should encourage victims to talk about their experiences and should listen nonjudgmentally. Explaining that domestic violence is common, that everyone has a right to live without IPV, and that help is available are some important first steps in counseling. The American College of Emergency Physicians (ACEP) has a policy that endorses screening for DV in the ED. However, many physicians not only feel inadequately trained to discuss the issue but also are frustrated by the absence of a clear solution.

It is important to conduct a safety assessment and to discuss safety planning with the patient. The patient may be in the ED because the abuse has been escalating, because of new or more severe physical threats, or because she is afraid to go home. Discharge planning will be influenced by the patient's perception of safety. Victims are often not ready to leave their abusers at the time that IPV is detected. Safety planning is advisable should the patient need to leave home quickly. She should be encouraged to think ahead and to plan for such an event. Safe storage of items, including extra car keys, copies of identification, money, and court documentation, is essential. The patient should be encouraged to plan where she could stay and what resources would be available in the event of an emergency. The patient should be informed that the medical record (including photographs) from the ED visit can be used as evidence at a future date.

Additional information about the present case revealed that the patient's ex-girlfriend had been taken to another facility and found to have injuries consistent with attempted strangulation. After completion of the laceration repair, the police officer accompanying the patient took him into custody. This illustrates the phenomenon that many male abusers present themselves as victims after a DV incident. The details of this case are far less important than the recognition that DV is pervasive in the United States and that victims rarely present with a chief complaint of IPV.

Clinical Pearls

1. DV is a common public health problem and likely to be seen in the ED.
2. Talking about IPV may have a positive effect on the patient's willingness to seek help.
3. It is the role of the emergency physician to ensure the patient's safety and to educate about safety planning.

REFERENCES

1. Rennison CM, Welchans S for the Bureau of Justice Statistics: Intimate partner violence. NCJ 178247, 2000.
2. Rounsaville B, Weissman MM: Battered women: A medical problem requiring detection. Int J Psych Med 78:191–202, 1977.
3. American College of Emergency Physicians: Domestic Violence Policy 400286. Accessed April 2003 at www.acep.org
4. Muelleman R, Burgess P: Male victims of domestic violence and their history if perpetrating violence. Acad Emerg Med 5:866–870, 1998.
5. Eisentstat S, Bancroft L: Domestic violence. N Eng J Med 341:886–892, 1999.

Linda Brown, MD
Richard Scarfone, MD

PATIENT 16

A 6-week-old boy with vomiting, diarrhea, and cyanosis

A 6-week-old boy is brought to the emergency department because of frequent vomiting and diarrhea. For the past 2 days he has had an average of 12 watery, nonbloody stools and three episodes of nonbloody and nonbilious emesis that is not projectile. The parents are not able to quantify his urine output. He is fed a premixed, soy-based formula. He has not had a fever or rash but has had decreased activity.

Physical Examination: Temperature 37.4°C; pulse 150; respiratory rate 58; blood pressure 75/40. General: ill-appearing, dusky, cyanotic infant with sunken anterior fontanelle (see figure). Mucous membranes are dry and capillary refill is 3–4 seconds. Chest: clear. Cardiac: tachycardia without murmur, rub, or gallop. Pulses: palpable.

Laboratory Findings: Hematocrit 31%, WBC 17, 400/μl, platelets 289,000/μl. Electrolytes notable for: Na 148 mEq/L, HCO_3 11 mEq/L. Room air oxygen saturation 93%; ABG (room air): pH 7.13, $PaCO_2$ 26 mm Hg, PaO_2 86 mm Hg. Chest x-ray: no infiltrates, normal heart size. ECG: within normal limits for age.

ED Course: The patient's cyanosis was not improved after administration of 10 L/min of supplemental oxygen via a non-rebreathing facemask. During venopuncture, his blood was noted to be dark brown in color (see figure).

Question: What is the most likely diagnosis?

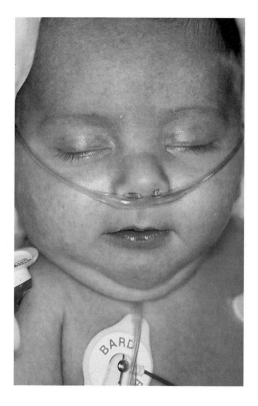
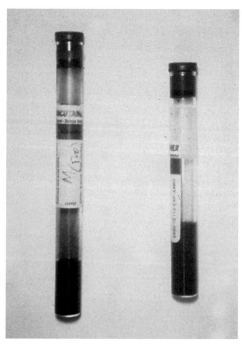

Diagnosis: Methemoglobinemia

Discussion: Methemoglobinemia occurs when the iron located within the hemoglobin molecule, normally in the ferrous (Fe^{++}) state, is oxidized to the ferric (Fe^{+++}) state. As a result, the newly formed methemoglobin loses its ability to carry oxygen, and the oxygen carried by the nonoxidized hemoglobin subunits is more tightly bound. This results in a left-shift of the hemoglobin-oxygen saturation curve, with less oxygen released to the tissues.

This alteration of hemoglobin most often occurs when an individual is exposed to an oxidizing compound. Common agents that may induce methemoglobinemia include nitrites, nitrates, benzocaine, sulfonamide antibiotics, aniline dyes, and naphthalene (mothballs). Dietary nitrates, especially those found in well water, may also cause methemoglobin to develop. Genetic forms of methemoglobinemia, resulting from a deficiency of either cytochrome b_5 or cytochrome b_5 reductase, are usually inherited in an autosomal recessive manner.

Methemoglobinemia may also be found in infants who present with a metabolic acidosis, usually as a result of diarrhea and dehydration. In one study, among infants younger than 6 months old with more than 24 hours of diarrhea, 64% had elevated methemoglobin levels. There was no correlation between the methemoglobin level and the severity of acidosis, but infants in this study with weights at or below the 10th percentile were at greatest risk for methemoglobinemia. The cause of methemoglobinemia in this setting is unclear, although there may be an association with nitrite-forming enteric bacteria, such as *Escherichia coli* and *Campylobacter jejuni*. Also, fetal hemoglobin is more easily oxidized than adult hemoglobin and infants have lower levels of cytochrome b_5 reductase, an enzyme that reduces iron to the ferrous state. Thus, the development of methemoglobinemia in infants with diarrhea may be multifactorial.

Clinical manifestations of methemoglobinemia are directly related to methemoglobin levels. Patients with levels below 10% are asymptomatic. Cyanosis is noted with levels of 10 to 30%, and with 30 to 50%, patients may present with tachycardia, dyspnea, anxiety, headache, and fatigue. Levels of 50 to 70% are usually associated with coma, acidosis, seizures, and arrhythmias, and levels greater than 70% may lead to cardiac arrest.

As noted above, cyanosis is a relatively early manifestation of methemoglobinemia. One diagnostic clue is that the oxygen saturation recorded by the pulse oximeter may not be consistent with degree of the patient's cyanosis. A pulse oximeter can determine the concentration of only two hemoglobin species: reduced hemoglobin and oxyhemoglobin. Methemoglobin, which aborbs light at different wavelengths than either of these two hemoglobin species, is not detected by standard pulse oximetry. This results in the pulse oximeter overestimating true arterial oxygen saturation. The patient's PaO_2 should be normal, since this is a measure of dissolved gas and not the amount of oxygen bound to hemoglobin.

The diagnosis may be established by measuring the methemoglobin level with cooximetry. Also, a simple bedside test is to place a drop of the patient's blood on filter paper; methemoglobin will give it a chocolate brown appearance.

Methylene blue is the treatment of choice for methemoglobinemia. The dose is 1 to 2 mg/kg (0.2 ml/kg of 1% solution), and it is infused intravenously over 3 to 5 minutes. The methylene blue is metabolized to leukomethylene blue, which acts as a reducing agent to convert the methemoglobin. Treatment is usually advised for all patients with levels greater than 30%. For children with levels between 20 and 30%, efforts should be made to remove the oxidant stress and correct any existing acidosis. In addition, methylene blue may be used for symptomatic children with levels in this range or for those not responding to these other measures. Lower thresholds for methylene blue therapy should be considered for patients with medical conditions resulting in impaired oxygen delivery. Methylene blue may not be effective for patients with G6PD deficiency. In addition, these patients may develop a paradoxical worsening of their methemoglobinemia as well as a hemolytic anemia with methylene blue therapy.

The present patient had diarrhea, significant dehydration, and duskiness. Further, his color did not improve with the administration of supplemental oxygen and his blood was noted to be dark brown in color. The diagnosis was confirmed with co-oximetry showing a methemoglobin level of 34%. The patient was successfully treated with intravenous fluids and methylene blue.

Clinical Pearls

1. Methemoglobinemia should be considered as a diagnosis in a cyanotic patient who does not improve with supplemental oxygen.
2. Infants with diarrhea and dehydration are at risk for developing methemoglobinemia.
3. Pulse oximetry is not helpful for estimation of oxygen saturation in patients with methemoglobinemia.
4. Patients with G6PD deficiency may not respond to treatment with methylene blue and are at higher risk for complications from this therapy.

REFERENCES

1. Price D: Methemoglobinemia. In Goldfranck LR et al (eds): Goldfranck's Toxicologic Emergencies, 7th ed. New York, McGraw-Hill 2002, pp 1438–1447.
2. Wright RO, Lewander WJ, Woolf AD: Methemoglobinemia: Etiology, pharmacology, and clinical management. Ann Emerg Med 34:646–656, 1999.
3. Tilman Jolly B, Monico EP, McDevitt B: Methemoglobinemia in an infant: Case report and review of the literature. Pediatr Emerg Care 11:294–296, 1995.
4. Pollack ES, Pollack CV: Incidence of subclinical methemoglobinemia in infants with diarrhea. Ann Emerg Med 24:652–656, 1994.
5. Barker SJ, Tremper KK, Hyatt J: Effects of methemoglobinemia on pulse oximetry and mixed venous oximetry. Anesthesiology 70:112–117, 1989.

Charlene An, MD
C. Crawford Mechem, MD
Jill Baren, MD, FACEP, FAAP

PATIENT 17

A 23-year-old man with nausea, vomiting, and fatigue

A 23 year-old man without significant past medical history presents with several days of nausea, vomiting, and general fatigue. The patient also complains of several days of productive cough, rhinorhea, polyuria, and a 10-pound weight loss over 1 month.

Physical Examination: Temperature 38.1°C, pulse 116, respiratory rate 30, blood pressure 125/68. General: thin, tired-appearing, tachypneic male. Skin: warm and dry, no rashes. HEENT: dry mucous membranes, fruity odor of breath. Neck: supple, no lymphadenopathy. Lungs: shallow breaths, clear, no wheezes or rales. Cardiac: tachycardia regular, no murmurs, rubs, or gallop. Abdomen: normal active bowel sounds, soft, nondistended, mild epigastric tenderness, no rebound or guarding. Neurologic: awake, alert, fully oriented, no focal weakness or sensory deficits.

Laboratory Findings: CBC: normal. Electrolytes: Na 129 mEq/L, K 6.3 mEq/L, HCO_3 14 mEq/L, Cl 95 mEq/L, BUN 24 mg/dl, Cr 1.2 mg/dl, glucose 676 mg/dl. Anion gap 20 (normal 10–12). Urinalysis: large ketones, large glucose, no leukocytes. ABG: 7.29, PCO_2 30 mm Hg, PO_2 96 mm Hg. ECG: sinus tachycardia, nonspecific T-wave flattening, no ST changes consistent with ischemia. Chest x-ray: normal.

Questions: What syndrome can explain this patient's signs and symptoms? What is the initial treatment?

Diagnosis and Treatment: Diabetic ketoacidosis (DKA). Initial therapy should include rehydration, insulin administration, and correction of electrolyte abnormalities.

Discussion: Diabetic ketoacidosis develops in the setting of inadequate levels of endogenous or exogenous insulin, which in turn leads to decreased uptake of glucose into muscle, liver, and fat cells. The body's metabolism shifts into a starvation state. To compensate, the counterregulatory hormones, glucagon, growth hormone, and catecholamines, are released into the general circulation. These hormones promote the breakdown of triglycerides into free fatty acids, which undergo beta-oxidation to yield acetone, beta-hydroxybutyric acid, and acetoacetic acid. Metabolic acidosis develops. These hormones also stimulate gluconeogenesis, which causes hyperglycemia. Elevated serum glucose results in an osmotic diuresis, causing dehydration and electrolyte abnormalities. These are exacerbated by vomiting and diarrhea, common complaints among patients with DKA.

DKA usually develops in patients with insulin-dependent diabetes mellitus; however, it may also rarely develop in cases of non-insulin-dependent diabetes. It is generally triggered by noncompliance with a prescribed insulin regimen or by a physiologic stressor. Examples of stressors are infection, acute myocardial infarction, trauma, stroke, pregnancy, or alcohol or drug abuse. DKA may also be the initial presentation of previously undiagnosed diabetes.

The initial evaluation of a patient with DKA includes a careful history focused on medications, medication noncompliance, and any symptoms suggestive of a stressor that may have precipitated the episode. The patient should be asked about dyspnea, polyuria, polydipsia, polyphagia, nausea, vomiting, diarrhea, abdominal pain, depressed mental status, or seizures. The physical examination should include careful search for evidence of dehydration (dry mucous membranes, poor skin turgor, sunken eyes, and depressed fontanelles in infants). Other significant findings include a fruity smell to the breath, rapid, shallow (Kussmaul) respirations, abdominal tenderness, altered mental status, focal neurologic deficits, or focal infection such as pneumonia, pyelonephritis, or cellulitis.

Initial laboratory studies are necessary to assess hydration status, identify electrolyte and other metabolic abnormalities, and look for underlying precipitants of DKA. In most patients, a CBC, electrolyte panel with calcium, phosphate, and magnesium, and serum ketone measurement are recommended. In addition to hyperglycemia, common laboratory abnormalities include an elevated anion gap metabolic acidosis, attributable to the formation of ketoacids. Hyponatremia in DKA is a direct result of the hyperglycemia. The measured serum sodium level drops by 1.6 mEq/L for every 100 mg/dl increase in glucose above 100 mg/dl. Extracellular shift of potassium in response to metabolic acidosis produces hyperkalemia, but most patients in DKA almost uniformly have a total body potassium deficiency. Hypophosphatemia may also develop. Other laboratory studies that are valuable in patients with DKA include urinalysis, urine and blood cultures, electrocardiogram, and chest radiograph.

The most important initial treatment is rehydration, followed by insulin administration and correction of electrolyte abnormalities. At the same time, any precipitants should be identified and managed. The usual adult fluid deficit is 6 to 10 liters. Rehydration alone will cause a drop in glucose levels. In adults without significant renal or cardiac disease, the rate of normal saline infusion is 1 to 2 L of 0.9% normal saline over the first 2 hours, followed by 200 to 500 ml/hour of 0.45% normal saline. When the serum glucose drops below 300 mg/dl, the intravenous solution should be changed to 5% dextrose in normal saline or 5% dextrose in water to provide the continued glucose substrate needed to resolve ketogenesis. Monitoring of urine output is essential to assess the effectiveness of rehydration. Regular insulin should be administered as an initial loading dose of 0.1 to 0.15 units/kg IV followed by a continuous infusion of 0.1 units/kg/hr. The goal should be to decrease serum glucose by 80 mg/dl/ hr. When serum glucose approaches 250 to 300 mg/dl, the rate of insulin infusion should be decreased but continued until the anion gap normalizes and serum ketones become undetectable.

It is important to monitor the electrolytes closely, checking them every hour initially, then every 2 to 4 hours as the acidosis and anion gap resolve. Potassium should be repleted as levels approach 5.3 mEq/L, as long there are no ECG changes suggestive of hyperkalemia. Phosphorus and magnesium should be monitored and repleted when indicated (see table).

Serum pH will normalize with hydration and insulin administration. In severe cases of DKA, it may be necessary to monitor electrolytes and ABG on an hourly basis initially. Calculating Winter's formula [$PaCO_2 = 1.5 \times (HCO_3) + 8 (+/-2)$] helps ascertain whether the patient is appropriately compensated for the metabolic acidosis. The present patient is appropriately compensated. His measured $PaCO_2$ is 30 and calculated $PaCO_2$ is 29.

SERUM K (MEQ/L)	KCL OR KPHOS (MEQ) ADDED TO IV FLUIDS
>5.5	None
5.0–5.5	10
4.5–5.0	20
4.0–4.5	30
3.5–4.0	40
<3.5	>40

Phosphate: Replete IV or PO if level < 1.0 mg/dL

The use of sodium bicarbonate to correct the metabolic acidosis of DKA is controversial because of the possibility of worsening intracellular acidosis. Its use should be restricted to the most severely acidotic patients.

Cerebral edema is one of the most serious complications of DKA. Signs and symptoms include bradycardia, rapid decline in mental status, or failure of mental status to improve with treatment of DKA. Although the cause is not entirely clear, it may be due to overly aggressive rehydration or too rapid correction of glucose, causing a rapid change in osmolarity and movement of fluid from the vasculature into cerebral tissue. Treatment of cerebral edema involves lowering intracranial pressure with mannitol 1 g/kg IV, and hyperventilation.

The present patient developed DKA for two reasons: He was an undiagnosed diabetic and he had left lower lobe pneumonia, as demonstrated by his follow-up chest radiograph on admission. The infiltrate did not appear on the initial chest radiograph because of dehydration. Initial serum ketones were present at a dilution of 1:16 and resolved after intravenous fluid and insulin administration. The patient received intravenous antibiotics, was changed to a subcutaneous insulin regimen, and was eventually discharged home after diabetes management education.

Clinical Pearls

1. The initial priority in the management of of a patient with DKA is fluid replacement followed by insulin replacement.

2. The use of sodium bicarbonate to treat acidosis has not been shown to improve outcome and may even have a deleterious effect. Consider its use in cases of severe acidosis (pH <6.9) and if the patient is hemodynamically unstable.

3. Monitor closely for signs of cerebral edema, especially in the first few hours of therapy.

4. Remember acute coronary syndromes when identifying the precipitants of DKA.

REFERENCES
1. Inward CD, Chambers TL: Fluid management in diabetic ketoacidosis. Arch Dis Childhood 86:443–444, 2002.
2. Viallon A, Zeni F, Lafond P, et al: Does bicarbonate therapy improve the management of severe diabetic ketoacidosis? Crit Care Med 27:2690–2693, 1999.
3. Graber TW: Diabetes mellitus and glucose disorders. In Rosen P, Barken RM (eds): Emergency Medicine Concepts and Clinical Practice, 3rd ed. St. Louis, Mosby-Year Book, 1992, pp 2180–2187.

Joseph J. Zorc, MD

PATIENT 18

A 5-year-old girl with wheezing and dyspnea

A 5-year-old girl is brought to the emergency department for cough, wheezing, and dyspnea. These symptoms began approximately 3 months ago, and have progressively increased in severity. About 3 weeks ago, she saw her regular physician and was started on albuterol and a short course of prednisone, with some improvement. Subsequently, the symptoms have worsened again and are increased with exertion and lying flat at night. For the past week, she has experienced low-grade fevers and occasional post-tussive, nonbilious emesis and loose, nonbloody stools. She has had no weight loss or hemoptysis, and her past medical history is unremarkable. There is no family history of asthma or respiratory disease.

Physical Examination: Temperature 39°C; pulse 140; respiratory rate 30; blood pressure 112/73; pulse oximetry 97% in room air. General: mild increased work of breathing but alert and able to verbalize while sitting up. Head and neck: shotty anterior cervical adenopathy. Chest: decreased breath sounds bilaterally with faint expiratory wheeze diffusely. Heart: regular rate and rhythm with no murmur or rub. Abdomen: soft, no hepatosplenomegaly or masses.

Laboratory Findings: Hemoglobin 10.6 g/dl, WBC 7200/μl, platelets 404,000/μl, potassium 4.4 mmol/L, uric acid 5.7 mg/dl. Chest radiograph and computed tomography (CT) scan: see figures.

Questions: What is your diagnosis? What are the principal diagnostic considerations? What immediate treatment is indicated?

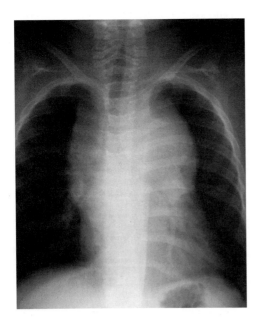

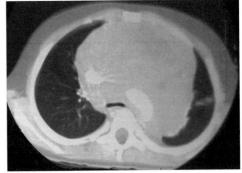

Diagnosis: The images show a large anterior mediastinal mass with compression of the distal trachea.

Discussion: The presentation of a mediastinal mass in a child is a potentially life-threatening emergency that raises a number of diagnostic and management issues. Masses are categorized by their anatomic location in the middle (adjacent to the heart, great vessels, and trachea), anterior, or posterior mediastinum. Overall, most mediastinal masses in children are benign, although the presence of acute symptoms suggests a malignancy. Symptomatic anterior and middle mediastinal masses in children are most commonly due to lymphoma, whereas posterior masses are usually neurogenic in origin. Compression of nearby structures may result in airway or vascular obstruction (superior vena cava [SVC] syndrome) that can be evaluated by CT and echocardiography.

A patient with a mediastinal mass may present with wheezing, cough, dyspnea, and other respiratory symptoms that mimic asthma. The potential for misdiagnosis raises the question of whether a chest radiograph should be obtained for every child with a first episode of wheezing. An early retrospective study found a low yield for routine radiography in this setting (6%) and suggested that the presence of clinical factors, including fever, severe tachypnea (>60 breaths/min) or tachycardia (>160 beats/min), or focal findings on lung examination could identify 95% of children with abnormal radiographs. A subsequent, large, prospective study was unable to achieve this level of accuracy, however. Thus, this question remains controversial, and a low threshold for imaging a child with a first episode of wheezing is appropriate. For a child with established asthma, radiographs are unnecessary unless specific findings suggest pneumonia, pneumothorax, or another alternative diagnosis.

Airway management of a mediastinal mass requires caution and should be individualized based on symptoms and the degree of airway obstruction observed on CT. If movement affects symptoms, the patient should be allowed to remain in a position of comfort. Sedation, muscle paralysis, and positive pressure ventilation may alter respiratory dynamics and cause complete airway obstruction. Inability to lie flat or obstruction of greater than 50% of the trachea are considered contraindications to endotracheal intubation. Early biopsy is important, as initiation of corticosteroids, radiation, or chemotherapy may cause rapid lysis of the tumor and complicate the diagnosis. Airway obstruction may initially worsen with therapy because of local swelling. Tumor lysis syndrome, pericardial tamponade, and pneumothorax are other potential complications of therapy.

In the present patient, a biopsy specimen was obtained by thoracotomy under local anesthesia and showed T cell lymphoblastic lymphoma. Initiation of chemotherapy and corticosteroids led to rapid regression of the mass and improvement of symptoms.

Clinical Pearls

1. Consider obtaining a chest radiograph in a child with a first episode of wheezing.
2. Imaging of the chest in children with established asthma is usually unnecessary unless specific clinical findings suggest an abnormality.
3. Airway management of a mediastinal mass should be approached with caution, as intubation may worsen obstruction.

REFERENCES

1. Hogarty MD, Lange B: Oncologic emergencies. In Fleisher GR, Ludwig S (eds): Textbook of Pediatric Emergency Medicine, 4th ed. Philadelphia, Lippincott Williams & Wilkins, 2000, pp 1157–1190.
2. National Asthma Education and Prevention Program: Expert panel report: Guidelines for the Diagnosis and Management of Asthma. NIH pub # 98–4051. Bethesda, MD, National Institutes of Health, 1997.
3. Walsh-Kelly CM, Kim MK, Hennes HM: Chest radiography in the initial episode of bronchospasm in children: Can clinical variables predict pathologic findings? Ann Emerg Med 28:391–395, 1996.
4. Shamberger RC, Holzman RS, Griscom NT, et al: CT quantitation of tracheal cross-sectional area as a guide to the surgical and anaesthetic management of children with anterior mediastinal masses. J Pediatr Surg 26:138–142, 1991.
5. Gershel JC, Goldman HS, Stein REK, et al: The usefulness of chest radiographs in first asthma attacks. N Engl J Med 309: 336–339, 1983.

Jill M. Baren, MD, FACEP, FAAP

PATIENT 19

A 15-year-old boy with weight loss, bradycardia, and hypothermia

A 15-year-old boy is sent to the emergency department from his pediatrician's office, where he was noted to be cold with a slow heart rate. His parents report a 17-pound weight loss over the last 18 days. He has also been constipated. The patient admits to feelings of sadness and hopelessness but denies suicidal ideation. He denies any fever, chills, night sweats, rash, or swellings. On further questioning, it is determined that he has had severe weight fluctuations over the last year.

Physical examination: Temperature 33.6°C; pulse 42; respiratory rate 18; blood pressure 115/63. Weight 49.8 kg. General appearance: emaciated, pale, and tearful. HEENT: eyes sunken, mucous membranes dry. Chest: clear bilateral breath sounds. Cardiac: bradycardic without murmur. Abdomen: scaphoid, nontender, diminished bowel sounds.

Laboratory Findings: Hemoglobin 15.2 g/dl; WBC 4400/μl. Platelets 271,000/μl. Serum electrolytes: elevated BUN 23, phosphorus 2.6, the remainder within normal limits. A growth curve from the patient's pediatrician was obtained (see figure).

Question: What diagnosis can explain the patient's weight loss and the complications of hypothermia and bradycardia?

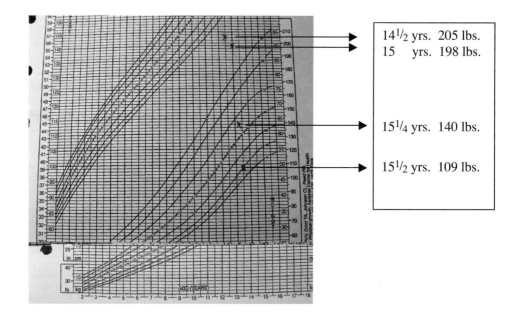

14½ yrs. 205 lbs.
15   yrs. 198 lbs.

15¼ yrs. 140 lbs.

15½ yrs. 109 lbs.

Diagnosis: Anorexia nervosa

Discussion: Anorexia nervosa is an eating disorder that can be difficult to diagnose because of the complex medical and psychosocial issues involved. The prevalence of this disease is estimated to be about 0.5 to 1% of teens, and only 5 to 10 % of those affected are male. Anorexia most often manifests in the early or middle years of adolescence. Although white, female, affluent individuals are believed to be at higher risk, the disease is seen in patients of all ethnic, cultural, and socioeconomic backgrounds.

Several factors are thought to contribute to the development of anorexia. Certain adolescents have difficulty accepting the normal weight gain that occurs with puberty, and anorexia may be an attempt to control this situation. With dieting, underlying hypothalamic dysfunction may become unmasked or exacerbated, and this may lead to psychiatric changes, which perpetuate the disease. There are genetic, personal, and familial influences as well. Anorexic individuals often come from families who are rigid and overprotective with poor ability to resolve conflict. Finally, the media and society often equate thinness with beauty and portray unrealistic ideals of body habitus, which creates pressure for young individuals.

To make the diagnosis of anorexia nervosa, several criteria must be fulfilled: (1) Refusal to maintain body weight above what is normal for age and height, (2) intense fear of gaining weight or becoming fat, (3) disturbed body image or denial of one's serious underweight condition, and (4) at least three cycles of amenorrhea in postmenarchal girls.

Evaluation of a patient with a suspected or known eating disorder should begin with a careful history and physical examination. The goal is to rule out any life-threatening medical complications and to determine whether inpatient or outpatient therapy is appropriate. Symptoms that relate to recurrent vomiting, caloric deprivation, or fluid restriction should be elicited, for example, esophagitis, muscle weakness, constipation, dizziness, or syncope. Patients should be fully undressed for the physical examination, as clothing often hides the extremely emaciated body habitus. Physical findings that are consistent with anorexia are hypothermia, orthostatic hypotension, bradycardia, lanugo hair on the arms and back, hypercarotenemia, hyperpigmentation of the chest and abdomen, and loss of pubic or scalp hair, all from severe malnutrition.

The differential diagnosis of a patient with suspected anorexia nervosa should include the other primary eating disorder, bulimia nervosa. Bulimia patients usually have a history of more vomiting or laxative abuse, have less weight loss, and are slightly older. Medical conditions that also need to be differentiated from anorexia are inflammatory bowel disease, diabetes mellitus, malignancy, thyroid conditions, Addison's disease, and substance abuse. A large number of anorexic patients have concomitant affective disorders, particularly depression.

Laboratory tests can help exclude other causes of severe weight loss and reveal complications of the disease and are recommended as part of the ED evaluation. A CBC should be obtained, as patients are often anemic and leukopenic. Electrolytes are especially important if a patient is vomiting recurrently or abusing laxatives or diuretics. Liver function tests and endocrine studies are helpful in establishing other diagnoses. An ECG should be performed to look for electrophysiologic disturbances (heart block, prolonged QT) and arrhythmias.

It is crucial for the ED physician to determine the safest form of treatment for anorexic patients. Although the mortality rate of this disease is only about 5%, the most common cause of death is suicide, followed by cardiac arrhythmias and electrolyte disturbances. The following medical conditions mandate inpatient treatment: bradycardia, orthostatic hypotension, hypothermia, altered mental status, dehydration, electrolyte disturbance, and suicidal ideation or attempt. Inpatient treatment is also necessary for patients who have dropped below 30% of their normal body weight, those who have persistent weight loss while enrolled in outpatient treatment, and those with a history of rapid weight loss over the preceding 3 months. Effective treatment occurs when an interdisciplinary team of providers from psychiatrists to nutritionists is involved in the patient's care. Overall, the prognosis is variable but often improved with aggressive early treatment.

Hospital Course: The present patient was started on strict meal rules with nutritional guidance. His caloric and fluid intake increased daily and he received phosphorus and vitamin supplementation. Refeeding resulted in an increase in body temperature and heart rate. He was started on sertraline after psychiatric consultation and was discharged to an inpatient treatment program for eating disorders when his weight reached 51 kilograms.

Clinical Pearls

1. Anorexia nervosa affects patients of all ethnic and socioeconomic backgrounds and is easily missed if stereotyping is applied.

2. Eating disorders and depression often coexist; patients with anorexia should be screened intensively for suicidal ideation, as this is their most common cause of death.

3. Indications for hospitalization are medical complications, particularly cardiac complications, rapid weight loss, suicidal ideation, and failure of outpatient treatment.

REFERENCES

1. Lavelle J: Adolescent emergencies. In Fleisher GR, Ludwig S (eds): Textbook of Pediatric Emergency Medicine, 4th ed. Philadelphia, Lippincott Williams & Wilkins, 2000, pp 1735–1738.
2. Steiner H, Lock J: Anorexia nervosa and bulimia nervosa in children and adolescents: A review of the past 10 years. J Am Acad Child Adolesc Psych 37:352–359, 1998.
3. Yagar J: Eating disorders. Psych Clin North Am 19:639–859, 1996.

Cynthia J. Mollen, MD, MSCE

PATIENT 20

A 6-year-old girl with genital lesions

A previously healthy 6-year-old girl was seen in an outside emergency department for constipation. During her physical examination, the treating physician noted a rash in the genital area. She was referred to the accepting emergency department for evaluation of possible sexual abuse. The patient, during a private interview with the physician and social worker, denies any inappropriate contact. She is in first grade. Her mother and grandmother care for her the majority of the time; her father and stepmother share custody and care for her every other weekend. She does not have a regularly scheduled babysitter. All four caregivers are with her in the ED. They all deny having concerns about potential abuse; no one reports noting any unusual or changed behavior. The patient has a several-year history of constipation and has been treated with medications for this intermittently in the past. Her last bowel movement was 5 days ago and was hard; she has had several episodes of bowel incontinence since, with release of small amounts of watery stool. She has not had any recent fever, abdominal pain, vomiting, vaginal discharge, or vaginal bleeding. Her parents note that over the last 3 days, she has intermittently complained of burning with urination; she has not had urinary frequency or urgency.

Physical Examination: Vital signs: temperature 37.2°C orally; pulse 100; respiratory rate 20; blood pressure 109/71 mm Hg. General: well-nourished, well-developed young girl in no acute distress. HEENT: normal. Chest: clear to auscultation. Cardiac: RRR without murmur. Abdomen: soft, nontender, nondistended, no masses, no hepatosplenomegaly, no rebound or guarding, normoactive bowel sounds. Genitourinary: (see figure) Tanner 1 pubic hair; area of hypopigmentation over vulva with several erythematous ulcerations; intact, normally pigmented, annular hymen with smooth edges. Rectum: Normal rugae; no fissures or tears; small amount of brown stool visible; guaiac test negative. Extremities: normal. Skin: no other rashes. Neurologic: normal.

Laboratory Findings: None.

Questions: What is the patient's diagnosis? Should child protective services be notified?

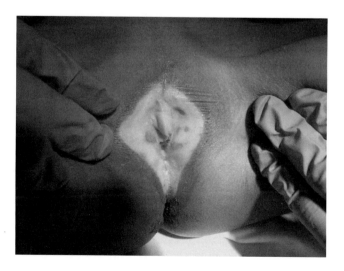

Diagnosis: Lichen sclerosis et atrophicus. This diagnosis in not necessarily associated with sexual abuse; in this case, since there was no history of abuse from the patient or concern from the parents, there is no need to notify child protective services.

Discussion: Lichen sclerosis et atrophicus (LSA) is a chronic condition affecting the epidermis and the dermis. It is characterized by ivory or white macules that form homogeneous, hypopigmented areas. Over time, the skin becomes thinned and the area may appear wrinkled. The true incidence of the disorder is unknown.

LSA is most common in women in the fifth and sixth decades and is six to 10 times more common in females than males. Approximately 15% of cases occur in children, most commonly grade-school-aged and adolescent girls. The anogenital area is most commonly affected. LSA is often described as having a "figure of eight" pattern when the vulva and the perianal areas are involved. The hymen is spared. In boys, LSA may cause phimosis. The disorder has been linked to an increased risk of vulvar squamous cell carcinoma in adult women, and there are anecdotal reports of men developing penile squamous cell carcinoma. There does not appear to be an increased risk of malignancy in extragenital lesions.

Although the cause of LSA is unknown, there are reported associations with trauma (including sunburn and pressure from waistbands) and autoimmune disorders. Similarly, the details of the pathophysiology are unknown. Some experts have reported decreased melanin production, a block in the transfer of melanosomes to keratinocytes, and melanocyte loss.

Clinically, patients can present with dysuria, itching and burning of the skin, painful defecation, constipation, and encopresis. On physical examination, the skin can be atrophic and very thin, and ulcerations and excoriations can be superimposed on the hypopigmented tissue. Fissures and subepidermal hemorrhages occur with minor trauma. Labial adhesions may occur as well. The diagnosis is usually made clinically; skin biopsy can be performed if the diagnosis is in doubt. Some authors have reported improvement in symptoms by puberty without treatment, although this is controversial, and the long-term risks for symptom recurrence and carcinoma in these patients are unknown. Patients are often treated with low-potency topical corticosteroids, and some authors advocate for short-term use of high-dose topical steroids. Topical lubricants may provide relief from burning and itching.

LSA is often mistaken for sexual abuse. Children should be questioned for possible abuse, because the conditions can coexist; in fact, it is possible that the trauma of sexual abuse may bring out LSA in predisposed individuals. However, LSA is not pathognomonic for abuse, and in patients with no history and an otherwise normal examination, the diagnosis of abuse does not need to be pursued.

The present patient received an enema in the ED for her constipation and was discharged on a topical lubricant, 1% hydrocortisone cream, and a stool softener. The family was instructed to follow-up with her primary care provider for ongoing management.

Differential Diagnosis	Distinguishing Features
LSA	Atrophic skin, white color, papular lesions
Localized scleroderma	Thickening of the skin
Sexual abuse	History; possible abnormal hymen
Tinea versicolor	Multiple, oval macules with a fine scale; usually on neck, chest, upper back, shoulders, and upper arms
Irritant dermatitis	Usually erythematous; if postinflammatory hypopigmentation, will see irregular mottling
Vitiligo	Lack of pigmentation with normal skin texture and thickness
Lichen planus	Atrophic areas with purple, papular border

Clinical Pearls

1. Lichen sclerosis et atrophicus is often mistaken for child abuse.
2. Patients should avoid local irritants and tight-fitting clothes.
3. Long-term follow-up is crucial to monitor for progression of disease and for psychosocial issues.

REFERENCES

1. Carlson JA, Grabowski R, Mu XC, et al: Possible mechanisms of hypopigmentation in lichen sclerosus. Am J Dermatopath 24:97–107, 2002.
2. Immobile and hypermobile skin. In Weston WL, Lane AT, Morelli JG (eds): Color Textbook of Pediatric Dermatology, 3rd ed. St Louis, Mosby, 2002, pp 264–269.
3. Bays J: Conditions mistaken for childe sexual abuse. In Reece RM, Ludwig S (eds): Child Abuse: Medical Diagnosis and Management, 2nd ed. Philadelphia, Lippincott Williams & Wilkins, 2001, 287–306.
4. Powell JJ, Wojnarowska F: Lichen sclerosis. Lancet 353:1777–1783, 1999.
5. Kellogg ND, Parra JM, Menard S: Children with anogenital symptoms and signs referred for sexual abuse evaluations. Arch Pediatr Adolesc Med 152:634–641, 1998.
6. Fischer G, Rogers M: Treatment of childhood vulvar lichen sclerosus with potent topical corticosteroid. Pediatr Dermatol 14:235–238, 1997.
7. Warrington SA, de San Lazaro C: Lichen sclerosis et atrophicus and sexual abuse. Arch Dis Child 75:512–516, 1996.

Charles V. Pollack, Jr., MD, MA

PATIENT 21

A 58-year-old man with chest pain

A 58-year-old man presents after resolution of 45 minutes of chest pain. The pain was described as a "pressure" sensation. It radiated down his arms and into his jaw, was associated with palpitations and dyspnea, and occurred while raking leaves. The pain resolved after he rested for about 20 minutes. There were three prior episodes of similar pain today, each lasting approximately 20 minutes, one of which occurred at rest and the others with minimal exertion. The patient denies nausea, vomiting, diaphoresis, cough, or change in the pain with inspiration or movement. Past medical history is significant for diet-controlled diabetes, hypertension, and remote use of tobacco. He denies illicit drug use. He currently takes hydrochlorathiazide. Family history is significant for a sister with acute myocardial infarction at age 55 years. While the patient is in the emergency department, the pain returns.

Physical Examination: Temperature 37.1°C; pulse 86; respiratory rate 21; blood pressure 150/85. General: anxious, thin. Skin: diaphoretic, pale. HEENT: unremarkable. Neck: no jugular venous distension. Chest: clear to auscultation, chest wall nontender to palpation. Cardiac: regular rate and rhythm, no murmurs, gallops, or rubs. Abdomen: normal. Extremities: no edema. Neuromuscular: normal.

Laboratory Findings: Room air pulse oximetry: 94%. CBC: normal. Electrolytes and renal function: normal. Chest radiograph: normal. ECG: ST-segment depression of 1.5 mm in anterior and lateral leads (see figure). Bedside cardiac troponin I: positive.

Questions: What are the patient's high-risk features for an acute coronary syndrome? What medical therapy should be immediately considered in the ED? Should the patient receive a fibrinolytic agent? What is the optimal overall management strategy?

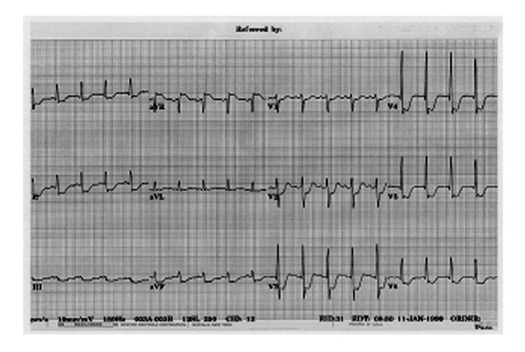

Diagnosis: Non-ST-segment-elevation (NSTE) acute coronary syndrome (ACS). The patient's ST segments are depressed, but this is not required to make the diagnosis of "NSTE" ACS. The terminology simply separates this clinical syndrome from that associated with elevation of the ST-segment, which prompts a different management approach. Because this patient's cardiac troponin test result is positive, he has, by definition, a non-ST-elevation myocardial infarction (NSTEMI); in the absence of a positive biomarker, NSTE ACS is termed *unstable angina.*

Discussion: There are recently published evidence-based guidelines for the management of NSTE ACS. Clinical and electrocardiographic features associated with the highest risk of adverse outcomes in NSTE ACS are ST-segment depression of at least 1 mm and chest pain at rest. This patient's ECG and his recurrence of pain in the ED clearly place him at high risk of mortality and major cardiovascular morbidity.

Pharmacologic management for high-risk NSTE ACS patients in the ED is described as "triple" therapy: anti-ischemic, antithrombotic, and antiplatelet. Nitroglycerin should be used to reverse ischemia, and morphine sulfate can be added for pain relief if needed. An antithrombin agent, either the low-molecular-weight heparin enoxaparin or unfractionated heparin by continuous intravenous infusion, should be started. The patient should receive aspirin as well. In addition, because he is at high risk for ACS, a platelet glycoprotein IIb/IIIa receptor antagonist should be considered along with the administration of oral clopidogrel (withheld if the patient is being transferred to the cardiac catheterization laboratory within 24 to 36 hours). There is no role for fibrinolytic therapy in patients with NSTE ACS.

Patients who meet high-risk criteria are optimally managed with early (24–36 hours) coronary angiography and revascularization (either percutaneously, as with balloons and stents, or with bypass grafting in the operating room) as indicated. If not available on-site, arrangements should be made for prompt transfer of high-risk patients from the ED to an institution with cardiac catheterization capability.

Clinical Pearls

1. Patients may have ACS even if they do not manifest diagnostic ST-segment changes on ECG.

2. "Unstable angina" and "non-ST-elevation MI" manifest as the same clinical syndrome; it is only the presence of a positive cardiac biomarker that distinguishes the NSTEMI from unstable angina.

3. Patients with high-risk features and ACS should receive aggressive medical therapy in the ED, including advanced antithrombotic and antiplatelet therapy. Optimal management for these patients includes early intervention in the catheterization laboratory.

REFERENCES

1. Pollack CV Jr, Roe MT, Peterson ED: 2002 update to the ACC/AHA guidelines for the management of patients with unstable angina and non-ST-segment elevation myocardial infarction: Implications for emergency department practice. Ann Emerg Med 41(3):355–369, 2003.
2. Braunwald E, Antman EM, Beasley JW, et al: ACC/AHA guidelines for the management of patients with unstable angina and non-ST-segment elevation myocardial infarction: A report of the American College of Cardiology/American Heart Association Task Force on Practice Guidelines (Committee on the Management of Patients with Unstable Angina). J Am Coll Cardiol 36:970–1062, 2000. Updated March 15, 2002, at *www.acc.org* and *www.americanheart.org.*
3. Pollack CV, Gibler WB: 2000 ACC/AHA guidelines for the management of patients with unstable angina and non-ST-segment elevation myocardial infarction: A practical summary for emergency physicians. Ann Emerg Med 38:229–240, 2001.
4. Pollack CV, Gibler WB: Advances create opportunities: Implementing the major tenets of the new unstable angina guidelines in the emergency department. Ann Emerg Med 38:241–248, 2001.
5. Greenbaum AB, Harrington RA, Hudson MP, et al, for the PURSUIT Investigators: Therapeutic value of eptifibatide at community hospitals transferring patients to tertiary referral centers early after admission for acute coronary syndromes. J Am Coll Cardiol 37:492–498, 2001.

PATIENT 22

A 40-year-old man with fever, chills, cough, and seizure

A 40-year-old man without significant past medical history is brought by ambulance from home after a witnessed seizure. He began to feel sick 2 nights ago, with productive cough, fever, chills, nausea, and nonbloody, nonbilious emesis. He awoke with nausea and anorexia and several hours later had a seizure. The patient drinks approximately 1 case of beer a day, often more.

Physical Examination: Vital signs: temperature 37.5°C (oral), pulse 116, blood pressure 126/90, respirations 12. General: thin, no respiratory distress, mildly diaphoretic. HEENT: oropharynx with dry mucous membranes, no thrush, mild tongue fasiculations. Neck: normal. Cardiac: normal. Chest: diminished breath sounds at the right base. Abdomen: protuberant, no fluid shift, nontender, nondistended, normal bowel sounds, nontender liver edge palpable 1 cm below costal margin. Extremities: mild tremor of hands bilaterally. Neurologic: agitated, scratches self vigorously, states "I'm infested."

Laboratory Findings: Room air pulse oximetry 93%, dextrose-stick 98. CBC: normal. Blood chemistries significant for an HCO_3 17, anion gap 27; the remainder is normal. Liver enzymes normal. ECG: sinus tachycardia at 116, normal axis and intervals. Chest radiograph: Large right lower lobe infiltrate.

ED Course: Two large-bore IV lines are started, and the patient is given diazepam for agitation. A liter of normal saline containing 100 mg of thiamine, 1 mg of folate, 2 g of $MgSO_4$ and multivitamins is infused. The patient's agitation requires physical restraint. Repeat vital signs showed a tachycardia of 136 and a respiratory rate of 22. The patient is diaphoretic and is speaking animatedly to the IV pole. The alcohol level is 95 mg/dl.

Question: What diagnosis can explain the patient's agitation, hallucinations, and vital sign abnormalities?

Diagnosis: Ethanol withdrawal syndrome

Discussion: Due to widespread use, abuse, social acceptance, and accessibility, ethanol is involved in a wide range of medical, social, and legal situations. Physicians are confronted daily with the sequelae of ethanol abuse. However, rarely will a patient state that they are withdrawing from ethanol. Ethanol withdrawal is often precipitated by, or masked by, more common complaints such as trauma or infection.

Although the exact mechanism is unknown, a current theory that explains some of ethanol's effects is as follows. The brain is in a balance between excitation and inhibition. Ethanol is a depressant. In cases of chronic abuse, the brain attempts to return to a baseline level of alertness by decreasing the amount of inhibitory neurotransmitter, while at the same time increasing the amount of excitatory neurotransmitter. This has the net effect of increasing alertness, leading to tolerance of the chronic ethanol exposure, and chaos when the ethanol is removed. The spectrum of symptoms of ethanol withdrawal stem from this imbalance between "on" and "off." The primary goal of treatment is to restore the balance between excitation and inhibition.

Ethanol withdrawal is a spectrum of illness, ranging from tremulousness to psychomotor hyperactivity to autonomic instability, all resulting from progressive central nervous system excitation and lack of inhibition. There is no characteristic order in which symptoms manifest. One can be tremulous and have a seizure without progressing into delirium tremens (DT). Conversely, one can have tremulousness and rapidly deteriorate into DT with tachycardia, hyperthermia, and other autonomic manifestations. The different states are best broken into those with intact mental status (hallucinosis, tremulousness) and those with altered mental status (seizures, delirium tremens.)

Ethanol withdrawal tremulousness, or "the shakes," is often an important visual clue to the diagnosis. It can be best visualized with outstretched arms. One can also visualize serpentine tongue fasiculations. It is often accompanied by tachycardia, diaphoresis, and nausea and vomiting. It is present in a majority of patients with ethanol withdrawal, and is often thought of as "early" withdrawal. Most importantly, the patient maintains an intact mental status.

Ethanol withdrawal hallucinosis is primarily visual. The hallucinations are characterized by a clear sensorium and otherwise normal mental status. A specific kind of hallucinosis is formication, or the visual and tactile sensation of insects crawling on the skin. It can often be accompanied by impressive excoriations. In both instances, the patient can have normal vital signs.

Ethanol withdrawal seizures are characteristically single, generalized tonic-clonic seizures that rarely progress to status epilepticus. They are often brief and self-limited, with a return to clear mental status without prolonged postictal period. Focal seizures should prompt a search for another cause. Approximately 30% of patients who develop DT have had an ethanol withdrawal seizure, and therefore seizure is a poor prognostic indicator.

Delirium tremens, or "the DTs," is the most serious of the ethanol withdrawal states, manifested by autonomic hyperactivity and delirium or altered mental status. DT has previously been associated with a very high mortality rate. Advances in management and treatment have reduced the mortality rate to less than 5%, which is primarily due to the underlying conditions leading to the withdrawal state, such as infection and trauma.

The mainstay of treatment involves restoring the inhibitory tone of the central nervous system using benzodiazepines. Owing to the severity of symptoms and the variable clinical course, oral medications are not recommended, unless symptoms are very mild or the patient has improved dramatically. Secondly, diazepam is often recommended over other agents, primarily because its active metabolites allow a longer duration of clinical effect and less frequent dosing needs. Patients should be medicated to sedation and then treated as necessary for symptoms, rather than on a standing schedule and dose.

Doses needed to control withdrawal symptoms are larger than doses commonly used in other clinical settings. Barbiturates also have efficacy in management and are often used when the patient is refractory to the effects of benzodiazepines. Additionally, propofol may be used in extreme cases but will require advanced airway management.

Beta-blockers and clonidine treat the symptoms of withdrawal, i.e. the increased sympathetic outflow, but do nothing to treat the withdrawal itself. They mask the response to therapy and should not be used as standard treatment. Neuroleptic agents, such as haloperidol and the phenothiazines have been shown to reduce the seizure threshold and increase mortality and should also be avoided.

Therapy is not limited to the pharmacologic management of the withdrawal. Patients need to be protected from physically harming themselves or others. Temperature, nutritional, and electrolyte abnormalities must be corrected. Chronic ethanol abusers are often malnourished, eschewing food for drink. They are often protein depleted and have deficiencies in important vitamins and minerals. The regular administration of thiamine, folate, and multivitamin solution has become commonplace in the ED. Serum electrolytes often show magnesium deficiency, and this also should be repleted.

The differential diagnosis of ethanol withdrawal includes other sedative hypnotic withdrawal states (benzodiazepines, barbiturates, opioids, and gamma-hydroxybutyrate), sympathomimetic intoxication (cocaine, methamphetamine), acute psychosis or hallucinosis, encephalitis, meningitis, structural central nervous system lesions, sepsis, and electrolyte imbalances such as hypoglycemia.

Hospital Course: The patient was administered diazepam in multiple doses, up to a total of 420 mg over the course of a few hours, with minimal effect on his agitation. Phenobarbital was added to his regimen, and he received a total of 260 mg in two separate boluses. After the second bolus, he required endotracheal intubation for airway protection. He was placed on a propofol infusion and admitted to the ICU. A noncontrast computed tomography scan of the head was negative, as was a lumbar puncture. He was continued on appropriate antibiotic coverage for his pneumonia and slowly weaned off of propofol. He was extubated on hospital day 3 and discharged to an alcohol rehabilitation facility on hospital day 5.

Clinical Pearls

1. Ethanol abuse crosses all socioeconomic boundaries; early identification is the key to treatment of withdrawal, as is identifying the reason for withdrawal.

2. Mental status is the key determinant of the spectrum of ethanol withdrawal syndrome.

3. Ethanol withdrawal still carries a mortality rate of approximately 5%, usually from concurrent illness.

REFERENCES

1. Hamilton RJ: Substance withdrawal. In Goldfrank LR, et al (eds): Goldfrank's Toxicologic Emergencies, 7th ed. New York, McGraw Hill, 2002, pp 1059–1074.
2. Jaeger TM, Lohr R, Pankratz VS: Symptom-triggered therapy for alcohol withdrawal syndrome in medical inpatients. Mayo Clin Proc; 76:695–701, 2001.
3. Mayo-Smith MF: Pharmacological management of alcohol withdrawal: A meta-analysis and evidence-based practice guideline. JAMA 278:144–151,1997.
4. Lohr R: Treatment of alcohol withdrawal in hospitalized patients. Mayo Clin Proc; 70:777–782, 1995.
5. American Psychiatric Association: Diagnostic and Statistical Manual of Mental Disorders, 4th ed. Washington DC, American Psychiatric Association, 1994, pp 198–199.
6. Gonzales RA: NMDA receptors excite alcohol research. Trends Pharmacol Sci 11:137–139, 1990.
7. Woo E, Greenblatt DJ: Massive benzodiazepine requirements during acute alcohol withdrawal. Am J Psychiatry 136: 821–823, 1979.

Robert Cloutier, MD

PATIENT 23

A 9-year-old boy with abdominal pain

A 9-year-old boy is brought to the ED with a 12-hour history of abdominal pain. The pain began gradually in the periumbilical region and is nonradiating, constant, and without precipitating or alleviating factors. The patient has vomited twice and is anorexic. His last normal bowel movement was yesterday. He denies urinary symptoms. While the patient was being driven to the ED, the pain became localized to the right lower quadrant and was exacerbated by bumps in the road. The child has no significant past medical history.

Physical Examination: Vital signs: temperature 38.5°C (oral); pulse 100; respiratory rate 21; blood pressure 105/63. General: young male in moderate discomfort. Chest: normal. Cardiac: normal. Abdomen: flat, nondistended, tender in the right lower quadrant, bowel sounds decreased, no organomegaly. Rectal: soft brown heme-negative stool; tenderness with palpation of the right side of the rectal vault.

Laboratory Findings: Urinalysis: pH 7.0, specific gravity of 1.025, negative leukocytes, nitrites, protein, glucose, and ketones. Abdominal radiograph: normal.

ED Course: Surgical consultation was requested and further imaging studies were discussed, but it was decided that the patient should go directly to the operating room.

Questions: What is the most likely diagnosis? What supporting evidence is required to establish this diagnosis?

Diagnosis: Acute appendicitis

Discussion: Acute appendicitis is the most common nontraumatic pediatric surgical emergency. There is slight male preponderance and a peak incidence between the ages of 9 and 12 years. Cases among children younger than 2 years of age, while rare, are among the most challenging to diagnose and have perforation rates as high as 90%. Evaluation in children, is fraught with pitfalls made difficult by a dynamic differential diagnosis that depends on the age of the patient. One of the cardinal rules of pediatric acute appendicitis is that atypical presentations are typical and contribute to the fact that morbidity and mortality are greater in pediatric patients than in adults. Rates of misdiagnosis vary between 28% and 57%.

Localization of pain to the right lower quadrant occurs in only approximately 50% of patients older than 12 years. In infants and children younger than 2 years of age, clinical signs can be vague and misleading. They may include generalized abdominal pain, vomiting, diarrhea, irritability, cough or rhinitis, grunting respirations, and right hip complaints with gait disturbance. Children between the ages of 2 and 5 more commonly present with right lower quadrant abdominal pain as opposed to generalized tenderness. Vomiting, anorexia, and fever are frequent in this age group; vomiting occasionally precedes the onset of abdominal pain. Nonspecific tests such as CBC can be misleading, and reliance on them as decision-making tools should be limited. Rather, laboratory values should be used as adjuncts in the larger clinical picture. Right lower quadrant ultrasonography or CT of the abdomen have become the diagnostic tests of choice, if needed.

The clinical approach involves an orderly elimination of other potential causes of abdominal pain. Most of these may be ruled out with a thorough history and physical examination coupled with a few basic diagnostic studies. Genitourinary causes and other gastrointestinal causes must be considered, such as testicular torsion, ectopic pregnancy, pelvic inflammatory disease, and urinary tract infection. Infectious gastroenteritis, including *Campylobacter jejuni* and *Yersinia enterolitica,* may closely mimic appendicitis with fever and right lower quadrant pain. Mesenteric adenitis is a consideration when peritoneal signs are not present. In younger children, intussusception and Meckel's diverticulitis cannot be overlooked. Lower lobe pneumonia, constipation, and diabetic ketoacidosis may be other important causes of symptoms mimicking appendicitis.

The present patient has a fairly typical presentation for appendicitis, with fever, vomiting, anorexia, and right lower quadrant pain, and was managed definitively in the operating room with removal of the inflamed appendix. The decision to pursue further imaging such as CT or ultrasonography is largely dependant on institutional preferences and consultant practices. Both modalities have respectable levels of sensitivity and specificity and are valuable adjuncts in cases in which the diagnosis remains unclear.

Clinical Pearls

1. Atypical and benign presentations occur frequently—misdiagnosis rates approach 50%.

2. Although rare, acute appendicitis may occur in children younger than 2 years of age. The younger the patient, the more difficult the diagnosis and the higher the perforation rate.

3. No single diagnostic test will diagnose appendicitis. CT and ultrasonography are important adjuncts to a well-developed clinical suspicion.

REFERENCES
1. Cantor RM, Callahan JM: Common abdominal emergencies in children. Emerg Med Clin North Amer 20:139–153, 2002.
2. Fleisher GR, Ludwig S, Henretig FM, et al: Appendicitis. In Textbook of Pediatric Emergency Medicine, Baltimore, Williams & Wilkins, 2000. pp 1515–1517.

Karen O'Connell, MD
George A. Woodward, MD, MBA

PATIENT 24

An 8-year-old victim of an auto versus pedestrian incident

An 8-year-old boy is brought to a community hospital emergency department immediately after being struck by a moving vehicle. He is awake and reporting mild shortness of breath and pain involving the left chest, left lower leg, and abdomen. The closest pediatric trauma center is approximately 80 miles away.

Physical Examination: Temperature 37.6°C; pulse 160; blood pressure 110/70; respiratory rate 36; oxygen saturation on room air 90%; Glasgow Coma Scale score 14; trauma score 14. General: awake and alert but mildly confused, no respiratory distress. Skin: acyanotic; small left parietal contusion; abrasions on left chest wall, abdomen, left hip, and bilateral knees. HEENT: pupils equally round and reactive, extraocular movements intact, oropharynx clear. Chest: slight decrease in breath sounds on left, clear to auscultation on right. Cardiac: regular tachycardia without a murmur. Abdomen: guarded and diffusely tender, nondistended. Extremities: hips tender to palpation but stable, left lower leg with deformity, no lacerations, normal distal pulses. Neuromuscular: able to move all four extremities with normal sensation throughout.

Laboratory Findings: CBC and blood chemistries: normal. ABG (room air): pH 7.37, $PaCO_2$ 26 mm Hg, PaO_2 60 mm Hg. Chest x-ray: small left pneumothorax without mediastinal shift (see figure). Pelvis x-ray: nondisplaced fracture of left and right pubic rami. Extremity x-ray: displaced left tibia and fibula fractures. Head CT: normal. Chest and abdomen CT: small pneumothorax and lung contusion on left; grade 3 liver laceration, no pneumoperitoneum; small fluid in paracolic gutters.

Questions: When should you consider transferring care of this patient to a trauma center? What are the legal responsibilities involved in patient transfer?

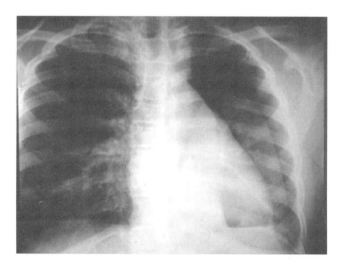

Answers: This young boy's grade 3 liver laceration, pneumothorax with decreased oxygen saturation, and orthopedic injuries complicate his case and make him a potentially unstable patient. Transferring him to a specialized pediatric trauma center with intensive care observation and intervention would optimize outcome. The referring hospital and physician are responsible for assessing the patient, initiating medical care, and arranging for transport to a facility that can offer specialized or advanced care. It is the referring medical team's responsibility to ensure that the patient is stable for transport and that the quality of care during transport does not represent a decrease in level of service.

Discussion: Emergency physicians in community hospitals may be the initial medical contact for some pediatric trauma patients. Identification of one's experience with and capabilities of caring for pediatric trauma patients are crucial steps in the optimal care of these patients. Guidelines for patient transfer should be standardized, available, and referred to as soon as possible after recognizing and stabilizing a critical patient. Important information to relay to the transport command center when arranging transport include demographics and location of patient, patient's stability, current level of medical care and type of intervention needed, urgency of need for advanced medical care, options available in the local medical community, and consent from patient or parent to transfer care.

The goals of interfacility transport are to provide the patient with the highest quality of care to meet his or her unique medical needs and to deliver that patient to a receiving facility in stable or improved condition. The Emergency Medical Treatment and Active Labor Act (EMTALA) outlines the legal responsibilities of both referring and accepting hospitals. The referring hospital and physician are responsible for assessing the patient and initiating medical care. When limitations of current medical care are recognized, the referring physician should arrange for transport to a facility that can offer specialized or advanced care. It is the referring medical team's responsibility to ensure that the patient is stable for transport and that the quality of care during transport does not represent a decrease in level of service. Consent for transport must be obtained by the referring facility. In cases in which a parent is unavailable, the referring physician can consent for transport, if it is in the patient's best interest. The receiving hospital is required to accept a patient if the space is available and the facility has the ability to provide the appropriate level of care required. Financial ramifications and/or reimbursement cannot be considered in the decision to transfer or accept a patient.

Communications regarding the safe transfer of patients can be optimized by the transport service by way of a specialized communication center. There should be a central access number, triage system, and command physician who can super-vise and participate on-line with the transport. The command physician must be available at all times to answer questions regarding patient care and give advice when stabilizing interventions are needed. An open line of communication should be maintained between referring and accepting medical personnel. The transport service should be immediately made aware of any changes in patient status.

There are three major modes of transport used in patient transfer: ground ambulance, helicopter, and fixed-wing aircraft. Each carries its own unique risks and benefits. The referring physician makes a decision based on the stability of the patient, level and expertise of intratransport observation needed, support equipment required, and options available. Ground transportation via ambulance involves a variety of levels of patient care and offers varying types of transport personnel. Ambulances can be staffed with volunteer, Basic Life Support, Advanced Life Support, critical care, and pediatric specialty personnel. Ground transportation has the advantage of direct patient transport from the referring to receiving facility. This mode involves relatively low expense, few weather restrictions, back-up availability if needed, and the ability to accommodate parents and additional staff. However, accident risk, traffic and road considerations, noise interference, and motion sickness need to be considered.

Helicopter use may be a more rapid transport option that requires only one third to one half the time of ground transportation. This mode is effective for transporting critical patients within a 100- to 150-mile radius. Helicopter transport avoids traffic and allows for access to difficult locations; however, a landing zone or helipad is required. There are more weather restrictions and interferences from noise and vibration. The space in which patient care is administered is smaller, allowing less room for interventions. One must also keep in mind the special altitude considerations involving pressure and gas laws. Certain patient conditions may worsen with the pressure changes and hypoxia induced by altitude.

Fixed-wing transport has the advantage of speed and is good for long-distance transfer. It is frequently the preferred method of transport for distances over 100 miles, as it is more economical with regard to time and expense than helicopter transport. The cabins can be pressurized, allowing for fewer problems related to altitude changes. Weather conditions interfere even less with the ability to carry out a transport. To use this form of transportation, a proximate airport needs to be available. The patient will experience multiple transfers during the process, which increase the time and risks involved. Each transfer poses a risk of equipment and tubing failure or dislodgement.

A major consideration in the decision regarding mode of transport is whether the patient needs immediate specialized pediatric intensive care intervention or observation. Pediatric critical care transport services are available to meet these needs. Specialized pediatric transport personnel include physicians, registered nurses, nurse practitioners, paramedics, and respiratory therapists. All personnel must have specific training and experience with the care of critically ill children and be familiar with the specific transport environment.

The present patient has multiple traumatic injuries and a potentially destabilizing liver laceration. He would benefit from specialized care and intensive monitoring during transport. Time of transport by ambulance, if traffic permits, would be approximately 1.5 hours. If helicopter transport is used, the patient could arrive at the accepting hospital in approximately 40 minutes. Given the severity of our patient's injuries and potential for deterioration, and urgency of need for advanced medical care, a speedy transfer by helicopter, with the appropriate ALS staff, is chosen.

Of the many risks involved in the transport of this patient, altitude physiology and how it will affect his small pneumothorax and respiratory status en route should be addressed. Most patients can acclimate to the alterations in gas and pressure properties that occur with changes in altitude. Those with more severe respiratory disease or low respiratory reserves are more adversely affected by the stresses of air transport. The medical personnel should be aware of each patient's individual condition so that preparation is made and potential problems identified prior to flying. Two laws of physics should be kept in mind when evaluating patients for air transport:

Boyle's Law: $P_1V_1 = P_2V_2$ (P_1 and V_1 represent initial pressure and volume and P_2 and V_2 are the resultant pressure and volume). Boyle's law states that at a constant temperature, the volume of a gas varies inversely with pressure. As altitude increases, barometric pressure decreases, resulting in an increase in the volume of a gas. Conversely, as one descends from altitude, the barometric pressure increases and gas volume decreases. The properties of this law may pose a problem for air in enclosed spaces, such as artificial air pockets in equipment (endotracheal tubes, blood pressure cuffs, mast trousers), potential or real in vivo air pockets (pneumothorax, pneumocephalus, pneumoperitoneum), and native body airspaces (ears, sinuses, bowel). When gas expands with ascent, the effects may range from mild discomfort in natural air spaces, to tissue compression and/or a tourniquet effect from equipment, to clinical compromise and deterioration with gas expansion in potential spaces.

Dalton's Law: $P_T = P1 + P2 + P3...$ This law states that the total pressure of a gas (P_T) is the sum of its individual pressures in that mixture (P1 + P2 + P3...). This law is reflective in oxygen availability as altitude changes. Hypoxia is the most dangerous stressor for air transport. Pressure changes determine the amount of ambient oxygen available for inspiration. The oxygen concentration in air is always 21% and does not change with altitude. What does change is the density of air. With increasing altitude, air density decreases, making the oxygen molecules farther apart and less available to the patient. The easiest way to overcome this problem is to provide supplemental oxygen.

The present patient has a small pneumothorax on x-ray. Gas trapped between the lung parenchyma and thorax will expand with increasing altitude and could potentially create a tension pneumothorax. There is a 20% increase in gas volume between sea level and 5000 feet and a 100% increase in volume between sea level and 18,000 feet. Given the lower altitude at which helicopters fly (approximately 500–1000 feet above ground level) and the local, direct route specific to this case, this patient's transport by helicopter should not cause significant pressure/volume changes. As this patient is currently stable, chest tube placement may not be necessary at this time. His pneumothorax could be managed with supplemental oxygen alone, preferably a 100% non-rebreather, with preparations made to immediately intervene with needle or tube decompression if indicated. However, if travel required large altitude changes, he could experience a compromise in respiratory function with even a small pneumothorax. In that case, ideal preparation before transport would include chest tube placement to relieve potentially increasing pressure of the entrapped air.

Fixed-wing aircrafts fly at higher altitudes and cabins must be pressurized. "Cabin" altitude could be pressurized between 0 and 8000 feet. At 8000 feet pressurization, there is a 33% increase in the volume of gas, potentially posing a problem for patients with entrapped air. A specific request should be made to the pilot to maintain the cabin altitude at a safe level.

Other risks to consider in this patient include bleeding at the site of liver laceration with excessive movement, potential destabilization of his pelvic fractures with multiple transfers, worsening of his long bone fracture with possible compromise of neurovascular integrity with malpositioning, and the potential for loss of intravenous access or other tube dislodgements with transfers. This patient's liver laceration and pelvic fractures are potential sources of continued blood loss. As hemoglobin is essential for oxygen transport and delivery to tissues, it is crucial that his hemoglobin level remain stable, with a level of 7 g/dl being the lower limit tolerated for safe air transport. A drop in hemoglobin will result in a drop in oxygen-carrying capacity. Oxygen tension in the blood should be maintained with supplemental oxygen.

Clinical Pearls

1. Open communication between the referring and the receiving caretakers and active participation and guidance from a qualified command physician are crucial for safe patient transport.

2. Patient stability, current level of medical sophistication, and urgency of need for advanced medical care are key factors in timing of transport.

3. Decisions surrounding mode of transport are based on patient's clinical status, characteristics of the specific disease process, need for immediate specialized care, environmental factors, traffic and road conditions, staffing requirements, and availability.

4. Proper preparation and anticipation of potential adverse effects that may occur during transport will help ensure patient safety.

REFERENCES

1. Woodward GA, Vernon DD: Aviation physiology in pediatric transport. In Jaimovich DG, Vidyasagar D (eds): Handbook of Pediatric and Neonatal Transport Medicine, 2nd ed. Philadelphia, Hanley & Belfus, 2002.
2. Williams A: Outpatient Department EMTALA Handbook 2002. Aspen Law and Business, Aspen Publishers, 2001.
3. Bitterman RA: Providing Emergency Care under EMTALA. American College of Emergency Physicians, 2000.
4. Woodward GA, King BR: Transport medicine. In Fleischer GR, Ludwig S (eds): Textbook of Pediatric Emergency Medicine, 4th ed. Philadelphia, Lippincott Williams & Wilkins, 2000.
5. Brink LW, Neuman B, Wynn J: Air transport. Pediatr Clin North Am 40:439–456, 1993.
6. Graneto JW, Soglin DF: Transport and stabilization of the pediatric trauma patient. Pediatr Clin North Am 40:365–380, 1993.
7. Pon S, Notterman DA: The organization of a pediatric critical care transport program. Pediatr Clin North Am 40: 241–261, 1993.

PATIENT 25

A 19-year-old woman with pelvic pain and vaginal bleeding

A 19-year-old woman arrives by ambulance with the report of acute onset of severe pelvic pain and vaginal bleeding for 30 minutes. She is sexually active and does not use contraception. She has had amenorrhea for 1 month.

Physical Examination: Temperature 37°C; pulse 120; respiratory rate 18, blood pressure 90/46. Skin: cool and diaphoretic. HEENT: normal. Chest: clear to auscultation. Cardiac: tachycardiac, no murmurs or rubs. Abdomen: distended, tender, decreased bowel sounds with diffuse rebound and guarding. Pelvic: scant amount of bright red blood in the vaginal vault, no clots or tissue, cervical os closed, cervix tender with motion, bilateral adnexal tenderness.

Laboratory Findings: Urine pregnancy test: positive. CBC: hemoglobin 12.6; platelets 144,000. Pelvic ultrasonography: see figures.

Questions: What life-threatening condition could be causing the patient's symptoms? How should management proceed? What is the clinical significance of a normal hemoglobin in the setting of blood loss?

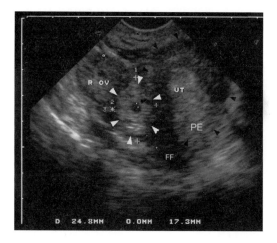
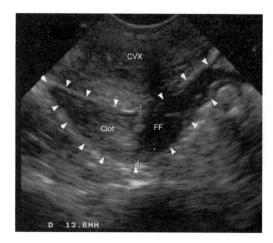

Diagnosis and Treatment: Ruptured ectopic pregnancy. The patient requires emergency surgical intervention. Volume resuscitation should begin immediately with type-specific blood, if possible.

Discussion: Ectopic pregnancy is defined as any pregnancy that occurs outside of the uterine cavity. In an ectopic pregnancy, the fertilized egg has implanted in the abdomen, cervix, peritoneal surface, ovary or, most commonly, the fallopian tube. It is the most common life-threatening cause of first trimester bleeding and can be difficult to diagnose. Undiagnosed ectopic pregnancy can progress to rupture and significant hemorrhage. The most common factors associated with ectopic pregnancy are in vitro fertilization, tubal surgery, history of pelvic inflammatory disease, prior ectopic pregnancy, and history of diethylstilbestrol exposure.

The increasing occurrence of pelvic inflammatory disease has led to an increased incidence of ectopic pregnancy in the United States of 1 to 2 per 100 pregnancies. Although prompt recognition and intervention has decreased mortality rates, ectopic pregnancy remains the most common cause of maternal mortality in the first trimester of pregnancy.

Ectopic pregnancy can manifest with various clinical signs and symptoms. Prior to tube rupture, the most common symptoms are abdominal pain and vaginal bleeding, but patients may report only one of these. The signs of ectopic pregnancy can be subtle until rupture occurs. Once intraperitoneal bleeding begins, the patient develops peritoneal signs.

The use of high-resolution transvaginal ultrasonography has improved the ability to establish this diagnosis at an earlier gestational age. Abdominal ultrasonography should detect a gestational sac when the β-HCG is greater than 6500 IU/ml. Transvaginal ultrasonography is more sensitive and can detect a pregnancy at a β-HCG level of between 1000 and 1500 IU/ml. If no intrauterine gestational sac is detected at a β-HCG level of 1500 mIU/ml or higher during a transvaginal ultrasonographic examination, an ectopic pregnancy should be suspected.

In the present patient, the transverse image (see figures on previous page, *left image*) shows the ectopic mass as an echogenic structure surrounding a cystic cavity (*white arrowheads*). The mass lies between the uterus (UT; *black arrowheads*), with its hyper-echoic endometrium inside the darker encircling myometrium, and the ovary (R OV). The posterior wall of the uterus is hard to discern due to the posterior acoustical enhancement (PE) caused by the endometrium. A small amount of free fluid (FF) can be seen. The low longitudinal endovaginal view (*right image*) reveals free fluid (FF) and clot (*arrowheads*) in the cul de sac behind the cervix (CVX).

Unstable patients with ectopic pregnancy such as this patient require emergency hemodynamic support and prompt surgical intervention. Immediate infusion with type-specific blood is done while preparations are made to go to the operating room. As in hemorrhagic shock due to trauma, rapid blood loss does not allow time for equilibration of the hemoglobin. The hemoglobin measured during or shortly after a significant loss of blood may return as a normal value.

Clinical Pearls

1. Ectopic pregnancy must be considered in all pregnant women who present with vaginal bleeding and/or abdominal pain early in pregnancy.

2. The presence of hemodynamic instability and a suspicion of or finding of ectopic egg pregnancy requires emergency gynecologic consultation.

3. Ectopic pregnancies can have vague, nonspecific signs and symptoms until rupture occurs.

REFERENCES
1. American College of Emergency Physicians: Policy statements: ACEP emergency ultrasound guidelines–2001. Ann Emerg Med 38:470–481, 2001.
2. Hick JL, Rodgerson JD, Heegaard WG, Sterner S: Vital signs fail to correlate with hemoperitoneum from ruptured ectopic pregnancy. Am J Emerg Med 19:488–491, 2001.
3. Tenore JL: Problem oriented diagnosis: Ectopic pregnancy. Am Fam Physician 61:1080–1088, 2000.
4. Alexander JD, Schneider FD: Vaginal bleeding associated with pregnancy. Prim Care 27:137–151, 2000.

Karen O'Connell, MD
Frances Nadel, MD

PATIENT 26

A 4-month-old boy with forceful vomiting

A 4-month-old boy presents to the emergency department at 2 AM with 1 day of forceful, non-bloody, nonbilious vomiting. He has had a rectal temperature of 37.8°C and has not fed well over the past day. There is no diarrhea or upper respiratory symptoms. During a previous hospitalization for an apparent life-threatening event, he was diagnosed with gastroesophageal reflux and discharged on reflux medications and an apnea monitor. His mother is also concerned about a rash on his head. She reports no history of trauma or ill contacts.

Physical Examination: Temperature 38.0°C (rectally); pulse 166; respiratory rate 38; blood pressure 100/60; pulse oximetry 100% in room air. General: well-appearing, active infant. HEENT: normocephalic, anterior fontanelle flat. Chest: clear. Cardiac: RRR without murmur. Abdomen: soft, nontender, nondistended, bowel sounds present. Skin: right parietal scalp with linear petechiae. Neurologic: crying but consolable, alert, focuses on face and tracks 180 degrees.

Laboratory Findings: Hemoglobin 10.7 g/dl, WBC 19,600/μl (54% segmented neutrophils, 40% lymphocytes, 6% monocytes), platelets 490,000/μl. A skeletal survey reveals a nondisplaced linear parietal skull fracture and a head computed tomography (CT) scan shows bilateral subdural hemorrhages (see figure).

Question: What is the most likely diagnosis?

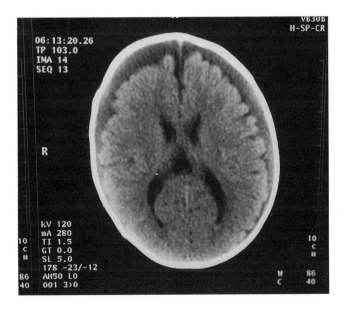

Discussion: Child maltreatment is defined as intentional harm or threat of harm to a child by someone acting in the role of a caretaker. An estimated 1.4 million children in the United States experience some form of maltreatment each year, with approximately 160,000 children suffering serious or life-threatening injuries. Some 1000 to 2000 children die each year from maltreatment, 80% of them under the age of 5 years and almost 40% in the first year of life. Physical abuse is the leading cause of serious head injury in infants, and head trauma is the most frequent cause of morbidity and mortality in abused children.

The detection of child abuse is often difficult because of vague histories and the lack of sensitive or specific signs and symptoms. One form of child abuse that can be the most subtle in its presentation is shaken-impact syndrome or shaken baby syndrome (SBS). Severe rotational cranial acceleration causes the distinctive head injuries as a result of violent shaking alone, impact alone or a combination of the two forces. The term *whiplash shaken baby syndrome* was originally coined in 1972 by John Caffey, a pediatric radiologist, to describe a specific constellation of clinical findings in infants that consists of retinal hemorrhages, subdural/subarachnoid bleeds, metaphyseal fractures, and little or no external evidence of trauma.

Shaken victims are usually younger than 3 years of age, with most cases occurring during the first year of life. The majority of victims are male, as are the perpetrators. Risk factors include young parents, unstable family situations, low socioeconomic status, disability or prematurity of the infant, and unrealistic caretaker expectations of the children. The trigger for shaking often results from tension and frustration generated by an infant's crying or irritability. Histories given for shaken infants are often vague and unreliable, such as a mild head injury from a simple fall from a bed or couch.

Common symptoms include lethargy, irritability, vomiting or poor feeding, breathing abnormalities, apnea, seizures, or changes in muscle tone. Symptoms can be acute or subacute, occurring intermittently for weeks before presentation as seen with chronic, sublethal episodes of shaking. The diagnosis of SBS requires a high index of suspicion. Many infants have multiple contacts with health care providers before the diagnosis is made. On work-up and evaluation of SBS victims, old intracranial hemorrhages are found in about 33% to 40% of all cases.

Head CT without intravenous contrast is considered the neuroimaging study of choice in the initial evaluation of a child with a traumatic brain injury. Magnetic resonance imaging (MRI) is of great value as an adjunct to CT, especially when one is further evaluating intraparenchymal brain lesions and in dating injuries. MRI is also superior in detecting small extra-axial hemorrhages. Subdural and subarachnoid hemorrhages are the most common intracranial injuries seen in SBS victims. Subdural hemorrhage is caused by the tearing of cortical bridging veins between the dura and arachnoid when shearing forces from shaking are applied. Hemorrhage tends to be most prominent in the interhemispheric fissure. Cerebral contusions are rare. Diffuse axonal injury and cerebral edema are more frequently found in severe cases of shaking. Diffuse axonal injury results from the sudden deceleration of the brain and rotational shearing forces that occur with shaking. Hypoxic-ischemic injury may result in cerebral edema and infarct. Common late findings, or those associated with chronic sublethal shaking, include extra-axial fluid collections, cerebral atrophy, and cystic encephalomalacia.

The most common differential diagnosis is accidental head injury. In cases of accidental head injury, the history is clear and consistent, the infant's symptoms reflect the forces described, and no unexplained skeletal injuries are noted. Subdural hemorrhages have been reported in infants after motor vehicle collisions or falls that involve significant height or angular deceleration. Skull fractures can occur with even minor falls onto a hard surface and can be associated with epidural bleeds. In infants and young children, household falls causing head injuries mainly involve low-velocity translational forces; rotational deceleration is extremely uncommon.

Unilateral or bilateral retinal hemorrhages are present in 75% to 90% of SBS victims. The number, size, and characteristics of hemorrhages vary with each case. More severe optic injuries that are pathognomonic for SBS include vitreous hemorrhage, optic nerve sheath hemorrhage, and nonhemorrhagic changes such as perimacular retinal folds and traumatic retinoschisis. Retinal hemorrhages are seen in less than 3% of accidental head trauma cases. Some nontraumatic causes include subarachnoid hemorrhage from congenital malformations, sepsis, coagulopathy, galactosemia, severe hypertension, and carbon monoxide poisoning. All children with suspected abusive head trauma should undergo a dilated retinal examination by a trained ophthalmologist.

A skeletal survey is essential in the evaluation of a young child suspected to be the victim of abuse. Approximately 30% to 70% of abused children with head injuries also have extracranial evidence of inflicted trauma. A skeletal survey may reveal abusive injuries such as old fractures with callous formation, multiple fractures in different stages of healing, posterior rib fractures, and metaphyseal fractures. Skull fractures are more likely to be nonaccidental if they are multiple, bilateral, diastatic, or depressed or if they cross suture lines. For some patients, a bone scan or delayed repeated skeletal survey can be helpful in detecting healing fractures that were not seen on initial evaluation.

The most common physical manifestations of child abuse are skin lesions, including bruising. The health care provider must determine whether the bruises are consistent with normal age-appropriate activity. Sugar et al's catch phrase "those who don't cruise rarely bruise" emphasizes that bruising in young infants is likely to have been inflicted. Out of almost 1000 children studied who had no known medical cause for bruising and in whom abuse was not suspected, these investigators found bruises in only 0.6% of infants younger than 6 months of age and 2.2% of preambulatory infants.

There is an incredibly high incidence of morbidity and mortality among SBS victims. Approximately 25% to 60% of shaken infants die. Infants who are comatose at presentation are at high risk for severe neurologic deficits and death. Long-term outcome studies of those who survive, although few in number, reveal that outcome is poor in almost all SBS victims.

Diagnosing head trauma in an infant or young child is challenging, especially when no history of trauma is given and the patient presents with nonspecific clinical signs. Data regarding the nature and frequency of head trauma support the need for careful consideration of child abuse in the differential diagnosis when a child younger than 1 year of age presents with an intracranial injury. The single most common diagnosis mimicking SBS is accidental injury. The occurrence of intracranial hemorrhage in children younger than 1 year of age without a history of significant head trauma such as a motor vehicle collision or a fall from a significant height should alert the physician to the possibility of child abuse. Current child abuse reporting laws require only that a health care provider "have reasonable suspicion" and not proof to make a report.

The present patient was admitted to the hospital, the Department of Human Services was contacted, and suspected child abuse was reported. An MRI scan was performed, which confirmed the presence of subdural hemorrhage, extra-axial fluid collections, and cerebral atrophy.

Clinical Pearls

1. A high index of suspicion is needed to diagnose shaken baby syndrome because of the unreliable histories and vague symptoms.

2. Bruising in young infant and perambulatory children should raise concern regarding the mechanism of injury.

3. When abuse is suspected, further helpful diagnostic studies include skeletal survey, cranial imaging such as CT and MRI, skilled ophthalmologic examination, and bone scans.

4. Only a suspicion for abuse and not proof is indicated in the reporting of possible maltreatment.

REFERENCES

1. Alexander RC, Levitt CJ, Smith WL: Abusive head trauma. In Reece RM, Ludwig S (eds): Child Abuse: Medical Diagnosis and Management, 2nd ed. Philadelphia, Lippincott Williams & Wilkins, 2001.
2. American Academy of Pediatrics, Committee on Child Abuse and Neglect, 2000–01: Shaken baby syndrome: Rotational cranial injuries—technical report. Pediatrics 108:206–210, 2001.
3. Jenny C, Hymel KP, Ritzen A, et al: Analysis of missed cases of abusive head trauma. JAMA 281:621–626, 1999.
4. Sugar NF, Taylor JA, Feldman KW: Bruises in infants and toddlers: Those who don't cruise rarely bruise. Arch Pediatr Adolesc Med 153:399–403, 1999.
5. Duhaime AC, Christian CW, Rorke LB, Zimmerman RA: Current concepts: Nonaccidental head injury in infants—the "shaken-baby syndrome." N Engl J Med 338:1822–1829, 1998.
6. Wissow LS: Current concepts: Child abuse and neglect. N Engl J Med 332:1425–1431, 1995.
7. Caffey J: On the theory and practice of shaking infants. Am J Dis Child 124:161–169, 1972.

Anthony J. Dean, MD

PATIENT 27

A 32-year-old woman with blunt truncal trauma

A 32-year-old female motorcyclist is brought to the emergency department unconscious. Rescue personnel describe a patient who was found helmeted on the side of the road. Witnesses described the patient being thrown 30 feet after impact.

Physical Examination: The patient arrives on a backboard with a cervical collar and wearing an intact motorcycle helmet. She has an 18-gauge intravenous catheter with normal saline infusing in the right antecubital space. She is moaning, opening her eyes to vocal stimuli. She can localize painful stimuli. Helmet is removed with inline cervical immobilization. Blood pressure 86/40, heart rate 130, respiratory rate 26, O_2 saturation 92%. Chest: 12×10 cm ecchymosis in the mid- to anterior axillary line on the right. HEENT: normocephalic, atraumatic. PERRL (4 mm). No hemotympanum. No facial trauma. Neck examination deferred. Breath sounds equal bilaterally. Abrasions on the back from the right deltoid to the buttock. Heart: tachycardiac, not muffled. Abdomen: abrasion and contusion over the left costal margin in the mid-axillary line, positive bowel sounds; soft, not distended. Pelvis stable. Rectal examination: good tone, heme negative. Extremities: grossly deformed left leg with 30 degrees valgus angulation and exposed bone.

Focused Assessment by Sonography in Trauma (FAST) Examination: Free fluid (*FF*) in the right pleural space and left splenorenal space (see figures).

Trauma Management: The patient is placed on 100% oxygen, a second large-bore intravenous line is placed, and Ringer's lactate is infused "wide open." The patient's oxygen saturation increases to 100%. A right chest tube is placed and immediately drains 500 ml of blood, which is collected in the cell saver. The patient continues to be tachycardiac with a blood pressure of 94/74. With free fluid identified in the peritoneum and persistent hypotension, the decision is made to take the patient to surgery for laparotomy. The patient is intubated using rapid sequence induction with the Sellick maneuver and continued inline cervical immobilization. Chest x-ray confirms good endotracheal and chest thoracostomy tube placement. The patient is transferred to the OR 17 minutes after her arrival in the ED.

Questions: Why was this patient taken to the operating room without performance of a computed tomography (CT) scan? How do the roles of CT and bedside ultrasonography complement one another in the management of the blunt trauma victim? How accurate is bedside ultrasonography in the detection of intraperitoneal hemorrhage?

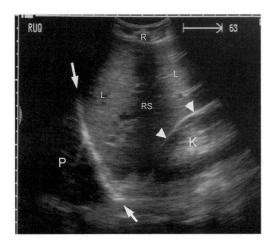
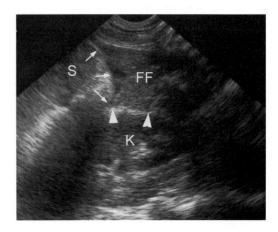

Diagnosis: Shattered spleen

Discussion: Mortality from blunt truncal trauma with an intact airway is usually due to internal hemorrhage. Rapid identification of internal bleeding leads to the best chance of successful operative control and repair. The first diagnostic test to identify peritoneal bleeding was the diagnostic peritoneal lavage developed in the 1960s. This test can be rapidly performed at the bedside and is highly sensitive in the detection of peritoneal blood. However, it is an invasive test, does not show the source of the blood, and sometimes detects bleeding that is not clinically significant. In the 1980s, the CT scan became widely available. CT provides detailed anatomic information about organ injuries and demonstrates the extent and location of internal hemorrhage. However, CT is time consuming, requires significant expenditures of personnel resources, and necessitates removal of frequently unstable patients from the resuscitation area. As a result, prior to the advent of bedside ultrasonography, it was often necessary to perform diagnostic peritoneal lavage prior to CT to identify patients who were potentially too unstable to go to the CT scanner.

Bedside ultrasonography in the evaluation of trauma was developed in Germany in the 1980s. Like other applications of emergency medicine bedside ultrasonography, the FAST examination is performed by the treating physician (emergency physician or surgeon) at the bedside, as an integrated component of the patient's management and care. The FAST examination does not interrupt other aspects of the patient's resuscitation and does not necessitate the patient's removal from the resuscitation area. It is now recommended by the American College of Surgeons in the Advanced Trauma Life Support manual as a component of the secondary survey.

Unlike ultrasonographic examinations performed by radiologists under more leisurely circumstances, the primary focus of the FAST examination is *not* the identification of specific visceral organ injuries but rather the rapid identification of blood in body cavities. The primary focus is on the peritoneum, but attention is also directed to the pleura and the pericardium. It usually takes between 1 and 5 minutes to perform a complete FAST examination. This reflects the exigencies of critically ill trauma patients as well as the limitations of time and equipment typically available in the ED. In this case, the FAST examination did not show the extent of the patient's splenic damage.

The FAST examination reliably detects 650 ml of free fluid. Thus, if performed very soon after trauma or in patients with slow internal bleeding, it may fail to identify hemorrhage. In patients with hemodynamic evidence of blood loss (hypotension or tachycardia), however, the volume of blood loss necessary to cause such findings is almost invariably sufficient to be detected by the FAST examination. Thus, a hypotensive trauma patient with a normal FAST examination finding mandates a search for blood loss in other locations, such as the retroperitoneum or thigh, or consideration of other causes of shock. An additional advantage of the FAST examination is that it can be repeated, especially in patients with changes in clinical status. As noted above, the FAST examination usually does not give information about the source of the hemorrhage or solid organ injury. For this reason, patients with free peritoneal fluid who are stable are usually taken to the CT department for anatomic delineation of their internal injuries. A patient with a negative FAST finding who is hemodynamically stable and for whom there is low clinical suspicion of significant internal organ injury may not need to undergo CT scanning. Such a patient can be managed clinically with serial observation (including, if necessary, serial FAST examinations) and, if appropriate, can be discharged.

The present patient was hemodynamically unstable with a positive FAST examination finding. The left image is a sagittal view of the right upper quadrant showing fluid in the pleural space (*P*) appearing dark, therefore hypoechoic. The diaphragm is a hyperechoic structure (*white,* between the *arrows*). Between the liver (*L*) and the kidney (*K*) is the potential hepatorenal space (*arrowheads*), which appears white, indicating the absence of free peritoneal fluid in this location. A rib (*R*) casts a shadow artifact (*RS*). The right image is a roughly sagittal view of the left upper quadrant (the left side of the image is cephalad, the right side caudad) showing the spleen (*S, small arrows*) and kidney (*K, arrowheads*). Between the two is a heterogeneously echogenic mass representing clotted blood. It can be distinguished from bowel by its lack of shadowing and its characteristically "pointy" shape.

The patient was taken to the OR, where a shattered spleen was identified and removed. Her blood pressure stabilized, and orthopedic surgeons copiously lavaged and reduced the compound left tibial and fibula fractures. Postoperatively, a CT scan of the head revealed bilateral frontal contusions. The patient made an uneventful recovery without neurologic deficit.

Clinical Pearls

1. Occult hemorrhage (usually abdominal) is the leading cause of morbidity and mortality in blunt trauma victims who survive to arrival in the ED.

2. The FAST examination can be integrated with the trauma resuscitation and reliably detects significant intraperitoneal or pleural hemorrhage.

3. Most stable patients with free intraperitoneal hemorrhage (positive FAST examination finding) require further delineation of injuries with CT scan.

REFERENCES

1. Ma OJ, Kefer MP, Mateer JR, Thoma B: Evaluation of hemoperitoneum using a single-vs. multiple-view ultrasonographic examination. Acad Emerg Med. 2(7): 581–6, 1995. Biffl WL, Moore EE, Kendall J: Postinjury torso ultrasound: FAST should be SLOH. J. Trauma, 48(4): 781–2, 2000.
2. Scalea TM, Rodriguez A, Chiu WC, et al (FAST Consensus Conference Committee): Focused assessment with sonography for trauma (FAST): Results from an international consensus conference. J Trauma 46:466–472, 1999.
3. Rozycki GS, Ballard RB, Feliciano DV, et al: Surgeon performed ultrasound for the assessment of truncal injuries: Lessons learned from 1540 patients. Ann Surg 228:557–567, 1998.
4. Porter RS, Nester BA, Dalsey WC, et al: Use of ultrasound to determine the need for laparotomy in trauma patients. Ann Emerg Med 29:323–330, 1997.
5. Ma OJ, Mateer JR, Ogata M, et al: Prospective analysis of a rapid trauma ultrasound examination performed by emergency physicians. J Trauma 38:879–885, 1995.
6. Jehle D, Guarino J, Karamanoukian H: Emergency department ultrasound in the evaluation of blunt abdominal trauma. Am J Emerg Med 11:342–346, 1993.
7. Liu M, Chen-Hsen L, P'eng F: Prospective comparison of diagnostic peritoneal lavage, computed tomographic scanning, and ultrasonography for the diagnosis of blunt abdominal trauma. J Trauma 35:267–270, 1993.

Thomas J. Lydon, MD, PhD
Francis DeRoos, MD

PATIENT 28

A 22-year-old woman with an ingestion

A 22-year-old woman with unknown past medical history is brought in by ambulance. She was found wielding a knife in the kitchen. Paramedics reported that there was an empty bottle of acetaminophen at the scene.

Physical Examination: Temperature 36.9°C; pulse 93; respiratory rate 26; blood pressure 117/76. General: sobbing, lethargic, strong odor of alcohol on breath. HEENT: 3 mm pupils, reactive. Chest: clear to auscultation. Cardiac: no murmurs, rubs, or gallops. Abdomen: soft, nontender, nondistended, normal bowel sounds. Extremities: no edema; multiple scratch marks in right anticubital fossa; well-healed, 4-cm, horizontal scar on volar surface of the right wrist. Neuromuscular: oriented to person only; unwilling to cooperate with examination.

Laboratory Findings: Blood chemistries: Na 141 mEq/L, K 3.1 mEq/L (normal 3.5–5.0), Cl 101 mEq/L, bicarbonate 24 mEq/L, BUN 9 mg/dl, Cr 0.8 mg/dl, glucose 94 mg/dl. CBC: normal. Liver function tests: AST 25 U/L, ALT 16 U/L, Tbili 0.3 mg/dl, Dbili 0.1 mg/dl, alkaline phosphatase 99 U/L. Special chemistries: Ethanol level 233 mg/dl, salicylate level 0, acetaminophen level 171 µg/mL (normal <5). Coagulation studies: normal. Urine pregnancy test: negative. Urine toxicology: positive for ethanol. ECG: normal sinus rhythm, normal axis, intervals, and wave-forms. Chest x-ray: normal.

Questions: Does this patient have a toxic level of acetaminophen? How should this patient be treated?

Diagnosis and Treatment: Acetaminophen overdose. The decision about whether to administer the antidote, *N*-acetyl cysteine (NAC), requires a more complete history. The patient also has ethanol intoxication.

Discussion: Knowledge of the metabolism of acetaminophen (*N*-acetyl-p-aminophenol, or APAP) is crucial in the understanding of toxicity and treatment. APAP metabolism occurs primarily through glucuronide and sulfate conjugation in the liver. A small fraction of APAP is metabolized via the mixed function oxidase system (P-450) forming *N*-acetyl-p-benzoquinoneimine (NAPQI), a highly reactive hepatotoxin. Typically, NAPQI combines with hepatic glutathione, which effectively detoxifies the metabolite. In the case of an overdose, the sulfation and glucoronidation pathways become saturated, resulting in an increased fraction of APAP being metabolized by the P450 system and significantly greater amounts of NAPQI. The overproduction of NAPQI depletes the inherent glutathione stores of the liver, leaving NAPQI free to react with hepatocyte lipid membranes and proteins. If the accumulation of NAPQI is unchecked, cell death ensues rapidly.

On a microscopic level, hepatocellular injury can occur within hours of ingestion; however, patient symptoms may not become apparent for many hours. The clinical course of acute acetaminophen poisoning is described in terms of four phases. Initially, the patient may present with nausea, vomiting, and diaphoresis or may be completely asymptomatic. Symptoms typically resolve within a few hours. By 18 to 24 hours, gastrointestinal symptoms may recur and some patients develop right upper quadrant tenderness. Laboratory finding's during this second phase may include increased AST, ALT, and bilirubin.

If poisoning is severe, within 72 to 96 hours the patient progresses into the third phase of toxicity, with fulminent hepatic failure, jaundice, severe coagulopathy, and encephalopathy. Transaminase levels typically rise into the 10,000 U/L range, and acute renal failure may develop due to renal P-450 production of NAPQI. If the third phase is survived, the patient recovers and regains normal hepatic function.

The management of patients with acetaminophen overdose relies on a quantitative serum acetaminophen level and an accurate determination of the time between ingestion and obtaining a serum level. The decision about whether to begin antidotal treatment is based on the Rumack-Matthew nomogram (see figure). A single serum level obtained between 4 and 24 hours after ingestion is compared to a treatment line. A serum acetaminophen concentration to the right of the treatment line requires initiation of the antidote, NAC. Because of similarities in chemical structure, NAC prevents hepatic necrosis by serving as both a reservoir for glutathione synthesis and as a glutathione substitute, which can rapidly bind and "detoxify" the destructive NAPQI. Oral NAC treatment begins with a loading dose of 140 mg/kg followed by 70 mg/kg every 4 hours for 17 doses. In Europe, Canada, and parts of the United States, an intravenous regimen of NAC has reduced therapy to 48 hours.

The present patient's sister was contacted to provide additional details of the suicide attempt. The patient arrived home at 2:00 AM and was last seen in the bathroom. A search of the bathroom uncovered an empty bottle of acetaminophen. The initial serum level was obtained at 6:30 AM. Using the nomogram, a serum level of 171 μg/mL at 4.5 hours after ingestion indicates that NAC treatment is needed. The patient received an initial dose of 9.8 g via nasogastric tube and was admitted for 17 subsequent doses of 4.9 g every 4 hours. The patient developed nausea and vomiting soon after admission, which resolved over 24 hours. On the morning of day 3, the patient developed mild right-upper quadrant abdominal pain, and laboratory values showed an AST of 90, an ALT of 47, and an INR of 1.4. The pain resolved after 2 hours, and all laboratory values returned to normal limits within 12 hours. The patient was discharged on hospital day 4.

Clinical Pearls

1. Treatment of any patient with overdose requires a clear timeline of events; when the patient is unable to give a history, one should attempt to contact family, friends, or other possible witnesses.

2. Overdose patients often ingest more than one substance.

3. In the case of acetaminophen toxicity, a lack of patient symptoms with the first 48 hours post-ingestion cannot be used to guide treatment or determine prognosis.

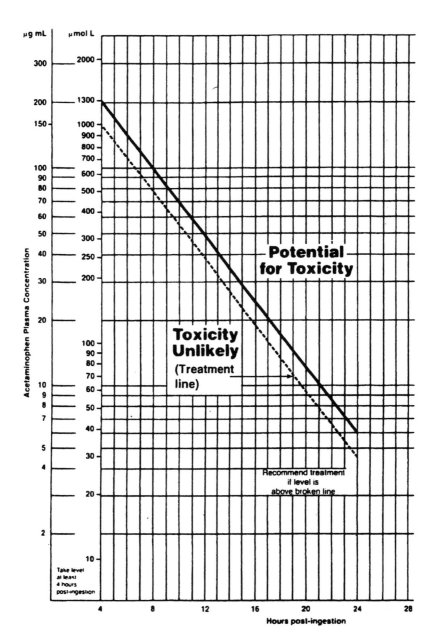

Rumack-Matthew nomogram. (From Goldfrank LR, Flomenbaum NE, Lewin NA, et al: Toxicologic Emergencies, 7th ed. New York, McGraw-Hill, 2002; with permission. [Originally from Management of Acetaminophen Overdose. McNeil Consumer Products Co., 1986.])

REFERENCES

1. Goldfrank LR, Flomenbaum NE, Lewin NA, et al: Toxicologic Emergencies. New York, McGraw-Hill, 2002, pp 480–505.
2. Rumack BH, Peterson RC, Koch GG, Amara IA: Acetaminophen overdose. Arch Intern Med 141:380–385, 1981.
3. Rumack BH, Matthew MD: Acetaminophen poisoning and toxicity. Pediatrics 55:871–876, 1975.

Evaline Alessandrini, MD, MSCE

PATIENT 29

A 9-month-old boy with fever and petechiae

A 9-month-old boy presents to the emergency department with a fever of 24 hours and a rash over most of his body. He has had diarrhea for 2 days, decreased oral intake for 1 day, and increased fussiness over the past 12 hours. His mother denies that he has had any travel, insect bites, bleeding, or easy bruising. He is otherwise healthy and his immunizations are up to date.

Physical Examination: Alert boy with periods of fussiness easily consoled by his mother. Temperature 39.8°C rectally; pulse 168; respiratory rate 40; blood pressure 85/56. Skin: Multiple 1–2 mm nonblanching erythematous lesions on face, trunk, upper and lower extremities; capillary refill brisk (see figure). HEENT: mucous membranes moist, tympanic membranes clear. Neck: supple without adenopathy. Chest: No work of breathing, clear breath sounds. Cardiac: tachycardiac without murmurs, gallops, or rubs. Abdomen: normal. Extremities: rash as noted, otherwise no abnormalities. Neurologic: nonfocal examination with good muscle tone.

Laboratory Findings: CBC: WBC 17,200/μl with 68% segmented neutrophils and 12% bands, platelets 371,000, hemoglobin and hematocrit normal. Blood chemistries: normal. Coagulation profile: PT 11.1, PTT 30. Cerebrospinal fluid: 2 WBCs, 2 RBCs, normal protein and glucose, Gram stain shows no organisms or white blood cells. Blood and cerebrospinal fluid cultures pending.

Questions: What is the most likely cause of the patient's fever and petechiae? What potential etiologic organism is associated with the highest morbidity and mortality? What management strategy should be instituted for this patient?

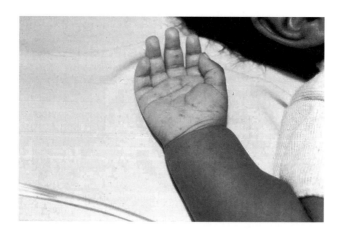

Diagnosis and Management Strategy: The most likely cause of the patient's illness is a viral agent causing fever and disruption of vascular integrity with subsequent development of petechiae; *Neisseria meningitides*, as a bacterial source, is associated with the highest morbidity and mortality rates and must therefore be considered. The management strategy includes hospitalization and therapy with broad-spectrum antibiotics after a full sepsis work-up.

Discussion: Fever and petechiae in children may be caused by a wide array of infectious agents (see table). However, the clinician must be aware of factors pointing to an invasive bacterial disease (IBD). Several prospective studies have demonstrated an incidence between 2% and 17% of IBD in children with fever and a hemorrhagic rash. The single study, which limited its study population to children with petechiae (not purpura), demonstrated an 8% rate of invasive, culture-proven bacterial disease. In the post–*Haemophilus influenzae* type b immunization era, most children with fever and petechiae caused by an invasive bacterial organism have meningococcal disease. Overall, most patients with fever and petechiae have negative bacterial cultures and/or serologic tests and are presumed to have a viral cause. Approximately 15% of children have a defined viral illness, usually enterovirus or adenovirus infection. Another 10% have noninvasive bacterial infection, nearly all of which are due to streptococcal pharyngitis. Infrequently, fever and petechiae are the presenting symptoms of other diseases such as Henoch-Schönlein purpura, idiopathic thrombocytopenic purpura, or leukemia, which are usually evident via clinical characteristics or laboratory results.

It is clearly important for clinicians to be able to identify children with fever and petechiae who are likely to have IBD. The fatality rate of invasive meningococcemia is estimated to be between 7% and 20%. Associated morbidity includes loss of limbs, neurologic sequelae, and sloughing of skin, necessitating grafting. Although no one factor is 100% sensitive in identifying children with IBD, a constellation of factors is useful in identifying children with fever and petechiae in whom IBD is unlikely. Multiple studies have demonstrated that well-appearing children with a normal white blood cell count (WBC between 5000 and 15,000/μl), a normal absolute neutrophil count (ANC between 1500 and 9000), an absolute band count of less than 500, and petechiae limited to the area above the nipple line are exceedingly unlikely to have an invasive bacterial infection. A recent European study demonstrated that no children with a C-reactive protein level less than 6 mg/dl had IBD.

The management of children who are ill appearing and have meningismus or purpura is straight forward. These children warrant a full sepsis evaluation, admission to the hospital with parenteral antibiotics, and fluids and vasoactive infusions to maintain normal hemodynamics. Prudent antibiotic choices would be those effective against meningococcal and streptococcal disease, including third-generation cephalosporins such as cefotaxime or ceftriaxone. Doxycycline should be administered if rickettsial disease is considered. Vancomycin should be administered in addition to cefotaxime or ceftriaxone to children with suspected pneumococcal meningitis. Furthermore, since sporadic as opposed to epidemic cases of meningococcemia appear to occur in children in the first 2 years of life, and these children have less competent immune systems in fighting encapsulated organisms, many experienced clinicians recommend full sepsis evaluations and admission for all children in this young age group.

Still, all children with fever and petechiae do not receive lumbar punctures or get admitted to the hospital. Well-appearing children with fever and petechiae should have a CBC with differential, blood culture, and PT and PTT. After a several-hour period of observation, children who remain

---

*Infections Associated with Fever
and Petechiae*

Bacterial

Neisseria meningitidis
Streptococcus pneumoniae
Haemophilus influenzae type b
Staphylococcus aureus
Streptococcus pyogenes
Escherichia coli

Viral

Enterovirus
Adenovirus
Influenza
Parainfluenza
Epstein-Barr virus
Rubella
Respiratory syncytial virus
Hepatitis viruses

Rickettsial

Rickettsia rickettsii
Ehrlichia

---

well appearing, who are not tachycardiac, whose petechiae have not progressed, and whose laboratory studies are normal may be considered for management as outpatients. Empiric antibiotic use should be decided on a case-by-case basis. There are no studies investigating the efficacy of antibiotic therapy in the outpatient management of patients with fever and petechiae. However, this author advocates the use of parenteral ceftriaxone, as the most likely bacterial pathogen in this circumstance carries such a high morbidity and mortality rate. In the event that outpatient management is chosen, it is imperative that patients receive excellent discharge instructions, are seen by their health care practitioner in 12 to 24 hours, and are instructed to return sooner if they become more ill or have any progression of their petechiae. The well-appearing child with fever and petechiae and a positive streptococcal antigen test may be treated as an outpatient with antistreptococcal antibiotics.

In the present patient, a 9-month old fussy infant, a full sepsis work-up was warranted. Parenteral antibiotics were administered and the infant was admitted to the hospital. Bacterial cultures were negative in this instance, but a stool culture grew enterovirus. The patient was discharged to home after 48 hours of negative bacterial cultures.

Clinical Pearls

1. The most common invasive bacterial disease causing fever and petechiae in children in the 21st century is infection with *Neisseria meningitidis*.

2. Viruses are the most common overall cause of fever and petechiae in children.

3. Well-appearing children older than 2 years of age with a normal white blood cell count (between 5000 and 15,000/μl), a normal absolute neutrophil count (between 1500 and 9000/μl), an absolute band count less than 500, and petechiae limited to the area above the nipple line may be considered for outpatient management after a period of observation in which they have normal vital signs and no progression of petechiae.

REFERENCES

1. Neilsen HE, Andersen EA, Andersen J, et al: Diagnostic assessment of haemorrhagic rash and fever. Arch Dis Child 85:160–165, 2001.
2. Wells LC, Smith JC, Weston VC, et al: The child with a non-blanching rash: How likely is meningoccal disease? Arch Dis Child 85:218–222, 2001.
3. DiGiulio GA: Fever and petechiae: No time for a rash decision. Clin Ped Emerg Med 1:132–137, 2000.
4. Mandl KD, Stack AM, Fleisher GR: Incidence of bacteremia in infants and children with fever and petechiae. J Pediatr 131:398–404, 1997.
5. Cohen AR: Rash: Purpura. In Fleisher G, Ludwig S (eds): Textbook of Pediatric Emergency Medicine. Baltimore, Williams & Wilkins, 1993, pp 430–438.
6. Baker RC, Seguin JH, Leslie N, et al: Fever and petechiae in children. Pediatrics 84:1051–1055, 1989.
7. Nguyen QV, Nguyen EA, Weiner LB: Incidence of invasive bacterial disease in children with fever and petechiae. Pediatrics 74:77–80, 1984.

M. Bradley Falk, MD
Jill M. Baren, MD, FACEP, FAAP

PATIENT 30

A 44-year-old man with confusion

A 44-year-old man is brought to the emergency department after being found at a highway toll-booth "acting strange" and "talking jibberish." A friend reports he has had symptoms of an upper respiratory infection for 2 weeks and was evaluated at another ED 24 hours previously. At that time he was "confused." She reports that he had a negative head computed tomography (CT) scan and was discharged home. She has not seen him again until this point.

Physical Examination: Vital Signs: temperature 37°C, heart rate 82, respiratory rate 18, room air pulse oximetry 98%. General: emotionally labile, crying. HEENT: pupils equally round/reactive (4 → 3 cm), extraocular movements intact, moist mucous membranes; clear rhinorrhea and nasal congestion. Neck: supple, nontender. Chest: normal. Cardiac: normal. Abdomen: normal. Extremities: no edema or rash. Neurologic: alert, oriented to person only; follows basic one-step commands; intermittent receptive aphasia; unable to spell but writes legible letters; cranial nerves 2–12 grossly intact, no visual field deficit; motor strength 5/5, symmetrical; sensation intact to light touch throughout; no cerebellar deficits (good finger/nose, heel/shin); reflexes 2+ and symmetric; negative Babinski reflex bilaterally.

Labororatory Findings: Finger-stick glucose: 88. CBC: normal. Electrolytes, BUN, creatinine: normal. Liver function tests: normal. Urine toxicology: negative. ECG: normal sinus rhythm with normal axis, no acute injury pattern. Head CT (see figure): acute ischemic infarct involving the left insular region.

Questions: Is this patient a candidate for thrombolytic therapy? His friend asks you if he can sit up in bed to be more comfortable. How do you answer?

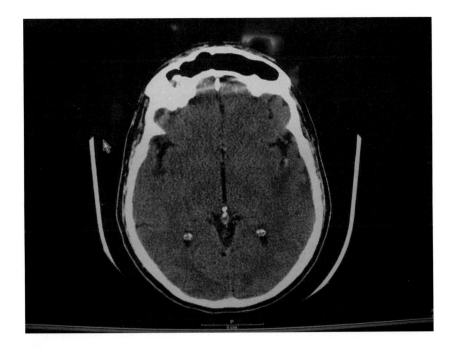

Diagnosis: This patient has suffered an ischemic stroke. He is *not* a candidate for lysis of a thrombus, as his last normal mental status was determined to be on the previous day. It is beneficial for him to remain in a supine position with his head flat.

Discussion: The patient's presentation invokes a broad differential diagnosis, including stroke (ischemic or hemorrhagic), traumatic brain injury, toxicologic process, encephalopathy, encephalitis, and acute psychosis. However, the findings on the head CT scan along with the aphasia led to the rapid diagnosis of ischemic stroke. Ischemic stroke occurs when insufficient blood flow to an area of the brain results in tissue ischemia and infarction. Surrounding the infarct zone is the *ischemic penumbra,* a term used to describe ischemic but potentially salvagable tissue. Whether this tissue survives depends on both the degree and the duration of ischemia. Time is essential in the management of the stroke patient. A faster time to diagnosis shortens the time to treatment. A useful sequence to remember for initial management of a suspected stroke is the following:

1. ABCs (airway, breathing, circulation), intravenous access, oxygen, cardiac monitor, fingerstick glucose.

2. Rapid history from *anyone* who can provide information. It is critical to determine when the patient was last seen acting at basline/normal, as this is a major determinant in the decision to give thrombolytics. Generally thrombolytics are not given if the patient arrives more than 3 hours from symptom onset (see table).

3. Pertinent brief neurologic examination to identify gross neurologic deficits (pupils, gaze palsy, facial droop, hemiplegia/paresis, major sensory deficits, aphasia, ataxia, visual field cut).

4. CBC, panel 7, coagulation studies.

5. Treat blood pressure >185/115.

6. Non-contrast-enhanced head CT as soon as possible.

7. If within the 3-hour time window, assess contraindications to thrombolytic therapy (see table).

If the head CT scan does not show intracranial hemorrhage, the patient has persistent symptoms, and exclusion criteria are absent, consider thrombolytic therapy. There is significant improvement at 3 months in patients treated within 3 hours of stroke onset.

The present patient is not a candidate, as he was last seen more than 24 hours prior to presentation. There is also an increased risk for subequent intracranial hemorrhage in the first 36 hours following thrombolytic therapy. Patients and/or families must be informed of both the benefits and the potential risks of thrombolytic therapy for stroke.

Cerebral perfusion pressure is necessary for adequate cerebral blood flow. Therefore, keeping

Exclusion Criteria for Thrombolytic Therapy (Tissue Plasminogen Activator [t-PA])

Symptoms >3 hrs duration

Seizure at stroke onset

Significantly resolving symptoms or isolated, mild neurologic deficits, such as ataxia alone, sensory loss alone, dysarthria alone, or minimal weakness.

Blood pressure >185/110 following intitial treatment, or any need for aggressive blood pressure control

Stroke or head trauma within past 3 months

ANY history of intracranial bleed

Surgery within 14 days

Gastrointestinal bleeding within 21 days

Recent myocardial infarction

Arterial puncture at a noncompressable site within 7 days

Use of oral anticoagulants or an INR >1.7

Use of heparin in past 48 hours and prolonged PTT

Platelets <100,000

Glucose <50 or >400

Thrombolytic therapy should not be given unless the emergent ancillary care and the facilities to handle bleeding complications are readily available.

Caution is advised before giving t-PA to persons with severe stroke (NIH Stroke Scale Score greater than 22).

the patient supine and euvolemic is paramount. Alterations in serum glucose and temperature instability have been shown to be harmful to the ischemic brain tissue and should be corrected early. Careful management of blood pressure is critical. As stated earlier, hypertension can exclude the use of thrombolytics. If blood pressure exceeds 185/110, intravenous labetolol can be used as initial therapy. Excessive blood pressure reduction should be avoided, as it can exacerbate ischemic symptoms. Anticoagulation with heparin is generally avoided because studies have shown an increased hemorrhagic transformation of ischemic stroke without any clinical benefit. Aspirin, however, should be given if the patient is *not* a thrombolytic candidate but avoided for 24 hours if thrombolytic therapy is given.

The patient was admitted to the neurology service. Over the next few days, he remained stable and was transferred to home for speech rehabilitation.

Clinical Pearls

1. Potential stroke patients should be appraoched with the "early early early" philosophy: early identification of symptom onset, early head CT, and early thrombolytics if the patient is a candidate.

2. Cerebral perfusion pressure can be maximized with patient positioning and pharmacologic control of blood pressure.

REFERENCES

1. Adams HP: Emergent use of anticoagulation for treatment of patients with ischemic stroke Stroke 33: 856–861, 2002.
2. Brott T, Bogousslavsky J: Treatment of acute ischemic stroke. N Engl J Med 343:10, 710–722, 2000.
3. Kasner SE, Grotta JC: Emergency identification and treatment of acute ischemic stroke. Ann Emerg Med 30:5, 642–653, 1997.
4. The NINDS t-PA Stroke Study Group: Generalized efficacy of t-PA for acute stroke: Subgroup analysis of the NINDS t-PA stroke trial. Stroke 28:2119–2125, 1997.
5. The NINDS t-PA Stroke Study Group: Intracerebral hemorrhage after intravenous t-PA therapy for ischemic stroke. Stroke 28:2109–2118, 1997.
6. American Heart Association Stroke Council: Guidelines for thrombolytic therapy for acute stroke: A supplement to the guidelines for the management of patients with acute ischemic stroke. Circulation 94:1167–1174, 1996.
7. The National Institute of Neurological Disorders and Stroke rt-PA Stroke Study Group: Tissue plasminogen activator for acute ischemic stroke. N Engl J Med 333:1581–1587, 1995.

Chirag Patel, MD
Stefanie Porges, MD

PATIENT 31

A 33-year old man with severe headache, neck stiffness, and photophobia

A 33-year old man without a significant past medical history presents to the ED with the worst headache of his life, which appeared while he was shoveling snow and reached maximal intensity within minutes. The headache is accompanied by photophobia, neck stiffness, nausea, and blurry vision. He denies fever, chills, recent upper respiratory infection, or any neurologic deficits.

Physical Examination: Temperature 36.4°C; pulse 78, respiratory rate 20, blood pressure 134/81. General: uncomfortable. HEENT: Fundi not visualized due to photophobia, otherwise normal. Chest: clear to auscultation. Cardiac: regular rate and rhythm without murmurs, gallops. Abdomen: normal. Extremities: without cyanosis or edema. Neuromuscular: alert and oriented. Cranial nerves, strength, sensation, gait, tandem walk, finger to nose, rapid alternating movements all normal, toes down-going, reflexes 2+ all extremities, normal gait, negative Romberg.

Laboratory Findings: CBC: normal. Blood chemistries: normal. Coagulation profile: normal. Electrocardiogram: normal sinus rhythm with normal intervals. CT scan of the head: see figure.

Questions: What is the most likely cause of the patient's headache and photophobia? If the CT scan were negative, what diagnostic test would be mandated?

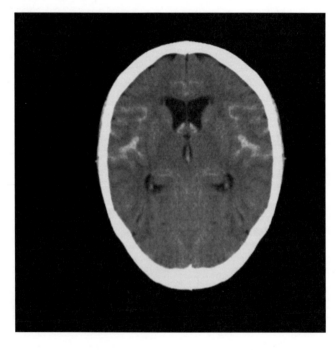

Diagnosis: Subarachnoid hemorrhage. A lumbar puncture is indicated if the CT scan is negative. Most nontraumatic subarachnoid hemorrhages are caused by ruptured saccular aneurysms.

Discussion: More than 1 million patients per year visit their primary care physician or ED with the report of headache. Of these, a small percentage need urgent diagnostic tests and treatment. Headache may be the initial symptom of a life-threatening cause such as a subarachnoid hemorrhage (SAH), other intracranial hemorrhage, mass lesion, encephalitis or meningitis, vasculitis, venous sinus thrombosis, or toxic metabolic disorder. Ten to 15% of patients with SAH die before reaching the hospital and 50% die within the first 6 months of diagnosis.

Rupture of an aneurysm causes arterial bleeding into the cerebrospinal fluid (CSF), which spreads quickly, causing elevated intracranial pressure. Although the bleeding lasts only a few seconds, rebleeding is common, especially within the first 12 hours. The typical patient has a severe headache (frequently described as the worst headache of his or her life) that develops during straining or exertion and rapidly reaches maximal intensity. The headache may or may not be accompanied by loss of consciousness, photophobia, nausea, vomiting, seizure, meningismus, diminished level of consciousness, or focal neurologic signs. Meningismus and back pain may develop in a few hours as the blood breaks down and causes aseptic meningitis. A warning leak from the aneurysm may occur in as many as 50% of patients several days to weeks prior to the hemorrhage. There are many deviations from this classic presentation.

A brand new or "worst" headache requires evaluation, as do headaches that deviate from an established pattern in a person with a headache disorder. The work-up consists of a CT scan without contrast. Current CT scan technology still fails to demonstrate the hemorrhage in up to 8% of patients within the first 12 hours and in 7–14% within 24 hours. It has a 50% failure rate within 5 days from the initial hemorrhage.

A lumbar puncture must be performed in a patient whose clinical presentation suggests SAH but in whom the CT scan is negative, equivocal, or technically limited. The opening pressure should be measured because it is often elevated in cases of SAH. Immediate centrifugation of the CSF differentiates true SAH from a traumatic tap. Xanthrochromia (pink or yellow tint of the CSF) represents SAH if it is present as early as 2 hours after the onset of symptoms; lumbar puncture before this time may fail to reveal xanthrochromia. Presence of red blood cells in the CSF that does not clear in sequential tubes may indicate hemorrhage, but CSF clearing in sequential collection tubes does not rule out old SAH. If both the CT scan and the lumbar puncture findings are normal, there is little evidence to suggest the need for angiography. These individuals may be referred to their primary care provider or neurologist.

If the CT scan or lumbar puncture reveals SAH, urgent neurosurgical consultation is required and further studies should be performed to determine the cause. Cerebral angiography is the most common study that reveals an aneurysm, but no angiographic cause is evident in 14 to 20% of cases. A nonaneurysmal pattern of hemorrhage may result from thrombosed aneurysms or angiographically occult vascular malformations, pial fistula, or prepontine vein rupture; these patients do not suffer the same degree of morbidity and mortality. Often, CT angiography is performed for rapid assessment in a patient who might require emergency craniotomy.

Once the diagnosis of SAH is made, aggressive medical management should be initiated, including aggressive correction of coagulopathy with fresh frozen plasma as necessary, central venous access, and decreasing elevated blood pressure. There is a high risk of rebleeding within 12 hours of the SAH. Decreasing the blood pressure reduces the chance of rebleeding but also increases the chance of infarction due to diminshed cerebral perfusion pressure, hydrocephalus, and tissue edema. Medication choices for high blood pressure are intravenous labetolol, nicardapine, or hydralazine. If unsuccessful, one can use a nitroprusside infusion. A goal of decreasing the mean arterial pressure to 90 mm Hg but not below will help to prevent infarction. Diminishing cognitive level represents decreasing cerebral perfusion requiring intracranial pressure monitoring. Acute hydrocephalus is decompressed with a ventriculostomy tube. Hypoxia, hypercarbia, and hypo- or hyperglycemia are noxious stimuli to cerebral tissue and should be corrected to avoid secondary brain injury.

Prevention of complications of SAH is also started once the diagnosis is made. SAH predisposes the patient to vasospasm around the third day post hemorrhage. The calcium channel blocker nimodipine has been shown to reduce vasospasm. Seizure prophylaxis with phenytoin, tegretol, or phenobarbital is also indicated. Definitive treatment is surgical or, in the right situation, with invasive neuroradiology techniques.

The present patient had a negative angiogram. The hemorrhage and hydrocephalus resolved in 4 days. The patient was discharged without any surgical treatment on nimodipine and anticonvulsants.

Clinical Pearls

1. The first or worst headache usually requires an evaluation, as do headaches that are different from the established pattern in a person with a headache disorder.

2. A negative CT scan does not rule out subarachnoid hemorrhage; a lumbar puncture is indicated. If both are unequivocally negative, the patient does not need angiography.

3. Hypertension should not be treated aggressively in a patient with SAH.

4. Calcium channel blockers should be started in the ED to prevent cerebral vasospasm if the SAH patient is diagnosed with anerysmal rupture.

REFERENCES

1. Jagoda AS, Dalsey WC, Fairweather PG, et al: Clinical policy: Critical issues in the evaluation and management of patients presenting to the emergency department with acute headache. Ann Emerg Med 39:108–122, 2002.
2. Edlow JA, Caplan LR: Avoiding pitfalls in the diagnosis of subarachnoid hemorrhage. N Engl J Med 342:29–35, 2000.
3. Vespa PM, Gobin YP: Endovascular treatment and neurointensive care of ruptured aneurysms. Crit Care Clin 15:667–684, 1999.
4. Charpentier C, Audibert G, Guillemin F, et al: Multivariate analysis of predictors of cerebral vasospasm occurrence after aneurysmal subarachnoid hemorrhage. Stroke 30:1402–1408, 1999.
5. Stieg PE, Kase CS: Intracranial hemorrhage: Diagnosis and emergency management. Neurol Clin 16:374–390, 1998.
6. Ruptured cerebral aneurysms: Perioperative management. In Ratcheson RA, Wirth FP (eds): Concepts in Neurosurgery, vol 6. Baltimore, Williams Wilkins, 1994.
7. Vermeulen M, Lindsay KW, Murray GD, et al: Antifibrinolytic treatment in subarachnoid hemorrhage. N Engl J Med 311:432–437, 1984.

Reza Daugherty, MD
Evaline Alessandrini, MD, MSCE

PATIENT 32

An 11-month-old boy with a choking episode

The mother of an 11-month-old boy brings her son to the emergency department because he had a choking episode approximately 30 minutes ago. The child was sitting on the kitchen floor while his mother was cooking dinner. She states that she heard him coughing and gasping for air. She looked down to find him "blue around the lips" but alert. She rushed over to pick him up and he immediately began to cry. She quickly placed him in the car and rushed to the hospital. There are no recent illnesses, vomiting, or fevers. No seizure activity was observed. He ate his usual dinner 30 minutes prior to the episode. He was born at full term with no complications. He was diagnosed with gastroesophageal reflux at 3 months of age because of recurrent episodes of "spitting up." He was placed on ranitidine and metoclopramide and has been symptom-free since. He has been growing well and has no other medical history.

Physical Examination: Vital signs: temperature 37.2°C rectally; pulse 135; respiratory rate 52; blood pressure 92/54. General: alert, with slightly hoarse cry and stridor when agitated. Intermittent dry cough and frequent crying episodes. Skin: pink, warm, and well perfused without rashes or hemangiomas. HEENT: no rhinorrhea. Oropharynx is unremarkable, without foreign body, erythema, or lesions noted. Chest: clear and equal breath sounds while quiet. Cardiac: RRR without murmur. Abdomen: normal. Neurologic: nonfocal and alert.

Laboratory Findings: Chest radiograph: trachea midline with normal caliber, no mediastinal shift, lungs without infiltrate, symmetric air expansion bilaterally, no foreign body noted. Lateral neck x-ray: see figure.

ED Course: The child was monitored in the ED with pulse oximetry. His respiratory rate remained in the 40s to 50s and his oxygen saturation remained normal. He had some crying episodes accompanied by occasional stridor, but no choking or cyanosis. He refused to drink from a bottle while in the ED.

Question: What further work-up, if any, would you do for this patient?

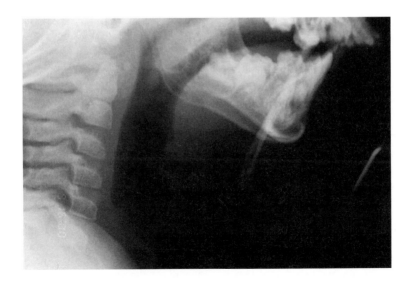

Discussion: In this patient, the rapid onset of symptoms in a previously well child strongly suggests the diagnosis of aspirated foreign body. The differential diagnosis of partial upper airway obstruction includes foreign body (FB) aspiration, epiglottitis, croup, bacterial tracheitis, retropharyngeal abscess, tonsillar/adenoidal enlargement, angioedema, and mechanical or chemical trauma. According to 1998 statistics from the National Center for Health Statistics, 142 children under the age of 5 years died as a result of suffocation from FB aspiration. Younger children are at greater risk because they tend to explore their environment by putting things in their mouth and do not have fully developed dentition with which to adequately chew. Boys account for a disproportionately higher percentage of victims than do girls, with nearly twice the likelihood in some studies. Children with neurologic problems and/or developmental delay are at particular risk and may present out of the typical age range. Food substances are by far the most commonly aspirated matter, accounting for 70% to 80% of episodes. In numerous studies, nuts, particularly peanuts, are the most common item found at the time of bronchoscopy, accounting for more than 70% of incidents alone. Of nonfood items, the leading offenders are plastic toy parts and pen caps. Overall, balloons have the highest associated risk of mortality, causing nearly one third of aspiration-associated deaths.

Classic symptoms of partial airway obstruction due to FB include an acute episode of choking with subsequent cough, stridor, dysphonia, drooling, and chest retractions. Some patients with small, subglottic foreign bodies may be asymptomatic and many patients present with none or only a few of these symptoms. The mechanism of this is theorized to be due to accommodation of cough receptors in the airway after persistent stimulation in as little as 15 minutes.

The diagnosis of total airway obstruction is made by history and physical examination. As immediate intervention is required, no other investigations are needed. Definitive relief of the obstruction must not be delayed by radiographic studies. A partial obstruction may become complete if the patient is forced to move from a position of comfort. If the diagnosis is uncertain, a person skilled in advanced airway management should accompany the patient to the radiology department for chest films and soft-tissue neck films to visualize the entire airway. Still, radiography usually plays a limited role in the diagnosis of children with suspected upper airway FB aspiration. Because most aspirated substances are food, they tend to be radiolucent. In some series, only 6% to 17% of aspirated FBs were radiopaque. At least one study found radiography to have a poorer sensitivity than history or physical examination and poorer specificity than history.

If the child is crying, coughing, or able to phonate, the airway is at least partially patent. These children should be approached with a calm demeanor and every attempt should be made to keep them from becoming more agitated. Oxygen saturation should be monitored with pulse oximetry and oxygen administered noninvasively by blow-by as needed. Children in whom there is a strong suspicion of FB aspiration should go directly to the operating room as quickly as possible for general anesthesia and rigid bronchoscopy. Prolonged delays in radiology should be avoided. The rigid bronchoscope has many advantages including (1) securing the airway definitively, (2) allowing continued ventilation of the patient throughout the procedure, and (3) permitting a wide variety of tools to be used to extract the FB. Several groups have reported recent success with the use of a flexible bronchoscope in removing FBs in children. Disadvantages in its use are that a rigid bronchoscope still needs to be present in case there is airway difficulty, and the flexible scope requires at least a size 4.5 mm endotracheal tube to pass. However, the flexible scope does have the advantage of being able to retrieve objects further down the bronchial tree. In very rare instances, less than 1% in some series, the object cannot be retrieved by either rigid or flexible bronchoscopy and necessitates open thoracotomy.

Children should generally be admitted to the hospital after removal of the FB for observation. Complication rates after rigid bronchoscopy range from 1% to 8%, and so these children should be monitored postoperatively. The risk of complications increases with the time the FB has been present in the airway due to surrounding tissue edema and tissue friability.

The present patient was taken to the operating room by a pediatric otolaryngologist. He was placed under general anesthesia uneventfully and a rigid bronchoscope was passed. A 1 cm × 1 cm flat blue foreign body was seen lying on top of the vocal cords, partially obstructing the airway. It was removed easily and found to be a plastic bread tie. The child remained in the hospital overnight for observation and was discharged the following day. This case represents a chilling prospect for the emergency physician. The child had a relatively benign physical examination and normal radiographic studies. The history was of concern but the unsuspecting physician may have attributed the episode to the child's history of reflux or the common childhood entity of viral croup.

Clinical Pearls

1. Children with upper airway foreign body aspiration may be relatively asymptomatic at presentation, and so the clinician must maintain a high index of suspicion given a suggestive history.

2. Plain radiography plays a limited role in the diagnosis of foreign body aspiration because of an unacceptably high false-negative rate.

3. Children with a history suggesting foreign body aspiration should have consultation by a specialist experienced in the use of bronchoscopy in children.

REFERENCES

1. Swanson KL, Prakash UB, Midthun DE, et al: Flexible bronchoscopic management of airway foreign bodies in children. Chest 121:1695–1700, 2002.
2. Rovin JD, Rodgers BM: Pediatric foreign body aspiration. Pediatr Rev 21:86–90, 2000.
3. Skoulakis CE, Doxas PG, Papadakis CE, et al: Bronchoscopy for foreign body removal in children: A review and analysis of 210 cases. Int J Pediatr Otorhinolaryngol 53:143–148, 2000.
4. Metrangelo S, Monetti C, Meneghini L, et al: Eight years' experience with foreign-body aspiration in children: What is really important for a timely diagnosis? J Pediatr Surg 34:1229–1231, 1999.
5. Zerella JT, Dimler M, McGill LC, Pippus KJ: Foreign body aspiration in children: Value of radiography and complications of bronchoscopy. J Pediatr Surg 33:1651–1654, 1998.
6. Muniz AE, Joffe MD: Foreign bodies, ingested and inhaled. Contemp Pediatr 14 pp: 78–98, 1997.
7. Rimell FL, Thome A Jr, Stool S, et al: Characteristics of objects that cause choking in children. JAMA 274:1763–1766, 1995.

Jill M. Baren, MD, FACEP, FAAP

PATIENT 33

A 22-year-old woman with sudden onset of shortness of breath

A 22 year-old woman with history of asthma attended a party in a crowded apartment heated by a wood-burning stove. She suddenly felt short of breath and realized she forgot her Albuterol metered-dose inhaler. She left the party, returned home, and administered an Albuterol treatment by home nebulizer. Fifteen minutes later, her husband found her severely short of breath and lethargic. She is brought to the emergency department by ambulance in marked respiratory distress. The patient's husband reports that she has long-standing asthma, is usually compliant with her medications (Albuterol as needed and fluticasone bid), and the last time this happened the patient almost died and was admitted to the intensive care unit for 2 weeks.

Physical Examination: Temperature afebrile; pulse 144; respirations 40; blood pressure 110/78; SaO_2 86% on room air. General: pale, diaphoretic, unable to speak more that one word at a time. HEENT: nasal flare. Neck: no jugular venous distension. Chest: paradoxical chest wall motion, decreased breath sounds in bilateral lung fields, faint wheezes. Cardiac: regular tachycardia. Extremities: cool with rapid, weak pulses. Neurologic: decreased level of consciousness but responds to painful stimuli with appropriate localization.

Laboratory Findings: Chest radiograph (see figure): hyperinflation, peribronchial thickening, no infiltrates.

Questions: What physical examination findings indicate the severity of the patient's asthma exacerbation? Which medications are immediately indicated? What are the therapeutic options if the patient does not respond to initial therapy?

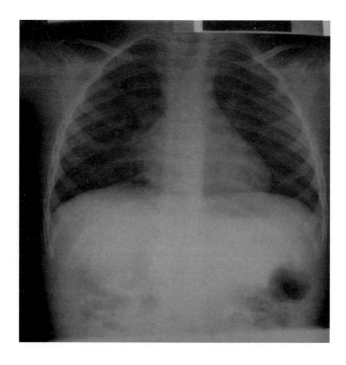

Diagnosis: Severe acute asthma exacerbation. The patient is severely dyspneic with paradoxical wall motion indicating severely increased work of breathing. Nasal flare, decreased level of consciousness, and poor perfusion indicate hypoxemia, hypercarbia, and impending respiratory failure. Aeration is poor, as wheezes are barely discernable. The patient requires immediate treatment with supplemental oxygen, nebulized albuterol, and intravenous corticosteriods. She should be placed on a continuous cardiac and pulse oximetry monitor. If she fails to respond, nebulized ipratropium and intravenous magnesium can be added to her therapy with preparation for possible intravenous beta-agonist therapy and intubation.

Discussion: Asthma is a common chronic disease in the United States. Of the 15 to 20 million persons affected, approximately 2 million seek care in the ED annually. Asthma deaths increased over a 10-year period from 1980 to 1990 and have since leveled off at about 5000 deaths per year, but hospitalization rates have continued to increase, particularly among pediatric patients. These statistics are disturbing in light of the fact that our knowledge of the pathophysiology and treatment of asthma has advanced considerably.

Asthma is a chronic inflammatory disease that is characterized by remissions and exacerbations. Many patients experience chronic low-level symptoms on a regular basis, such as wheeze, decreased exercise tolerance, and nocturnal cough. During an exacerbation, most patients will report of acute shortness of breath, cough, wheeze, or chest tightness due to bronchial inflammation, hyperactive smooth muscle activity, and airflow obstruction.

Typical physical findings during an asthma exacerbation include tachypnea, tachycardia, accessory muscle use (intercostal, subcostal, and supraclavicular retractions), wheezing, and other abnormal breath sounds with decrease in overall aeration. Absence of wheezing in the setting of respiratory distress indicated poor air entry and should alert the emergency physician to the presence of a severe exacerbation. Overall assessment of respiratory distress should reflect both oxygenation and ventilation. Tachypnea and accessory muscle use are indications of impaired ventilation, whereas inadequate oxygenation manifests as nasal flare, color change (pallor or cyanosis), and change in mental status (confusion, irritability, or lethargy). Oxygenation can also be directly assessed with pulse oximetry (noninvasive) or arterial blood gas. Markedly altered mental status indicates hypercarbia and hypoxia and signals that respiratory failure is imminent, with need for immediate intubation.

There are three goals for the approach to an asthma exacerbation in the ED: (1) accurate assessment with the recognition of hypoxemia and determination of the severity of the exacerbation; (2) reversal of airflow obstruction with quick relief (rescue medications) and anti-inflammatory and other medications; and (3) reduction of recurrent airflow obstruction with appropriate disposition and follow-up.

Most patients with a mild to moderate exacerbation do not require supplemental oxygen. According to national guidelines, pregnant patients, children, patients with comorbid diseases, and those with room air saturation less than 90% should be given supplemental oxygen. Pulmonary function tests in the setting of acute asthma exacerbation are used to determine severity whenever possible, as these tests are one of the few objective ways to do this. Clinical assessment findings are not highly correlated with true lung function. In the ED, the most common pulmonary function test performed is the peak expiratory flow. It requires consistent and correct positioning as well as patient effort, and the results must be interpreted within this context. If a patient has not been trained in the maneuver or does not know his or her personal best peak expiratory flow, 400 L/minute for adult females and 500 L/minute for adult males can be used as normal values.

Inhaled beta-agonists are the standard first-line therapy for the management of acute asthma and are the most effective rescue medications for relieving airflow obstruction. Their onset of action is within 5 minutes. The recommended dose of albuterol is 2.5–5.0 mg every 15 to 20 minutes in the first hour of therapy, however, it can be given more frequently, and even continuously as needed. It is also acceptable and often preferable to administer albuterol via metered dose inhaler at a rate of two to eight puffs every 5 minutes. The metered-dose inhaler delivers the drug more efficiently, but it may be difficult for some patients to coordinate their breathing with this apparatus when in distress.

Systemic corticosteroids are indicated for most patients with an asthma exacerbation. Corticosteroids speed the resolution of airflow obstruction, potentiate the effects of beta-agonist therapy, and decrease hospitalization rates for sicker patients. Oral doses of prednisone (40–60 mg) should be administered to all patients except those who have resolved their exacerbation symptoms entirely after one albuterol treatment. If a patient is unable to tolerate or is too ill to receive oral corticosteroids, they can be given intravenously. Ipra-

95

tropium bromide is an anticholinergic inhaled medication that works synergistically with albuterol to decrease airflow obstruction via vagally mediated pathways. It is recommended in the setting of moderate to severe asthma at a dose of 250 to 500 μcg per treatment.

Most asthma patients respond to inhaled beta-agonist, anticholinergic, and corticosteroid therapy. For the small percentage of patients who do not, there are other therapeutic agents that can be added. Magnesium sulfate has potential benefit to some patients with severe acute asthma and should be considered in patients who fail to improve with albuterol and ipratropium therapy and who show signs of progression to respiratory failure. It is given as an intravenous infusion of 2 g in 50 to 100 ml D_5W or NS over 10 minutes. Side effects include burning, flushing, lethargy, weakness, hypotension, and dysrhythmia. Systemic beta-agonists should also be considered in severely ill patients. Options include subcutaneous or intravenous administration of epinephrine or the more beta-selective drug terbutaline.

Ultimately, if no response is achieved with these aggressive measures, intubation may become necessary for respiratory failure, significant hypoxia, or mental status changes. In the ED, intubation of the asthmatic patient should proceed using a rapid sequence protocol. Ketamine (1–3 mg/kg IV) is an excellent drug for induction, as it causes bronchodilation. Etomidate, succinylcholine, and midazolam are good alternatives. A paralytic agent should follow. Ventilation of an intubated asthmatic patient is very challenging because of the prolonged expiratory phase leading to air trapping, hyperinflation, and barotraumas. To avoid this complication, permissive hypercapnea is often tolerated with slow rates of 8 to 12 breaths/minute to allow for adequate exhalation time.

The present patient received nebulized albuterol, ipratropium, intravenous methylprednisolone, and 100% oxygen by facemask. She became increasingly agitated and was given subcutaneous epinephrine, which resulted in increased cooperation. Repeat examination revealed loud coarse bilateral inspiratory and expiratory wheezes. She was placed on continuous albuterol and admitted to the intensive care unit. She was discharged 5 days later on a corticosteroid taper and with instructions to attend asthma education classes to learn about symptom recognition, trigger avoidance, and proper use of rescue medications.

Clinical Pearls

1. The younger the patient, the more likely increased work of breathing will be manifested as accessory muscle use (chest wall retractions) due to highly compliant chest wall mechanics. Therefore, an adult with paradoxical chest wall motion during an asthma exacerbation is likely in severe respiratory distress.

2. Absence of wheezing can be an ominous sign in a patient with poor aeration and indicates a severe asthma exacerbation.

3. Disposition from the ED should be based on an objective measure of airflow obstruction (peak expiratory flow) in addition to clinical assessment. In general, patients with peak expiratory flow rate of > 70% predicted can be safely discharged.

REFERENCES

1. Emond SD, Camargo CA Jr, Nowak RM: 1997 National Asthma Education and Prevention Program Guidelines: A practical summary for emergency physicians. Ann Emerg Med 31:579–589, 1998.
2. Lin RY, Pesola GR, Bakalchuk L, et al: Superiority of ipratropium plus albuterol over albuterol alone in the emergency department management of adult asthma: A randomized clinical trial. Ann Emerg Med 31:208–213, 1998.
3. National Asthma Education and Prevention Program: Expert panel report 2: Guidelines for the diagnosis and management of asthma. DHHS pub # NIH 97–4051, 1997.
4. Idris AH, McDermott MF, Raucci JC, et al: Emergency department treatment of severe asthma: Metered-dose inhaler plus holding chamber is equivalent in effectiveness to nebulizer. Chest 103:665–672, 1993 .
5. Rowe BH, Keller JL, Oxman AD: Effectiveness of steroid therapy in acute exacerbations of asthma: A meta-analysis. Am J Emerg Med 10:301–310, 1992.

Bruce D. Rubin, MD

PATIENT 34

A 68-year-old man with left flank pain

A 68-year-old man presents to the emergency department with a 2-day history of left-sided flank pain, which he describes as sharp, colicky in nature, and unrelated to exertion, movement, position, or eating. He has a history of high blood pressure, but has not seen a physician in 10 years or taken any medications. He denies chest pain, shortness of breath, back pain, or difficulty with urination.

Physical Examination: afebrile; pulse 86; blood pressure 185/90. General: well-nourished, well-developed man, appears uncomfortable. HEENT: normal. Chest: clear to auscultation. Cardiac: regular rate and rhythm, no murmurs. Abdomen: soft, nondistended, small pulsatile mass with mild tenderness to palpation at left mid-abdomen, no guarding or rebound. Rectal: brown stool, heme negative. Extremities: symmetrical +2 femoral pulses.

Laboratory Findings: Electrolytes: normal. CBC: normal. Urine dip: 2+ hemoglobin. ECG: normal. CT scan without contrast: see figure.

Questions: What is the abnormal finding on the CT scan? What size is considered normal for the abdominal aorta? What is the correlation between aortic size and risk of rupture? What should be done for patients with aortic aneurysms discovered radiographically?

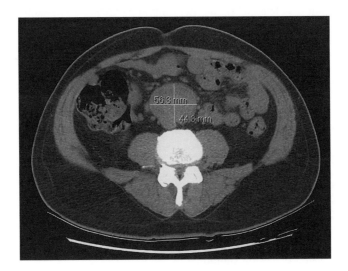

Diagnosis: Abdominal aortic aneurysm (AAA)

Discussion: AAA is the tenth leading cause of death in the elderly. 10,000 to 15,000 deaths per year occur from rupture. One third of abdominal aneurysms eventually rupture if left untreated, with an associated mortality rate of 80% in the acute setting. Nine percent of people older than 65 years of age have an unsuspected asymptomatic abdominal aortic aneurysm.

An aneurysm is defined as a dilation of all three layers of the arterial wall (in contrast to a dissection, which involves separation of the intimal layer from the media). Aneurysms arise from a chronic degenerative process that produces localized weakening of the aortic wall. The abdominal aorta is predisposed to aneurysmal formation due to high systolic and pulse pressures compared to the thoracic aorta. Risk factors for aneurysm formation include connective tissue disorders, family history, age older than 50 years, atherosclerotic disease, smoking, and hypertension.

AAA has a variety of clinical manifestations, including constant abdominal pain, often localized to left middle or lower quadrant with radiation to the back, and more atypical presentations, including bilateral or unilateral flank, costovertebral angle, or hip pain. Patients can also present with syncope, shock, or sudden death.

The diagnosis can be easily missed by ascribing the symptoms to a different condition such as musculoskeletal back pain, renal colic, or pancreatitis. The only physical examination finding of demonstrated value is direct abdominal palpation. The sensitivity of abdominal palpation for the detection of AAA ranges from 76% to 100%. Abdominal palpation is safe, and there have been no reports of precipitating rupture by its use. The examination should be done with the patient in a supine position with knees raised to relax abdominal muscles. The examiner should position both hands on the abdomen with palms down and index fingers extended. Deep palpation should be made to feel for pulsations, usually found just cephalad of the umbilicus (bifurcation of aorta). Index fingers should be placed on either side of pulsations to measure the distance.

Plain radiography is generally unhelpful in confirming the diagnosis of AAA. Approximately 65% of patients with symptomatic AAA have calcified aorta, but negative plain radiographs cannot exclude the presence of an aneurysm. The gold standard for diagnosis is angiography, but ultrasonography, and computed tomography also have a role and are often safer and easier to perform. Emergency medicine bedside ultrasonography (EMBU) has recently been studied and has shown close to 100% sensitivity for diagnosis of AAA. EMBU can be technically limited by obesity and bowel gas, making the study difficult to perform and ruptures difficult to visualize unless there is massive free fluid seen in Morrison's pouch. EMBU is particularly ideal for the unstable patient. Computed tomography (CT) scan without contrast can illuminate the true diameter of the aorta, while adding contrast helps to demonstrate anatomic details such as leakage or thrombus.

The appropriate treatment for AAA is surgical repair. Current recommendations for elective repair are for aneurysms of 4 to 6 cm (normal aorta less than 2.5 cm). The size of the aneurysm is directly related to the likelihood of rupture. Aneurysms smaller than 4 cm have a 0% risk of rupture per year, whereas those 4 to 4.9 cm have a 1% risk of rupture/year. There is a clear increase in risk of rupture with increase in size (see table).

The present patient was originally thought to have a renal calculus. He was scheduled for a CT scan without contrast, which showed a 5.6-cm AAA (see figure). He was evaluated by a vascular surgeon and taken emergently for repair in the operating room. His course was eventful for postoperative transient ischemic attack; otherwise, he recovered well.

One-Year Incidence of Rupture Based on Size of Aorta

SIZE OF AORTA (CM)	1 YEAR INCIDENCE OF RUPTURE (%)
5.5 – 5.9	9.4
6.0 – 6.9	10.2
7.0 – 8.0	32.5

Clinical Pearls

1. Always consider abdominal aortic aneurysm in patients 50 years or older who present with back, flank, or abdominal pain.

2. Abdominal palpation is useful in detecting large aneurysms (>5 cm), which are more likely to rupture, but is limited in larger patients and cannot entirely exclude the diagnosis of AAA.

3. Be careful when attributing chest, back, or abdominal pain to benign conditions in elderly patients.

REFERENCES

1. Thompson R: Detection and management of small aortic aneurysms. N Engl J Med 346:1484–1486, 2002.
2. Fink H, Lederle F, Roth C et al: The accuracy of physical examination to detect abdominal aortic aneurysm. Arch Intern Med 160:833–836, 2000.
3. Lederle F, Johnson G, Wilson S, et al: The aneurysm detection and management study screening program: Validation cohort and final results. Arch Intern Med 160:1425–1430, 2000.
4. Hallett J: Management of abdominal aortic aneurysms. Mayo Clin Proc 47:395–399, 2000.
5. Gillum RF: Epidemiology of aortic aneurysm in the United States. J Clin Epidemiol 48:1289–1298, 1995.
6. Lederle FA, Walker JM, Reinke DB: Selective screening for abdominal aortic aneurysms with physical examination and ultrasound. Arch Intern Med 148:1753–1756, 1988.
7. Ingoldby CJH, Wujanto R, Mitchell JE: Impact of vascular surgery on community mortality from ruptured aortic aneurysms. Br J Surg 73:551–553, 1986.

Amy L. Puchalski, MD

PATIENT 35

A 4-month-old girl with rhinorrhea and worsening cough

A previously healthy 4-month-old girl presents to the emergency department with a cough and coryza. The rhinorrhea started 2 weeks ago, and for the past week she has had episodes of constant coughing that last for about 1 minute. She seems to have trouble catching her breath while coughing but never becomes cyanotic. For the past 3 days, the coughing episodes have been followed by vomiting. She has no fever, seems well when she is not coughing, and has been drinking her usual amount.

Physical Examination: Temperature 37.4°C; heart rate 132, respiratory rate 28; blood pressure 84/56; pulse oximetry 98% in room air. She is alert and comfortable. HEENT: moist mucous membranes, small right subconjunctival hemorrhage, clear rhinorrhea. Respiratory: lungs clear to auscultation bilaterally, no retractions, witnessed 30-second episode of constant cough followed by emesis. Neurologic: alert, grossly intact cranial nerves, normal tone and strength in all extremities.

Laboratory Findings: WBC 29,000/µl with 84% lymphocytes. Chest radiograph: no focal infiltrates.

Questions: What is the likely diagnosis? How should this infant be managed?

Answers: The infant's clinical course and lymphocytosis are consistent with a diagnosis of pertussis. The baby was hospitalized for observation, empirically started on erythromycin, and 24 hours later the polymerase chain reaction results from her nasopharyngeal aspirate was positive for pertussis.

Discussion: The clinical syndrome of pertussis, or "whooping cough," is caused by *Bordetella pertussis,* an aerobic gram-negative rod. Since 1980, there has been a rise in the number of cases diagnosed yearly in the United States, with 7867 cases reported in 2000, more than half of which were in children younger than 5 years of age. Since the 1990s, there has been, unfortunately, an increase in the number of deaths from pertussis, particularly among infants. From 1997 to 2000, 90% of all deaths due to pertussis were in children younger than 6 months of age. There is a great deal of morbidity due to pertussis in this age group, as supported by the fact that 63% of those younger than 6 months were hospitalized from 1997 to 2000. In 1993, pertussis became the most common reportable vaccine-preventable disease in children under the age of 5. This trend is thought to be due to an increased susceptibility to pertussis in adults, as vaccination does not impart lifetime immunity. The disease often goes unrecognized in adults because of its milder course, and therefore this population serves as a reservoir for infection of infants and children.

Pertussis is a highly communicable disease with an estimated attack rate of 60% in children. The bacteria are spread primarily by inhalation, although some cases result from close contact with respiratory secretions. The bacteria infect respiratory epithelial cells directly, but toxin-mediated effects are primarily responsible for the clinical course of the illness. The toxins act to paralyze respiratory cilia as well as cause inflammation in the bronchi and peribronchial tissue. This inflammatory response results in airway obstruction, mucus plugging, and atelectasis.

The typical clinical course of pertussis follows three stages. First is the catarrhal stage, characterized by mild cough and rhinorrhea, sometimes along with fever and conjunctivitis. It typically lasts 1 to 2 weeks before progression to the second phase, the paroxysmal stage. This is usually the time when the diagnosis is suspected, as it is characterized by bursts of prolonged coughing spasms followed by a sudden, prolonged inflow of air that may sound like a "whoop." Young infants, however, may not produce the characteristic "whoop" after coughing spasms. Patients sometimes vomit after the coughing paroxysms, and infants may become cyanotic during the events, although between episodes they appear relatively well. This phase can last up to 6 weeks before progressing to the convalescent stage. There is a gradual recovery over this 2 to 3-week period, but patients may have coughing paroxysms with viral upper respiratory infections for the next several months.

Infants younger than 6 months of age are particularly at risk for complications of pertussis. Bacterial pneumonia is the most common complication, occurring in 11.8% of infants from 1997 to 2000, as well as the most frequent cause of death from pertussis. Neurologic complications, such as seizures and encephalopathy, are also found more frequently in infants, occurring in 1.4% and 0.2%, respectively. Other rare complications include pneumothorax, epistaxis, subconjunctival hemorrhages, subdural hemorrhages, and rectal prolapse. It is recommended that all infants under the age of 6 months with known or suspected pertussis be admitted to the hospital.

The laboratory diagnosis of pertussis can be achieved with nasopharyngeal culture, fluorescent antibody testing, or PCR. Children may exhibit a marked lymphocytosis on peripheral blood smear with an absolute lymphocyte count exceeding 20,000, but this is not typical in young infants or adults. A chest radiograph may demonstrate the characteristic "shaggy" right heart boarder but more often is negative. It is important to remember that the clinical course in adults and adolescents is much more mild than in children and is characterized by at least 7 days of a dry cough.

Treatment is primarily supportive, though a 14-day course of erythromycin can eradicate the organism from secretions and make the disease course less severe. Chemoprophylaxis with 14 days of erythromycin is recommended for all household and close contacts. Contacts under 7 years of age should complete their primary vaccination series, and those who have not been vaccinated in more than 3 years require a booster. The present patient did well during her hospitalization and was discharged after 5 days when her cough was improving.

Clinical Pearls

1. Pertussis is under-recognized in adolescents and adults, and the diagnosis of pertussis should be considered in those with more than 7 days of dry cough.

2. The characteristic lymphocytosis caused by pertussis is usually not seen in infants younger than 3 months old or in adults.

3. Infants younger than 6 months of age with pertussis should be admitted to the hospital, as they are at greater risk of cyanotic episodes, respiratory arrest, and other complications of pertussis.

REFERENCES

1. Centers for Disease Control and Prevention: Pertussis. Health Topics 2002, http://www.cdc.gov. Accessed July 2002.
2. Centers for Disease Control and Prevention: Summary of notifiable diseases—United States, 2000. MMWR Morbid Mortal Wkly Rep. 49: 1–102, 2002.
3. Fleisher GR: Infectious disease emergencies. In Fleisher GR; Ludwig S (eds): Textbook of Pediatric Emergency Medicine. Philadelphia Lippincott, Williams, & Wilkins, 2000.
4. Hoppe JE: Neonatal pertussis. Ped Infect Dis J 19:244–247, 2000.
5. Black S: Epidemiology of pertussis. Ped Infect Dis J 16:S85–89, 1997.
6. Qiushui H, Mertsola J: Epidemiology and prevention of pertussis. Curr Opin Ped 9:14–18, 1997.

Anthony J. Dean, MD

PATIENT 36

A 43-year-old woman with abdominal pain and fever

A 43-year-old woman presents with epigastric pain which has progressively worsened over the past 4 days. She denies previous episodes of similar pain. She is nauseated, with decreased appetite, and subjective fever. She has had no diarrhea or constipation. She has no history of abdominal surgery, no urinary or gynecologic symptoms. She denies prior gastrointestinal disease. She has a history of hypertension and hyperlipidemia for which she is taking hydrochlorothiazide, triamterene, and atorvastatin.

Physical Examination: Vital signs: temperature 37.7°C (confirmed rectally), heart rate 88, respiratory rate 18, blood pressure 148/94. General: obese, in apparent discomfort. HEENT: Moist mucous membranes, no icterus. Abdomen: bowel sounds present; diffuse epigastric tenderness, with some guarding. No masses, obturator, psoas, or Murphy's sign. Rectal examination with brown heme-negative stool. Physical examination otherwise normal.

Laboratory Findings: WBC 11,000/μl (73% polys, no bands), otherwise normal. Blood chemistry and urinalysis: normal. Emergency medicine bedside ultrasonography (EMBU): gallbladder with multiple stones, wall thickness of 8 mm, mural edema and irregularity; pericholecystic edema with a question of frank pericholecystic fluid (see figures); sonographic Murphy sign.

Questions: Does this patient have biliary colic or cholecystitis? How are these two conditions distinguished? What is the value of ultrasonography compared with other diagnostic modalities in evaluating biliary tract disease?

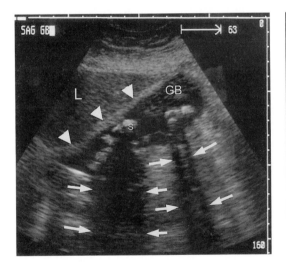 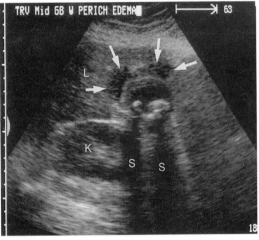

Diagnosis: The patient has gallstones with associated findings (mural irregularity and edema and pericholecystic fluid) to suggest acute cholecystitis.

Discussion: Although gallstones are often asymptomatic, and episodes of biliary colic are self-limiting, cholecystitis represents an acute inflammatory state that mandates hospital admission and surgical removal of the diseased gallbladder.

The lifetime incidence of gallstones for men and women in the United States is about 15% and 30%, respectively. Most gallstones are asymptomatic most of the time. A person with gallstones has a 1% to 3% chance of developing symptoms in any given year. The initial symptom is usually biliary colic. This waxing and waning pain is thought to be caused by an obstructing stone in the neck of the gallbladder causing distension and reflex spasmodic contractions. The pain resolves gradually after the stone either passes (leading to the possibility of common bile duct obstruction), or drops back into the fundus of the gallbladder. After the first bout of biliary colic, there is a 66% chance of a second attack within a year. If the offending gallstone is not dislodged, cholecystitis ensues, with a positive feedback loop of inflammation initiated by the noxious chemical properties of the bile under pressure, leading to mural distension, mucosal and mural edema, and ischemia. Secondary bacterial infection occurs in about 50% of cases.

The primary findings in patients with symptomatic gallstones are right upper quadrant(RUQ) pain/tenderness often exacerbated by meals and associated with fever. This classic picture is seen in the minority of patients. While 50% of patients with biliary disease do report RUQ pain, the pain in patients with gallstones is most often diffuse, epigastric, and can occur anywhere from the RUQ to the left iliac crest. Although 60% of patients with gallstones may report fatty food intolerance or a relationship with a meal, 40% of patients with nonspecific abdominal pain report the same. Vomiting, heartburn, dyspepsia, eructation, and stomach cramps are common but nondiscriminatory. Only 5% of patients are febrile.

The disposition of patients with acute biliary disease is based on the distinction of those with biliary colic (outpatient management) from those with acute cholecystitis (hospitalization). Biliary colic is classically described as well localized, sharp, waxing and waning RUQ pain. Patients are usually afebrile and have normal white blood cell counts. In contrast, acute cholecystitis is suggested by the presence of unremitting RUQ pain associated with low-grade fever, and mild leukocytosis. Clinical findings are often unreliable in distinguishing biliary colic from cholecystitis. Patients with biliary colic describe steady pain that can last for 16 hours, reaches peak intensity soon after onset, and gradually subsides. Conversely, many patients with proven cholecystitis do not have fever or leukocytosis. The distinction between cholecystitis and biliary colic therefore usually depends on further diagnostic testing.

Biliary disease should at least be considered in most patients presenting with abdominal pain. Since the vast majority of patients without gallstones do not have biliary tract disease, the next step is to rule in or to exclude the presence of gallstones. If gallstones are identified, a determination must be made as to whether the patient has acute cholecystitis. Diagnostic tests used to answer these questions include plain radiography, ultrasonography, radioisotope scans (HIDA, DIDA scans), oral cholecystography, endoscopic retrograde cholangiopancreatography (ERCP), and percutaneous transhepatic cholangiography (PTHC). Of this list, only the first two are available on a routine and timely basis in the ED. Plain radiographs are insensitive in the detection of gallstones, and only rarely give information about complications such as emphysematous cholecystitis. Ultrasonography is more than 95% sensitive in the detection of gallstones and has become the primary test of choice in the evaluation of biliary tract disease in almost all clinical settings, including the ED. If gallstones are identified, sonography can identify gall bladder wall abnormalities (especially thickening), pericholecystic fluid, and common bile duct enlargement to suggest the diagnosis of cholecystitis as opposed to biliary colic. The **sonographic Murphy's sign**—tenderness elicited by probe pressure on the gallbladder (and not elsewhere in the abdomen)—is a specific (90%) and fairly sensitive (60%) sign of gallstone disease. Sensitivity is much higher in patients with cholecystitis.

The left figure in this case is a longitudinal scan of the gallbladder. By convention, the left side of the image is cephalad, the right is caudad. Below the liver (*L*), the gall bladder wall (*arrowheads*) has blurry luminal and hepatic margins, suggesting inflammation. The gallbladder (*GB*) is filled with echogenic stones with posterior shadowing (*arrows*). The other figure is a transverse scan of the gallbladder, showing the liver (*L*) anterior to the gallbladder, which contains echogenic stones with posterior shadowing (*S*). Pericholecystic edema appears as dark areas in the hepatic parenchyma (*arrows*). The gallbladder wall again appears edematous, with loss of its usual crisp margins. The kidney (*K*) appears contiguous to the liver and gallbladder.

EMBU can be performed at the bedside by the treating physician, thus obviating the delays and expense involved in calling a technician or specialist in from home. EMBU is a *focused* and *limited* sonographic evaluation, with the goal of ruling in or out the disease under consideration. In the present situation, this is done by the identification of gallstones. With practice, however, it is not difficult for the emergency physician to identify the sonographic signs of cholecystitis. In addition, EMBU often provides information about other disease processes in the differential diagnosis of epigastric pain such as subphrenic, hepatic, or perinephric abscesses, or pancreatic pseudocysts. EMBU has the advantage that it can be performed rapidly at all hours, decreasing the time to diagnosis and disposition for patients with and without stones as the cause for their abdominal pain.

As a generally accepted therapeutic approach to gallstone disease, asymptomatic stones are not treated. Symptomatic stones are usually treated by cholecystectomy (elective or emergency), although there are nonoperative modalities available (e.g., prostaglandin inhibitors, ursodeoxycholic acid, lithotripsy) for patients without evidence of cholecystitis or cystic neck obstruction.

In the present case, the patient received intravenous hydration, and antibiotics to cover for typical bowel flora were given empirically. A surgical consultation was obtained, and the patient was admitted to the hospital, where cholecystectomy was performed the following day.

Clinical Pearls

1. The lifetime prevalence of gallstones is about 30% for females and 15% for males, the majority of which remain asymptomatic. Treatment is directed to the less than 25% of patients who develop symptoms.

2. The history and physical examination alone are unreliable for identifying patients with gallstone disease and, once gallstones are identified, are also unreliable in differentiating biliary colic from cholecystitis.

3. If gallstones are identified and thought to be the cause of the patient's symptoms, the emergency physician's primary goal is to distinguish patients with biliary colic, who can be managed on an outpatient basis, from those with cholecystitis, who require hospitalization.

4. Ultrasonography is the most useful single test in the evaluation of the biliary tract. EMBU can effectively exclude biliary disease by the absence of stones and often provides information to distinguish biliary colic from cholecystitis.

REFERENCES

1. Blaivas M, Harwood RA, Lambert MJ: Decreasing length of stay with emergency ultrasound examination of the gallbladder. Acad Emerg Med 6:1020–1023, 1999.
2. Gruber PJ, Silverman RA, Gottesfeld S, et al: Presence of fever and leukocytosis in acute cholecystitis. Ann Emerg Med 28:273–277, 1996.
3. Singer AJ, McCracken G, Henry MC, et al: Correlation among clinical, laboratory, and hepatobiliary scanning findings in patients with acute cholecystitis. Ann Emerg Med 28:267–272, 1996.
4. Attili AF, De Santis A, Capri R, et al: The natural history of gallstones: The GREPCO experience. Hepatology 21:656–660, 1995.
5. Traverso LW: Clinical manifestations of gallstone disease. Am J Surg 165:405–409, 1993.
6. Hopper KD, Landis JR, Meilstrup JW, et al: The prevalence of asymptomatic gallstones in the general population. Invest Radiol 26:939–945, 1991.
7. Diehl AK, Sugarek NJ, Todd KH: Clinical evaluation for gallstone disease: Usefulness of symptoms and signs in diagnosis. Am J Med 89:29–33, 1990.
8. Jorgenson T: Abdominal symptoms and gallstone disease: An epidemiological investigation. Hepatology 9:856–860, 1989.

Vivian Hwang, MD

PATIENT 37

A 33-year-old man with a history of chronic myelogenous leukemia presents with fever and chills

A 33-year-old man with a history of chronic myelogenous leukemia who is 1 week status post chemotherapy presents to the emergency department with acute onset of fever and chills 4 hours prior to arrival. He also reports headache, myalgias, and one episode of vomiting and diarrhea. He denies other symptoms.

Physical Examination: Vital signs: temperature 40.3°C orally; pulse 153; respiratory rate 20; blood pressure 94/58; room air pulse oximetry 97%. General: well-nourished and well-developed man, awake, with flushed appearance. HEENT: PERRLA, EOMI, oropharynx clear, no sinus tenderness, mucous membranes dry, tympanic membranes clear bilaterally. Neck: supple. Chest: clear to auscultation bilaterally, Hickman port site anterior left chest without erythema or tenderness. Cardiac: regular tachycardia, no murmurs. Abdomen: bowel sounds present, soft, nondistended, nontender, no hepatosplenomegaly. Extremities: normal. Genitalia: normal male genitalia, no lesions, no perirectal erythema or tenderness. Skin: no rashes. Neurologic: alert and oriented.

Laboratory Findings: CBC: WBC 600/μl, hemoglobin 12.0 g/dl, platelets 83,000 μL. Electrolytes: sodium 136, potassium 3.5, chloride 99, bicarbonate 27, BUN 26, creatinine 1.4, glucose 109. Electrocardiogram: sinus tachycardia, rate 130s, normal axis, normal intervals. Chest x-ray: no infiltrates, normal heart size. Urinalysis: normal.

Question: What oncologic complication does this patient have?

Diagnosis: Neutropenic fever

Discussion: Neutropenic fever is the most common oncologic emergency encountered in the emergency department. Patients should be evaluated and treated expeditiously, as infections are the most common cause of death in cancer patients.

Neutropenia is defined as an absolute neutrophil count less than 500/mm^3 or less than 1000/mm^3 with a predicted decline to less than 500/mm.^{3} Fever is defined in patients with malignancy as a single oral temperature reading greater than 38.3°C or a temperature of 38.0°C over at least 1 hour.

In the oncologic patient, the development of neutropenia is usually the result of the adverse effects of cytotoxic chemotherapy. The most vulnerable period is 7 to 15 days after chemotherapy. Neutropenia can also develop secondary to radiation therapy or can be the manifestation of neoplastic disease. The risk of infection increases with the degree of neutropenia, the length of neutropenia, and the rate of its development.

The clinical presentation of the neutropenic febrile patient varies widely. Often, patients may look and feel well. However, infection is present in more than 90% of patients. The remaining 10% have fever secondary to drugs, tumor, or transfusion of blood products.

When evaluating an oncologic patient with neutropenic fever, it is imperative to investigate all potential sources of fever. These include the oropharynx, ears, sinuses, perirectum, skin, and indwelling catheter sites. Initial laboratory testing should include a CBC with differential, two sets of blood cultures, urinalysis, urine culture, and chest x-ray.

Pathogens may be identified in only 30% to 40% of patients. Although gram-negative organisms such as *Escherichia coli, Klebsiella pneumoniae, Pseudomonas aeruginosa,* and *Enterobacter* species remain important causes of morbidity and mortality, there has recently been a shift toward gram-positive organisms, especially *Streptococcus viridans.* In addition to bacterial infections, neutropenic patients are also susceptible to fungal and viral infections.

The mortality rate in the first 48 hours of untreated neutropenia with fever is 50%. All patients with an absolute neutrophil count less than 1000/mm^3 should receive immediate empiric broad-spectrum intravenous antibiotics. Empiric antibiotic therapy should consist of either combination therapy with an antipseudomonal penicillin or third-generation antipseudomonal cephalosporin plus aminoglycoside or monotherapy with either carbapenem or a fourth-generation cephalosporin such as cefepime. There have been many studies comparing monotherapy with combination therapy; however, no method of therapy has shown an unacceptably high mortality rate. Vancomycin is added to empiric coverage in patients with severe mucositis, quinolone prophylaxis, colonization with methicillin-resistant *Staphylococcus aureus* (MRSA) or penicillin-resistant *Streptococcus pneumoniae,* an obvious catheter-related infection, or hypotension.

In addition to antibiotics, the use of leukocyte growth stimulants such as granulocyte colony stimulating factor and granulocyte-monocyte colony-stimulating factor have been used to stimulate bone marrow production of leukocytes. These have been shown to decrease morbidity and mortality in neutropenic patients with solid tumors. Their use at the onset of febrile neutropenia should be reserved for patients with a high risk of infectious complications.

Febrile neutropenic patients are admitted for further evaluation and management of fever. Recent studies have looked at the possibility of outpatient management of neutropenic fever in "low-risk" patients but until validated in large, randomized studies, it is prudent to admit these patients for intravenous antibiotics.

In the present patient, intravenous fluids and empiric antibiotic therapy were started in the emergency department. The patient was admitted to the intensive care unit for further management. His blood cultures grew out *Escherichia coli.* The patient did well and was discharged 3 days later on oral antibiotics.

Clinical Pearls

1. Despite well appearance, patients with neutropenic fever should be treated expeditiously with empiric intravenous antibiotics, as infection is present in 90% of patients.

2. There has been a recent shift toward infection with gram-positive organisms in febrile neutropenic patients, and therefore antibiotic coverage must include empiric choices to cover these organisms.

REFERENCES

1. Glauser MP: Neutropenia: Clinical implications and modulation. Intens Care Med 26:5103–5110, 2000.
2. Jones RN: Contemporary antimicrobial susceptibility patterns of bacterial pathogens commonly associated with febrile patients with neutropenia. Clin Infec Dis 29:495–502, 1999.
3. Ramphal R: Is monotherapy for febrile neutropenia still a viable alternative? Clin Infect Dis 29:508–514, 1999.
4. Zinner SH: Changing epidemiology of infections in patients with neutropenia and cancer: Emphasis on gram-positive and resistant bacteria. Clin Infect Dis 29:490–494, 1999.
5. Hughes WT, Armstrong D, Bodey GP, et al: 1997 Guidelines for the use of antimicrobial agents in neutropenic patients with unexplained fever. Clin Infect Dis 25:551–573, 1997.

Eron Friedlaender, MD

PATIENT 38

A 4-year-old girl with lethargy and abdominal pain

A previously healthy 4-year-old girl is brought to the emergency department with 2 weeks of progressive right-sided abdominal pain. She also has had intermittent nonbloody, nonbilious emesis but denies fever, diarrhea, or constipation. Her parents report marked lethargy, pallor, and decreased oral intake over the same time period, as well as some shallow, rapid breathing when reclining at night.

Physical Examination: Vital signs: temperature 37.8°C orally; pulse 123; respiratory rate 24; blood pressure 94/54. General: pale, irritable. HEENT: anicteric, moist mucous membranes, no lymphadenopathy. Chest: good aeration, slightly decreased breath sounds at the bases. Cardiac: tachycardiac, regular rhythm, normal S1 and S2, no murmur, faint gallop. Abdomen: liver edge palpable below umbilicus. Extremities: strong distal pulses, no edema.

Laboratory Findings: Hemoglobin 11.4 g/dl. Electrolytes and liver function tests within normal limits. Chest x-ray: cardiomegaly, bilateral pulmonary vascular congestion, small bilateral pleural effusions (see figure). Electrocardiogram: sinus tachycardia, left axis deviation, flattened T waves, slightly decreased voltages.

ED Course: The patient was placed on continuous cardiorespiratory monitoring and given 2 L of supplemental oxygen by nasal cannula. Two large-bore intravenous catheters were placed. Cardiology was consulted, and the echocardiogram showed mildly dilated left and right ventricles, markedly depressed left ventricular function, and shortening fraction of 16% (normal 30–45%). The patient was admitted to the cardiac intensive care unit on diuretics and inotropic support.

Question: What disease process is most likely responsible for this patient's condition?

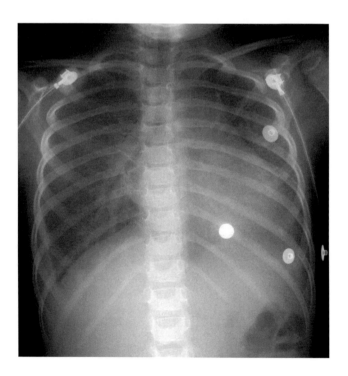

Diagnosis: Dilated cardiomyopathy

Discussion: Dilated cardiomyopathy refers to an acquired state in which the left or both ventricles are enlarged and hypocontractile, resulting in impaired systolic function. Depressed myocardial performance, quantified in terms of shortening fraction, ejection fraction, cardiac output, or cardiac index, translates clinically into congestive heart failure as the metabolic demands of the body exceed the heart's ability to adequately perfuse all vital organs and peripheral tissues.

This disease has a reported annual incidence of 2 to 8 cases per 100,000 people. There are many potential causes for the development of dilated cardiomyopathy. The most common identifiable cause is postinfectious myocarditis. Idiopathic diseases, along with nutritional deficiencies, inborn errors of fatty-acid oxidation, storage diseases, endocrinopathies such as thyrotoxicosis, chronic tachyarrhythmias, and familial variants account for the majority of the remaining cases.

Depressed myocardial activity triggers a series of compensatory neurohormonal responses aimed at improving oxygen delivery to the tissues of the body. As inotropic function declines, ventricular filling pressures, end-diastolic pressures, and end-diastolic volumes increase, causing the myocardium to hypertrophy and the ventricles to dilate. Decreased renal perfusion stimulates an up-regulation of the renin-angiotensin axis in an effort to conserve salt and water, thereby increasing blood volume and blood pressure. Hypotension and poor peripheral perfusion also signal the body to increase sympathetic tone; the elevated heart rate serves to increase cardiac output.

Patients with dilated cardiomyopathy become symptomatic as congestive heart failure develops. The same processes the body employs to increase afterload in the face of a weakened myocardium also create pulmonary congestion and peripheral edema and eventually increased myocardial metabolic needs to maintain the increased blood pressure. Typical symptoms include nausea, anorexia, dyspnea on exertion, orthopnea, chest pain, syncope, palpitations, and decreased exercise tolerance. On physical examination, patients appear pale with tachycardia, tachypnea, rales, and retractions. Cardiac evaluation demonstrates a displaced apical impulse, a narrow pulse pressure, and a gallop rhythm. Hepatomegaly and ascites may be appreciated. Peripheral pulses are often weak and extremities may be cool and edematous.

Noninvasive evaluation with radiographs, electrocardiograms, and echocardiography allows for an estimation of disease severity. The chest radiograph frequently reveals cardiomegaly, pulmonary vascular congestion, and pleural effusions. The electrocardiogram may demonstrate ventricular and atrial enlargement, a prolonged PR interval, nonspecific STT wave changes, low voltages, and tachyarrhythmias. Echocardiography confirms depressed contractility.

The treatment of patients with dilated cardiomyopathy is largely supportive care. Inotropes and digoxin may be used to enhance cardiac function, whereas diuretics, vasodilators, and positive pressure ventilation ameliorate symptoms associated with pulmonary edema. Antiarrhythmics are used for patients with evidence of myocardial irritability, and anticoagulants are administered liberally because a hypocontractile myocardium promotes intracardiac thrombus formation and places affected individuals at risk for embolic disease.

The prognosis for recovery from dilated cardiomyopathy depends in large part on the specific cause of the pathologic condition. In general, however, one third of patients do not survive, one third have stable disease with some cardiac dysfunction, and one third have complete recovery.

Clinical Pearls

1. The most common causes of dilated cardiomyopathy in children are idiopathic and postinfectious myocarditis.

2. Patients with dilated cardiomyopathy frequently present with signs and symptoms of congestive heart failure.

3. Patients with dilated cardiomyopathy are at risk for malignant arrhythmias and embolic disease.

REFERENCES

1. O'Laughlin M: Congestive heart failure. Pediatr Clin North Am 46:263–273, 1999.
2. Towbin J: Pediatric myocardial disease. Pediatr Clin North Am 46:289–312, 1999.
3. Gajarski R, Towbin J: Recent advances in the etiology, diagnosis, and treatment of myocarditis and cardiomyopathies in children. Curr Opin Pediatrics 7:587–594, 1995.
4. Stockwell J, Tobias J, Greeley W: Noninflammatory, noninfiltrative cardiomyopathy. In Nichols D, Cameron D, Greeley W, et al (eds): Critical Heart Disease in Infants and Children. St. Louis, Mosby, 1995.
5. Gilbert E, Bristow M: Idiopathic dilated cardiomyopathy. In Schlant R, Alexander R (eds.): Hurst's The Heart, 8th ed. New York, McGraw-Hill, 1994.
6. Manolio T, Baughman K, Rodenheffer R, et al: Prevalence and etiology of idiopathic dilated cardiomyopathy (Summary of a National Heart Lung and Blood Institute Workshop). Am J Cardiol 69:1458, 1992.

PATIENT 39

A 65-year old woman with flu-like symptoms and syncope

On a cool autumn day, a 65-year-old woman is brought to the emergency department by her husband after "passing out" at home. She states, "We both got the flu today." Her symptoms are headache, weakness, nausea, and vomiting.

Physical Examination: Temperature 37.5°C, heart rate 132, respiratory rate 22, blood pressure 142/88. General: awake, alert, oriented to person and time. HEENT: No evidence of trauma. Dry mucous membranes. Neck: Supple, no jugular vein distension or adenopathy. Chest: clear to auscultation and percussion. Heart: irregular tachycardia without murmur, rub, or gallop. Abdomen: normal. Extremities: no cyanosis, edema, or deformities. Neurologic: slight dysmetria, otherwise normal. Skin: slightly pale.

Laboratory Findings: CBC: WBC 11,800/μl, hemoglobin 12.5 g/dl, hematocrit 37.4%, platelets 340,000/μl. Blood chemistries: Na 140 mEq/L, K 4.0 mEq/L, Cl 102 mEq/L, HCO_3 23 mEq/L, BUN 15 mEq/L, creatinine 0.9 mEq/L, glucose 120 mEq/L. ABG (room air): pH 7.34, PCO_2 34, HCO_3 24, PO_2 92, O_2 saturation 96%. Cardiac isoenzymes: normal. ECG: atrial fibrillation. Chest radiograph: unremarkable.

Questions: What test should be ordered next? What is the presumptive diagnosis? What treatment should be initiated immediately?

Diagnosis and Treatment: A carboxyhemoglobin (COHgb) level is drawn and reported as 28%. High-flow oxygen by an aviator mask is initiated, and intravenous hydration is started while consultation with a hyperbaric physician is obtained.

Discussion: Carbon monoxide (CO) toxicity is the leading cause of morbidity and mortality due to poisoning worldwide, yet its diagnosis can elude even astute clinicians, owing in part to its manifestation with nonspecific symptoms. Historical data that may provide valuable clues can be found in the table.

Historical Factors that Suggest Carbon Monoxide Toxicity

- Similar symptoms in multiple patients in the same time and place
- Death or illness of small household pets
- Use of combustible fuels in poorly ventilated spaces (space heaters, oil burning equipment)
- Onset coincidental with colder weather or after a heavy snowfall

The physical examination is often unremarkable. Vital sign abnormalities include tachycardia and tachypnea, but normal vital signs are not uncommon early in the presentation. Obtunded patients may have persistent focal neurologic findings, but most patients have normal findings on examination or, at most, subtle findings. Signs of cerebellar dysfunction may presage cognitive sequelae. The legendary "cherry-red" skin hue is an autopsy finding, not a clinical one. Reports of experienced phlebotomists, nurses, or EMTs noting brighter than expected venous blood are at best unquantifiable.

The most common dysrythmia associated with CO poisoning is atrial fibrillation, but this is usually seen only in patients with underlying cardiovascular disease (often previously undiagnosed). Sinus rhythm is by far more likely. Leukocytosis is occasionally seen, and CO-mediated hypoxia can induce lactic acidosis resulting in an elevated anion gap. These findings are more likely in seriously poisoned patients but may be absent, especially if there is a delay in diagnosis due to lack of suspicion.

The affinity of hemoglobin for CO is 200 times greater than that for oxygen and results in tissue hypoxia as the primary insult. CO mortality is primarily cardiac; however, the most frequent clinical toxicity noted is delayed neurologic (cognitive) sequelae. These effects correlate poorly with COHgb levels, develop in up to 45% of poisoned patients from 2 to 42 days after exposure, and can occur even if the patient is treated expeditiously and aggressively.

Treatment has always focused on induction of hyperoxia to compete for hemoglobin binding sites and hasten CO dissociation. Non-rebreather masks commonly found in the ED deliver well below 50% FIo_2, so a tight-fitting mask should be used whenever possible. Increasing the partial pressure of oxygen above 1.0 atmosphere in a hyperbaric chamber reduces CO half-life more rapidly. However, the use of hyperbaric oxygen (HBO_2) therapy remains controversial, in part due to conflicting results reported in randomized clinical trials to date. Consultation and referral for HBO_2 therapy should at least be considered for patients with mental status and neurologic abnormalities, history of loss of consciousness, and COHgb level > 25% or base excess ≤ 2 mmol/L.

The present patient's diagnosis was suspected based on historical data. The findings of atrial fibrillation, leukocytosis, and partially compensated metabolic acidosis with elevated anion gap all support the diagnosis confirmed by the COHgb level. The patient had positive cerebellar findings and a history of syncope, which led to referral and treatment with HBO_2 therapy. Her atrial fibrillation converted spontaneously while she was in the chamber, and she was discharged after 16 hours of observation. She was well without sequelae at 6-week follow-up.

Clinical Pearls

1. CO poisoning should always be included in the differential diagnosis for vague systemic symptoms.

2. A careful history will often yield the requisite information to suspect CO toxicity. Physical examination and point-of-care testing may only provide confirmatory evidence.

3. Consider referral for hyperbaric oxygen therapy for patients with syncope, neurologic abnormalities, or elevated carboxyhemoglobin levels.

REFERENCES

1. Weaver LK, Hopkins RO, Chan KJ, et al: Hyperbaric oxygen for acute carbon monoxide poisoning. N Engl J Med 347:1057–1067, 2002.
2. Thom SR: Hyperbaric oxygen for acute carbon monoxide poisoning. N Engl J Med 347:1105–1106, 2002.
3. Raub JA, Mathieu-Nolf M, Hampson NB, Thom SR: Carbon monoxide poisoning: A public health perspective. Toxicology 145:1–14, 2000.
4. Hampson NB (ed): Hyperbaric oxygen therapy: Committee report. Kensington, MD: Undersea and Hyperbaric Medical Society, 1999.
5. Ernst A, Zibrak JD: Carbon monoxide poisoning. N Engl J Med 339:1603–1608, 1998.

Steven Larsen, MD

PATIENT 40

An 83-year-old man with a resting tachycardia and abdominal pain

An 83-year-old man, healthy except for borderline hypertension, presents to the emergency department complaining of a 2-week history of constant, diffuse abdominal pain. He has no fevers, chills, or sweats. His appetite is good and he has had no weight loss. Bowel movements are normal without bright red blood per rectum or melena. He denies any chest pain, shortness of breath, nausea, or diaphoresis.

Physical Examination: Temperature 36.2°C pulse 117 regular; blood pressure 113/89. Skin: warm and dry. HEENT: normal. Neck: supple with +2 carotids and no audible bruit or murmur. Chest: clear to auscultation with equal, bilateral breath sounds. Cardiac: No heave or thrill on palpation; regular rate with normal S_1, S_2, no S_3; no murmur, rub, or gallop. Abdomen: normal bowel sounds; no pulsatile mass; mild, diffuse tenderness on deep palpation; no guarding or rebound: Rectal examination: brown stool, heme-negative. Extremities: normal.

Laboratory Findings: CBC: normal. Chemistries: normal. Obstruction series: nonspecific bowel gas pattern without evidence of free air. Electrocardiogram: sinus tachycardia with normal intervals and axis; no evidence of ischemia.

Questions: Should the clinician be relieved by the absence of classic peritoneal findings on examination? Does the absence of a fever or elevated WBC count eliminate the possibility of occult infection in this elderly patient? What specific physical findings should heighten the clinician's concern that this patient has a significant medical condition that warrants further emergency evaluation?

Diagnosis and Treatment: Atypical presentation for an acute abdomen. Initial treatment should include intravenous fluid resuscitation, antibiotics, and surgical evaluation.

Discussion: The elderly patient with abdominal pain represents a diagnostic challenge for physicians. Because of the physiologic changes of aging, elderly patients with acute intra-abdominal pathology frequently fail to demonstrate classic physical findings such as peritoneal signs. Additionally, other indicators of infection, such as fever and/or elevated peripheral WBC counts are frequently absent. In elderly patients with acute cholecystitis, for example, only 30% to 55% have fever of 38°C or higher, only 50% present with leukocytosis, and 25% have no tenderness on examination. The atypical presentation of the elderly patient with an acute abdomen, coupled with a lack of physical evidence or laboratory abnormality, often leads to a delay in diagnosis and increased morbidity and mortality.

Physicians must maintain a heightened sensitivity for subtle, unexplained discrepancies in the elderly patient's presentation. Attention to vital signs may provide life-saving clues to the presence of infection or blood loss. With the natural aging process, there are changes in these parameters. For instance, the respiratory rate in an elderly patient frequently ranges from 16 to 25 respirations per minute. Systolic blood pressure frequently increases and the maximal heart rate decreases (maximum expected heart rate $= 230 -$ age). Blunted thermoregulatory mechanisms result in lower baseline core temperatures and less predictable responses to infection.

The most worrisome physical finding in this patient's presentation is his resting tachycardia. For an elderly patient, a sinus tachycardia of 117 is clinically significant. It is a warning sign for altered physiology and needs to be addressed promptly. In managing the patient with a sinus tachycardia, the clinician must identify the underlying cause and treat it accordingly. Sinus tachycardia can signify underlying physiologic stress such as pain, anxiety, hypoxia, hypovolemia, and/or fever. This patient's sinus tachycardia, taken in the context of abdominal pain, hypothermia, and low blood pressure, should alert the physician to a possible occult process of infection. The burden rests on the physician to identify a plausible explanation for these findings.

In the present case, the patient was initially considered stable for discharge because of lack of objective clinical and laboratory findings. However, the emergency physician elected to pursue a further evaluation. An abdominal computed tomography scan was obtained and demonstrated acute diverticulitis with a large abscess and evidence of microperforation. The patient was subsequently admitted to the hospital for intravenous antibiotics and bowel resection.

Clinical Pearls

1. Elderly patients frequently present with delayed or atypical manifestations of intra-abdominal pathology.

2. An elderly patient may be afebrile and lack leukocytosis in the setting of active infection.

3. Hypotension, tachycardia, and/or hypothermia may be the only clinical indicators of serious infection in the elderly patient.

REFERENCES
1. Woolard R, Becker B, Haronian T: Geriatric considerations. In Harwood-Nuss (ed): Clinical Practice of Emergency Medicine. Philadelphia, Lippincott pp 1769–1777, 2000.
2. Sanson T, O'Keefe K: Evaluation of abdominal pain in the elderly. Emerg Med Clin North Am 14:615–627, 1996.
3. Bugliosi T, Meloy T, Vukov L: Acute abdominal pain in the elderly. Ann Emerg Med 19:12, 1990.

Louis M. Bell, MD
Hillary Bogner, MD, MSCE

PATIENT 41

A 7-month-old boy with fever and decreased shoulder range of motion

A previously healthy 7-month-old boy presents to the emergency department with a 13-day history of decreased range of motion of his right shoulder and recurrent fevers. Initially, he had decreased movement in his entire right upper extremity and a fever of 40.2°C. He was taken to a nearby hospital's emergency department. Radiographs of the right shoulder were reported as normal. He was treated with antipyretics and discharged to home. The next day he was still febrile and was taken to another hospital's emergency department. He was transferred to a third hospital, where again radiographs of the right shoulder were obtained. No abnormalities were noted and after he become afebrile, he was sent home. He was not treated with antibiotics. Since then, the range of motion of his arm is reported to have improved, but he has not regained normal full range of motion of his shoulder. This morning, his mother noticed swelling and redness of his right shoulder. The patient's mother denies trauma, upper respiratory tract infection symptoms, vomiting, diarrhea, or any ill contacts. The patient has no significant past medical history. He is taking no medications other than antipyretics and has no known drug allergies. His immunizations are all up to date.

Physical Examination: Vital signs: temperature 37.6°C rectally; pulse 92; respiratory rate 28; blood pressure 90/60. General: well-nourished and well-developed child in no distress. Chest: clear to auscultation. Cardiac: RRR without murmur. Abdomen: soft with masses, no hepatosplenomegaly. Extremities: right shoulder is erythematous, indurated, and tender to palpation. There is pain with passive motion and decreased active motion; no other joints have abnormalities.

Laboratory Findings: Hemoglobin: 8.9 g/dl, WBC: 15,800/μl with 6% bands, 30% neutrophils, 52% lymphocytes, 6% monocytes, and 5% atypical lymphocytes, platelets 912,000/μl. ESR: 109 mm/hr. Blood cultures were obtained. Radiograph of right shoulder revealed a widened joint space, soft tissue swelling, and a lytic lesion in the proximal humerus (see figure).

Questions: What is the most likely diagnosis? What information in the history would help in determining both the most likely pathogen and the antibiotic regimen?

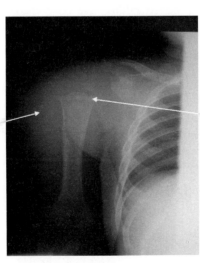

Soft tissue swelling of right shoulder

Lytic area in right proximal humerus

Diagnosis: Osteomyelitis of the right humerus and septic arthritis of the joint space. Information about pets in the household would reveal contact with snakes and raise the suspicion of *Salmonella* species as a possible pathogen in this case.

Discussion: In the present patient, arthrocentesis of the right shoulder was performed and revealed WBC 10,300 cells/µl with 86% neutrophils. A Gram stain demonstrated many WBCs and gram-negative rods. A magnetic resonance imaging (MRI) scan of the shoulder joint revealed joint effusion and bony inflammation consistent with osteomyelities (see figure below). The culture of the right shoulder joint fluid grew *Salmonella arizonae*. This isolate was susceptible to ampicillin. A bone scan was positive for uptake of technetium-labeled methylene diphosphate in the right proximal humerus. The child required two incision and drainage procedures during the hospital stay. On further questioning, his mother revealed that they had a "black snake" and two doves at home that were allowed to roam freely around the apartment. Although the patient had never been bitten by the snake, he had touched the snake on numerous occasions. A culture of the snake's feces grew *Salmonella arizonae*. A culture of the snake's mouth was negative for *Salmonella arizonae*.

In children, osteomyelitis most commonly develops after hematogenous spread of bacteria to the area of the growth plate of the growing child. This pathophysiology explains why the long bones are often involved. The most common bones affected are femur, tibia, and humerus. The most common bacterial pathogen isolated in immunocompetent children is *S. aureus*. In general, presumptive antibiotic therapy is therefore a penicillinase-resistant antibiotic such as oxacillin.

In this case, however, the history of exposure to a snake would have alerted one to the possibility of other potential bacterial pathogens associated with reptile exposures. Exposure to the *Salmonella arizonae* found in the feces of the pet snake led to bacteremia and then localized infection in the right humerus.

Various infections are caused by *Salmonella arizonae,* formerly known as *Arizona hinshawii*. The clinical spectrum of *Salmonella arizonae* infections is similar to that seen with other *Salmonella* infections. Infections include gastroenteritis, septicemia, pneumonia, meningitis, septic arthritis, and osteomyelitis. Foods such as egg powder, eggnog, ice cream, custards, and unpasteurized milk have been implicated in many outbreaks. Recently it has become known that contact with reptiles or the ingestion of rattlesnake meat or capsules made from dried and crushed rattlesnake and used as a folk remedy has been implicated in many solitary cases.

Most of the reported cases of *Salmonella arizonae* infection have been in adults with underlying diseases. These cases have included patients with neoplasms, acquired immunodeficiency syndrome, systemic lupus erythematosus, cardiac disease, and sickle cell anemia as well as patients treated with immunosuppressive agents such as prednisone. There have also been cases of *Salmonella arizonae* infection in children with underlying diseases. In an early report from 1953, a 2-year-old boy with Letterer-Siwe disease is described in whom both blood cultures and cultures of multiple bone lesions were found to be positive for

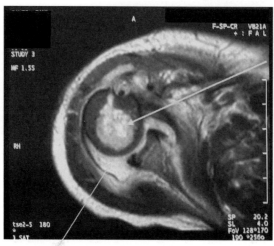

Boney inflammation of right proximal humerus

Joint right shoulder effusion

Salmonella arizonae. A report in 1973 described a 2½-year-old girl with sickle cell anemia and diffuse *Salmonella arizonae* osteomyelitis.

Reports of *Salmonella arizonae* infections in patients without underlying diseases are much more rare. However, many of the reports of *Salmonella arizonae* infection in seemingly normal patients have been in children. For example, an outbreak was reported among five children who developed severe gastrointestinal symptoms after the ingestion of homemade ice cream at a picnic lunch. Stool specimens from each of the six children grew *Salmonella arizonae.*

A case report by Croop et al. described an 11-year-old boy who developed *Salmonella arizonae* osteomyelitis of the hip after cleaning the cage of a pet snake. This was one of the first case reports to report that exposure to pet snakes could lead to *Salmonella arizonae* infections in humans. This parallels the transmission of *Salmonella* infections through contact with pet turtles or pet iguanas. Reptiles have been shown to be an important reservoir of salmonellosis and have repeatedly been implicated in the transmission of the infection to children and adults. Presumptive antibiotic therapy for suspected *Salmonella* infections (until antibiotic susceptibilities are known) are third-generation cephalosporins.

Clinical Pearls

1. Osteomyelitis in infants and children is hematogenous in origin. The long bones are most commonly affected.

2. The most common pathogen associated with osteomyelitis in children is *S. aureus.*

3. A careful history should always include exposures to exotic pets, even in young infants and toddlers, as this will raise the suspicion of *Salmonella* as a potential pathogen and inform decisions about presumptive antibiotic therapy.

REFERENCES

1. D'Aoust JY, Daley E, Crozier M, Sewell AM: Pet turtles: A continuing international threat to public health. Am J Epidemiol 132:233–238, 1990.
2. Noskin GA, Clark JT: *Salmonella arizonae* bacteremia as the presenting manifestation of human immunodeficiency virus infection following rattlesnake meat ingestion. Rev Infect Dis 12:514–517, 1990.
3. Riley KB, Antoniskis D, Maris R, Leedom JM: Rattlesnake capsule-associated *Salmonella arizonae* infection. Arch Intern Med 148:1207–1210, 1988.
4. Ewing WH: Edwards and Ewing's Identification of Enterobacteriaceae, 4th ed. New York, Elsevier Science, 1986.
5. Kelly J, Hopkin R, Rimsza ME: Rattlesnake meat ingestion and *Salmonella arizonae* infection in children: Case report and review of the literature. Pediatr Inf Dis J 14:320–322, 1985.
6. Croop JM, Shapiro B, Alpert G, et al: *Arizona hinshawii* osteomyelitis associated with a pet snake. Pediatr Infect Dis 3:188, 1984.
7. Marzouk JB, Josep P, Lee TY, et al: *Arizona hinshawii* septicemia associated with rattle snake powder. Calif Morbidity 1:25, 1983.
8. Fainstein V, Yancey R, Trier R, Bodey GP: Overwhelming infection in a cancer patient caused by *Arizona hinshawii:* Its relation to snake pill ingestion. Am J Infect Control 4:147–53, 1982.
9. Johnson H, Lutwick LI, Huntley GA, Vosti KL: *Arizona hinshawii* infection: New cases, antimicrobial sensitivities, and literature review. Ann Intern Med 85:587–592, 1976.
10. Hruby MA, Honig GR, Lolekha S, et al: *Arizona hinshawii* osteomyelitis in sickle cell anemia. Am J Dis Child 125:867–868, 1973.
11. Wolfe MS, Armstrong D, Louria DB, Blevins A: Salmonellosis in patients with neoplastic disease. Arch Intern Med 128:546–554, 1971.
12. Guckian JC, Byers EH, Perry JE: *Arizona* infection of man: Report of a case and review of the literature. Arch Intern Med 119:170–175, 1967.
13. Fisher RH: Multiple lesions of bone in Letterer-Siwe disease: Report of a case with culture of paracolon *Arizona* bacilli from bone lesions and blood, followed by response to therapy. J Bone Joint Surg Am 35:445–464, 1953.
14. Murphy WJ, Morris JF: Two outbreaks of gastroenteritis apparently caused by a paracolon of the *Arizona* group. J Infect Dis 86:255–259, 1950.

Sumeru Mehta, MD
C. Crawford Mechem, MD

PATIENT 42

A 45-year-old man with acute numbness and weakness

A 45-year-old man with a history of transient ischemic stroke 6 years ago and hypertension is brought in by ambulance with acute left-sided weakness, numbness, tingling, and slurring of speech beginning less than 1 hour prior to presentation.

Physical Examination: Temperature 36.7°C; pulse 95; respiratory rate 20; blood pressure 191/122. Skin: no lesions. HEENT: pupils round and reactive to light and accommodation. Chest: normal. Cardiac: normal. Abdomen: normal. Neurologic: motor strength 0/5 left upper extremity, 5/5 right upper extremity, 1/5 left lower extremity, 5/5 right lower extremity; sensation decreased to light touch on the left side; left facial droop with slurring of speech; alert and oriented to person, place, and time.

Laboratory Findings: CBC: normal. Blood chemistries: sodium 139 mmol/L, potassium 4.1 mmol/L, chloride 103 mmol/L, CO_2 content 21 mmol/L, urea nitrogen 35 mg/dL, serum creatinine 1.4 mg/dl, glucose 92 mg/dl. Sedimentation rate: 1 mm/h. Lactate dehydrogenase: 995 U/L. Coagulation studies: normal. ECG: sinus rhythm, inferior Q waves, minimally elevated ST segment isolated to lead V2, unchanged from previous ECG. Head CT (see figure): acute right-sided thalamic hemorrhagic stroke.

Questions: How are therapy and treatment different in hemorrhagic versus ischemic stroke? What is an acceptable target blood pressure in this clinical setting? Which drugs are used in the management of a spontaneous intracerebral hemorrhage?

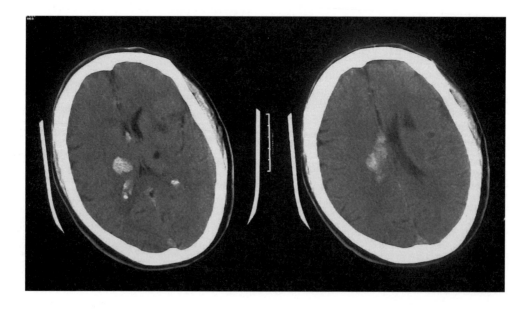

Diagnosis and Treatment: Spontaneous intracerebral hemorrhage; early management focuses on control of blood pressure and intracranial pressure and early neurosurgical evaluation. Anticoagulants such as aspirin, heparin, glycoprotein IIb/IIIa inhibitors, and thrombolytics are strictly contraindicated. Only severe hypertension (i.e., systolic blood pressure greater than 220 mm Hg, diastolic blood pressure greater than 120 mm Hg, or a mean arterial pressure [MAP] greater than 130 mm Hg) should be treated with labetolol or nitroprusside.

Discussion: Stroke is defined as an acute focal neurologic deficit resulting from vascular disease that lasts for more than 24 hours. Spontaneous (nontraumatic) intracerebral hemorrhage (ICH) is a common problem and accounts for 10% to 15% of all strokes. It is associated with a high mortality rate, with only 38% of affected patients surviving the first year. ICH is classified as either primary or secondary. Primary hemorrhage accounts for 78% to 88% of all cases and results from the spontaneous rupture of small vessels damaged primarily by chronic hypertension or other angiopathic process. Hypertension is still the leading cause of ICH and is responsible for approximately 55% of cases. Secondary ICH occurs in a minority of patients and is associated with vascular abnormalities, such as aneurysms, arteriovenous malformations, tumors, or coagulopathy. The most common sites of hemorrhagic stroke are the cerebral lobes, basal ganglia, thalamus, brainstem, and cerebellum. Extension into the ventricles may occur with large hemorrhages.

Hematoma formation leads to edema and neuronal damage in the surrounding parenchyma, which may last anywhere from 5 days to 2 weeks. Early edema results from the release and accumulation of osmotically active serum proteins from the clot; subsequently, vasogenic and cytotoxic edema results from disruption of the blood-brain barrier and neuronal death.

Clinical features of a large hemorrhagic stroke include a decreased level of consciousness due to increased intracranial pressure and direct compression of the thalamus, the brainstem, and the reticular activating system. Patients with a supratentorial ICH may present with contralateral sensory-motor deficits of varying severity as well as higher level cortical dysfunction, including gaze deviation, hemianopsia, and aphasia. Patients with an infratentorial ICH may present with brainstem dysfunction, including abnormalities of gaze, other cranial-nerve abnormalities, and contralateral motor deficits. Ataxia and dysmetria are prominent when the intracerebral hemorrhage involves the cerebellum. Other nonspecific symptoms include headache, vomiting, and meningismus resulting from blood in the ventricles. The 6-month mortality rate after spontaneous ICH ranges from 23% to 58%. Three factors, including low score on the Glasgow Coma Scale (less than 9), a large volume of the hematoma (more than 60

ml) and the presence of ventricular blood on the initial computed tomographic (CT) scan, have consistently predicted a high mortality rate.

Imaging of the brain is required to definitively distinguish between cerebral infarction and intracerebral hemorrhage. Given the availability of thrombolytic therapy, the early differentiation between ischemic and hemorrhagic stroke is imperative for early management. On the initial CT scan, the location and size of the hematoma and presence of ventricular blood and/or hydrocephalus should be noted. Selected patients should undergo conventional angiography to look for secondary causes of ICH.

The risk of neurologic deterioration and cardiovascular instability is highest during the first 24 hours after stroke onset. Any patient with a decreased level of consciousness or impairment of airway protective reflexes should be immediately intubated. An urgent neurosurgical consultation is required for any patient with rapid deterioration or clinical evidence of transtentorial herniation or hydrocephalus on CT scan. A mass effect from the hematoma, surrounding edema, and obstructive hydrocephalus, with subsequent herniation, is the chief secondary cause of death in the first few days after the hemorrhage. Treatment with osmotic agents (e.g., mannitol) and hyperventilation is recommended only in patients with impending herniation, with the option of intraventricular catheter placement for cerebrospinal fluid drainage until surgical decompression can be performed. Randomized trials have failed to demonstrate efficacy of corticosteroids in the treatment of patients with ICH.

Elevated blood pressure is common after hemorrhage and is associated with expansion of the hematoma and a poor outcome. It still remains unclear whether the hypertension is a consequence of the stroke and whether it causes expansion of the hematoma. Hypertension can also be a protective response (Cushing-Kocher response) by preserving cerebral perfusion pressure. While there is still significant controversy regarding the initial treatment of blood pressure after a stroke, current American Heart Association guidelines mandate intravenous antihypertensive treatment for mean arterial pressures greater than 130 mm Hg.

The goals of surgical evacuation of a hematoma are to reduce the mass effect, block the release of neuropathic products, and prevent prolonged interaction between the hematoma and the parenchyma. Currently, surgical evacuation is recommended for patients with cerebellar hemorrhage, those with hematoma diameter greater than 3 cm, and those with a Glasgow Coma Scale (score) less than 14. Evacuation should also be considered for young patients with moderate to large lobar hemorrhage and clinical deterioration, or patients with basal ganglion hemorrhage that is expanding and/or is associated with progressive neurologic deterioration.

Most stroke-associated seizures occur at the onset of the hemorrhage or within the first 24 hours and should be treated with intravenous anticonvulsants. The anticonvulsants may be discontinued after 30 days if no further seizure activity is noted.

The present patient was treated with intravenous labetolol for MAP greater than 130 and was admitted to the neurologic intensive care unit for further monitoring. Neurosurgical evacuation was not necessary because of the size of the hematoma and the hemodynamic stability of the patient. A repeat CT scan 1 hour after presentation showed no increase in the size of the hemorrhage. The patient was subsequently discharged to a rehabilitation facility.

Clinical Pearls

1. Aspirin therapy should be withheld until imaging of the brain is performed to definitively distinguish between cerebral infarction and intracerebral hemorrhage.

2. While still controversial, most studies recommend intravenous antihypertensives (labetolol and nitroprusside) for MAPs greater than 130 mm Hg.

3. Urgent neurosurgical consultation is required for any patient with rapid deterioration, clinical evidence of transtentorial herniation, or hydrocephalus on CT scan.

REFERENCES

1. Brown MM: Brain attack: A new approach to stroke. Clin Med 2:60–65, 2002.
2. Qureshi AI, Tuhrim S, Broderick JP, et al: Medical progress: Spontaneous intracerebral hemorrhage. N Engl J Med 344:1450–1460, 2001.
3. Broderick JP, Adams HP, Barsan W, et al: Guidelines for the management of spontaneous intracerebral hemorrhage: A statement for healthcare professionals from a special writing group of the Stroke Council, American Heart Association. Stroke 30:905–915, 1999.
4. Qureshi AI, Wilson DA, Hanley DF, et al: No evidence of ischemic penumbra in massive experimental intracerebral hemorrhage. Neurology 52:266–272, 1999.
5. MacKenzie JM: Intracerebral haemorrhage. J Clin Pathol 49:360–364, 1996.

PATIENT 43

A 13- year-old boy with knee pain

A 13-year-old boy presents to the emergency department with left knee pain. On the way to school today, he tripped on the steps and banged his left knee against a metal railing. In triage, the patient is noted to have a small bruise on his left knee and a mild antalgic gait. During further evaluation, the child denies any other trauma. The ibuprofen that he took a few hours ago helped his symptoms. There is no history of fever, rash, gastrointestinal symptoms, or recent illness. He does not have sickle cell disease. His appetite, energy, and activity have remained normal. The patient is not active in organized sports and has not started any new physical activities over the last several months. His mother states, however, that he has been complaining of knee pain over the last several months, and she has taken him to see the doctor for this several times. She states that his x-rays have all been normal and that the doctor told her that he had "growing pains."

Physical Examination: Vital signs: temperature 37.8°C orally; pulse 72; respiratory rate 20; blood pressure 128/72; weight 82 kg. General: well-appearing, obese male in no distress. There is a small ecchymosis on the medial aspect of the patient's left knee; there is no effusion, point tenderness, instability, or warmth noted about the knee. While lying flat, the affected leg is externally rotated. There is decreased internal rotation of the left hip. There is no other evidence of bone or joint disease on examination.

Laboratory Findings: Hip x-ray: see figure.

Question: What is the most likely diagnosis?

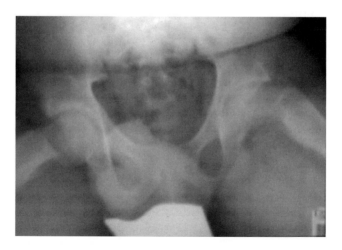

Diagnosis: Slipped capital femoral epiphysis

Discussion: Slipped capital femoral epiphysis (SCFE) is the most common hip disorder in adolescents. Early correct diagnosis of this syndrome is directly related to physician awareness that SCFE is part of the differential diagnosis. Although much is written about this disorder, physicians continue to miss this diagnosis. Thus, the scenario presented here is not uncommon. Many patients are evaluated for knee/thigh pain and have had normal knee x-rays or further diagnostic studies before the correct diagnosis is made. Delay in diagnosis results in more severe slippage and increased morbidity.

The annual incidence is approximately 2 cases per 100,000 population. It more commonly affects boys, and the majority of cases (78%) present during the adolescent growth phase. Boys present between 10 and 16 years of age, and girls between 9 and 15 years. Additionally, a delay in skeletal maturation is noted in a majority of those affected. Several investigators have reported an association with obesity, with weight-for-age noted to be greater than the 90th percentile in approximately two thirds of the patients. Bilateral symptomatic involvement occurs in 25% of all patients; approximately 50% have bilateral disease at presentation, and the remaining develop it over the following 1 to 2 years. The physeal plate at the femoral head widens because of an increase in the zone of hypertrophy. There is abnormal cartilage maturation and subendochondral bone formation as the femoral head slips posteriorly. The exact etiology remains unclear, but it is undoubtedly multifactorial. Proposed mechanisms include local trauma, obesity, variation of normal femoral anteversion, inflammatory processes, and endocrine diseases.

Patients with SCFE present with hip, groin, thigh or knee pain, and a change in the range of motion of the hip and may or may not have a gait abnormality. Pain from the hip joint can be referred to the medial aspect of the thigh and the knee via the femoral and obdurator nerves that also supply the hip joint. Pain is often described as aching and is exacerbated by walking and going up stairs. Rest and analgesics provide temporary relief. Remember that the pain can be bilateral. The findings of the knee examination are normal. Four patterns of presentation have been described: pre-slip, chronic, acute, and acute-on-chronic. During the pre-slip phase, patients report of intermittent groin, hip, or thigh pain that is more pronounced with exertion. Physical examination may show mild hip pain on rotation and perhaps a slight decrease in internal rotation. Plain radiographs usually do not reveal the abnormality at this time. The majority of patients present with chronic SCFE characterized by groin, medial thigh, or knee pain of greater than 3 weeks' duration, with an associated antalgic gait. The affected limb is held in external rotation, and there is pain and decreased internal rotation and adduction on hip examination. On passive flexion of the affected hip, the limb will automatically abduct and externally rotate. Acute-on-chronic presentation occurs when a patient has a previous history of hip or knee pain and presents with an acute increase in pain associated with decreased in range of motion. Acute presentations occur in less than 10% of patients and are characterized by acute onset of new, severe pain.

Diagnosis is made by examining two views of the hip, either an anteroposterior (AP) and lateral or an AP and frog-leg view. The frog-leg view should be avoided in any patient with severe pain to avoid further displacement. On the AP film, there is widening and irregularity of the physeal plate. A crescent-shaped density may be seen in the proximal portion of the femoral neck, known as the Blanch sign of Steel. This represents the displaced femoral head behind the femoral neck. A line (Klein's Line) drawn along the outer aspect of the femoral neck should intersect the capital physeal plate on the AP view. On the lateral view, posterior displacement of the femoral head can be seen. This view may be difficult to obtain in obese patients. The posterior, medial displacement of the femoral head is accentuated and thus more easily seen on the frog-leg view of the hips. Ultrasonography has been used for the diagnosis of SCFE and reveals atrophy of the quadriceps muscle. Computed tomographic scans may be used to confirm epiphyseal displacement in patients with suspected SCFE when plain radiographs are normal. There is some information to suggest that magnetic resonance imaging can identify abnormalities in the physeal plate even earlier than computed tomographic scanning can.

Immediate orthopedic consultation and non-weightbearing is indicated in patients with SCFE. Orthopedic surgeons often categorize patients into two groups: those with stable and those with unstable SFCE. Patients with stable slips are able to walk; those with unstable slips have severe pain and are unable to bear weight. Patients with an unstable slip are at increased risk of avascular necrosis of the femoral head. Stabilization is most often accomplished by percutaneous placement of cannulated screws that stabilize the epiphysis (see figure at right). A gentle reduction also is done. The patient is then discharged on crutches, and

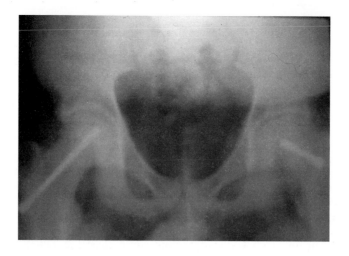

weight bearing is allowed after the pain resolves. No running or jumping is allowed until the physis fuses, which may take as long as 2 years. Important complications include avascular necrosis and osteoarthritis, which are related to the severity of the slip at the time the diagnosis is made.

Clinical Pearls

1. SCFE is the most common hip disorder in adolescents, and prompt diagnosis has great impact on patient outcome.

2. Hip pathology should always be considered in children and adolescents presenting with groin, thigh, or knee pain.

3. Immediate orthopedic referral and non-weightbearing is necessary to prevent further slippage at the epiphysis.

REFERENCES

1. Kehl DK: Slipped capital femoral epiphysis. In Morrissy RT, Weinstein SL (eds): Lovell and Winter's Pediatric Orthopedics, 5th ed. Vol 2. Philadelphia, Lippincott, 2001, pp 999–1033.
2. Matava MJ, Patton CM, Luhmann S, et al: Knee pain as the initial symptom of slipped capital femoral epiphysis: An analysis of initial presentation and treatment. J Pediatr Orthop 19:455, 1999.
3. Reynolds RAK: Diagnosis and treatment of slipped capital femoral epiphysis. Curr Opin Pediatr 11:80–83, 1999.
4. Ledwith CA, Fleisher GR: Slipped capital femoral epiphysis without hip pain leads to misdiagnosis. Pediatrics; 89:660, 1992.

PATIENT 44

A 2-year-old girl with lethargy

A 2-year-old girl is brought to the emergency department with a 2-day history of fever, irritability, vomiting, and poor eating. The child is ordinarily in day care but has not attended because of high fever and progressively listless behavior.

Physical Examination: Vital signs: temperature: 40.3°C rectally; pulse 178; respiratory rate 27; blood pressure 88/51; room air pulse oximetry 100%. General: listless toddler who responds sluggishly to painful stimuli. Pupils: equal and reactive. Mucous membranes: dry. Neck: bilateral cervical lymphadenopathy, marked irritability with flexion of the neck. Chest: clear to auscultation, no wheezes, rales, or rhonchi. Cardiac: tachycardiac without murmur. Abdomen: flat, nondistended, nontender. Skin: no petechial rash; cool with capillary refill 3 seconds. Neurologic: no gross motor or sensory deficits.

Laboratory Findings: CBC: WBC 44,000/μl, Hgb 13.1 g/dl, platelets 234,000/μl. Electrolytes: Na 129, K 3.9, Cl 97, BUN 34, Cr 0.9. Glucose 79 g/dl. PT 12.1 seconds. Urinalysis: negative. Chest x-ray: no infiltrates or cardiomegaly. CSF: WBC 4400/hpf, RBC 5/hpf, protein 111, glucose 29. CSF differential: 82 neutrophils, 19 lymphocytes. Urine, blood, and CSF cultures pending.

ED Course: An intravenous line is quickly placed and normal saline bolus of 20 ml/kg is given and repeated. A lumbar puncture is performed and intravenous antibiotics are started immediately thereafter. The patient is admitted to the pediatric intensive care unit for continued treatment.

Questions: What is the most likely diagnosis? What are the complications? What is appropriate empirical therapy?

Diagnosis: Bacterial meningitis

Discussion: Bacterial meningitis is becoming increasingly rare in the age of comprehensive childhood immunizations. Time to antibiotic therapy is crucial to avoid complications. Signs and symptoms are difficult to elicit in children younger than 2 years of age. Children up to the age of 2 years, particularly neonates, tend to present with nonspecific symptoms, including vomiting, fever, irritability, and somnolence. Clinical suspicion is of paramount importance in this vulnerable population. As children age, their symptoms progressively become more recognizable; however, not until the age of 2 years do presentations including headache, fever, neck stiffness, and decreased activity become more prevalent.

Causative organisms in the neonatal age group include group B *Streptococcus* and enteric gram-negative rods such as *Escherichia coli, Listeria monocytogenes, Streptococcus pneumoniae, Neisseria meningitides,* and *Salmonella* species. In general, in children older than 2 to 3 months, the predominant causative organisms change, with *Streptococcus pneumoniae, Neisseria meningitides,* and *Haemophilus influenzae* often responsible. Meningitis is often the result of hematogenous spread of the organisms to the central nervous system from colonized nasal mucosa or from bacteremia secondary to a distant source (e.g., middle ear infection).

The presentation of this patient is rather classic, with lethargy, neck stiffness, and fever. The lumbar puncture results are pathognomonic for meningitis. Cerebrospinal fluid (CSF) white blood cell (WBC) counts ranging from 200 to 20,000/mm^3 are expected. Protein levels are generally greater than 100. Polymorphonuclear leukocyte (PMN) predominance can be, but is not always, a distinguishing characteristic of bacterial meningitis from aseptic meningitis.

The patient's vital signs indicate an early shock state, requiring immediate fluid resuscitation and continuous intensive care monitoring. In addition to shock, other complications of bacterial meningitis include seizures, hypoglycemia, hyponatremia secondary to syndrome of inappropriate antidiuretic hormone secretion, and apnea.

Treatment includes supportive measures and timely administration of antibiotics immediately following or concurrent with the lumbar puncture. The use of steroids as adjunctive therapy is controversial and has not been entirely accepted as the standard of care. Empiric antibiotic coverage should include a third-generation cephalosporin such as ceftriaxone or cefotaxime and vancomycin if resistant *S. pneumoniae* is of concern. In the infant population (age <3 months), the use of an aminoglycoside or a third-generation cephalosporin with ampicillin is the empiric regimen of choice to cover previously discussed organisms.

Clinical Pearls

1. Meningitis, while rare, represents a true medical emergency but is amenable to treatment if addressed in a timely fashion.
2. Timely administration of antibiotics concurrently or immediately following lumbar puncture is vital. CSF cultures may be rendered sterile more quickly than is commonly thought.
3. CSF findings in bacterial and aseptic meningitis may both contain a PMN predominance, contrary to classic teaching.

REFERENCES

1. Kanegaye JT, Soliemanzadeh P, Bradley JS: Lumbar puncture in pediatric bacterial meningitis: Defining the time interval for recovery of cerebrospinal fluid pathogens after parenteral antibiotic pretreatment. Pediatrics; 108:1169–1174, 2001.
2. Fleisher GR, Ludwig S, Henretig FM, et al: Meningitis. Textbook of Pediatric Emergency Medicine. Baltimore, Williams & Wilkins, 2000, pp 731–735.
3. Negrini B, Kelleher KJ, Wald ER: Cerebrospinal fluid findings in aseptic versus bacterial meningitis. Pediatrics; 105:316–319, 2000.

PATIENT 45

A 27-year-old man with chest pain and shortness of breath after blunt trauma

A 27-year-old man ambulates into the emergency department after having been struck once in the left chest with a baseball bat during an assault. He complains of lower left-sided anterolateral chest pain and shortness of breath. The pain is much worse with inspiration. He denies any loss of consciousness or abdominal pain.

Physical Examination: General: mild distress, holding left lower lateral chest with hand for comfort. Vital signs: temperature 37.2°C, heart rate 122, respiratory rate 25 and shallow, blood pressure 130/72. *Primary trauma survey:* airway open and patent, breath sounds present bilaterally, trachea midline, symmetric strong radial pulses, no signs of external hemorrhage, awake and alert. *Secondary trauma survey:* head normocephalic, neck nontender, chest tender to palpation with contusion over the left lower chest at the anterior axillary line, abdomen soft and nontender. Repeat vital signs: heart rate 130, respirations 28, blood pressure 84/46. Breath sounds decreased on the left.

Laboratory Findings: CBC: normal. Chest radiograph (see figure): pulmonary contusion of the left lower lobe and a small apical pneumothorax.

Questions: What is the most likely cause of the sudden onset of hypotension? How should further interventions and studies be prioritized?

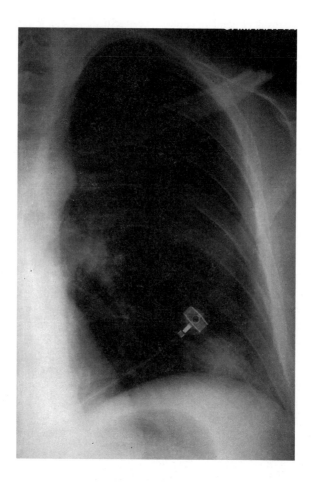

Diagnosis and Treatment: Pulmonary contusion, pneumothorax, and splenic laceration. Initial management should include supplemental oxygen, the placement of two large-bore intravenous lines, type and screen for blood, and decompression of the left chest with a needle thoracostomy followed by placement of a left chest tube.

Discussion: Hypotension is frequently encountered in both blunt and penetrating chest trauma. Because the chest contains the heart, lungs, and great vessels, the potential for catastrophic and potentially fatal injury is great. Traumatic causes of hypotension secondary to blunt chest trauma include aortic injury, tension pneumothorax, massive hemothorax, or direct cardiac injury. Aortic injuries result from shearing forces secondary to sudden deceleration and are often immediately fatal unless significant operative resources and a skilled surgeon are immediately available. Direct cardiac injuries that result in hypotension include cardiac rupture and cardiac tamponade. Uncontained cardiac rupture is catastrophic and quickly fatal. Myocardial wall injuries that are contained by the pericardium rapidly result in cardiac tamponade with associated hypotension and jugular vein distension. Trauma-induced tamponade requires prompt thoracotomy to facilitate direct repair of the cardiac injury to prevent death from cardiovascular collapse.

Tension pneumothorax is more easily treatable but also potentially fatal unless immediately suspected in a patient with chest trauma, hypotension, and decreased or absent breath sounds. Jugular vein distension and tracheal shift associated with tension pneumothorax are not always readily appreciable. Suspected tension pneumothorax should be immediately treated with needle thoracostomy in the second or third intercostal space on the midaxillary line of the affected side, followed by placement of a chest tube on the same side. Massive hemothorax is generally evident on chest radiograph and should be initially managed with a large-bore chest tube on the affected side. Initial chest tube output of greater than 1500 ml or persistent bleeding of more than 200 ml over 2 to 4 hours mandates operative intervention with thoracotomy.

Another potential source of hypotension in blunt chest trauma is bleeding from associated intra-abdominal injuries. Despite interventions, the present patient remained hypotensive, and an abdominal computed tomographic scan (see figure below) showed a splenic laceration and hemoperitoneum. The anatomic "overlap" of the abdominal and thoracic cavities is of crucial importance in the assessment and management of trauma. The actual position of the diaphragm at any given point is dependent on the phase of respiration. At maximal exhalation, the diaphragm is at the level of the nipples anteriorly. Any injury of the lower chest must be carefully evaluated for associated intra-abdominal injury. In this case, the force that produced the left lower lobe pulmonary contusion was also sufficient to lacerate the patient's spleen, the actual cause of hypotension.

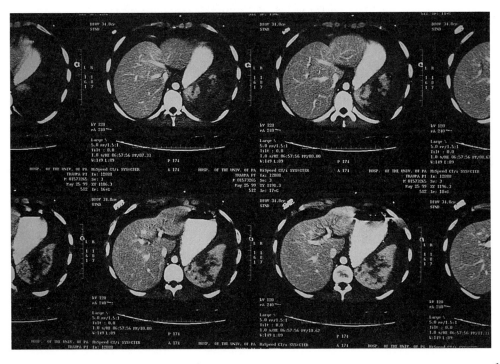

Clinical Pearls

1. Chest trauma is can be associated with intra-abdominal injuries. This is especially true in any case of blunt trauma inferior to the nipple line and in any case of penetrating trauma.

2. In the hypotensive blunt trauma patient, tension pneumothorax should be suspected even in the absence of jugular venous distension and tracheal shift.

REFERENCES

1. Peitzman AB, Rhodes M, Schwab CW, Yearly DM: The Trauma Manual. Philadelphia, Lippencott–Raven, 1998.
2. Advanced Trauma Life Support for Doctors–Student Manual. Chicago, American College of Surgeons, 1997.

Jane Lavelle, MD

PATIENT 46

A 14-year-old girl with abdominal pain for 2 days

A 14-year-old girl presents with the complaint of midline, lower abdominal pain starting 2 days ago. She describes the pain as constant and aching. She has noted a thin, whitish, foul-smelling vaginal discharge. She complains of dysuria but has no urgency or frequency. She has been eating and drinking normally. There is no report of vomiting, diarrhea, fever or chills, or abnormal vaginal bleeding. Her last menstrual period was approximately 3 to 4 weeks ago. She had unprotected sex 3 weeks ago. She has never been treated for a sexually transmitted disease before; and she has never been pregnant.

Physical Examination: Vital signs: temperature 37.8°C orally; pulse 110; respiratory rate 20; blood pressure 128/72. General: patient is alert but looks uncomfortable. Chest: clear, no CVA tenderness. Abdominal examination: bilateral lower quadrant tenderness, more severe on the right side; mild guarding but no rebound. Pelvic examination: thin grey discharge; uterine and left adnexal tenderness; no masses or ovarian enlargement.

Laboratory Findings: WBC 14,000/μl (76% segmented neutrophils, 16% lymphocytes, 7% monocytes), hemoglobin 12.9 g/dl, platelets 336,000/μl; ESR 30 mm/hr. Urinalysis: WBC 4–8/hpf, RBC 1–2/hpf, negative for nitrites. Urine HCG negative. Urine culture: no growth. Cervical ligase chain reaction for *Neisseria gonorrhoeae* and *Clamydia trachomatis* negative; Wet prep: negative for *Trichomonas*.

Questions: What is the most likely diagnosis? What further diagnostic test should be performed? What therapy should be instituted?

Diagnosis: Pelvic inflammatory disease

Discussion: Pelvic inflammatory disease (PID) is an ascending, polymicrobial infection of the upper genital tract that occurs in sexually active females. It is most often caused by *C. trachomatis* and *N. gonorrhoeae,* but other important pathogens have also been identified. It is challenging to diagnose because it manifests with a wide variety of symptoms. PID is a clinical diagnosis; when compared to laparoscopy, experienced practitioners make the correct diagnosis clinically approximately two thirds of the time. Prompt, accurate diagnosis is important in reducing long-term sequelae in patients. Perihepatitis (Fitz-Hughes-Curtis syndrome) is a form of PID characterized by acute right upper quadrant tenderness, often in the face of silent pelvic disease. Inflammatory material from the fallopian tube tracks up the paracolic gutter and localizes around the liver capsule. The complication of tubo-ovarian abscess (TOA) occurs when resolution of the upper genital tract infection is delayed or if there is tubal scarring (see figure). The true incidence of TOA in adolescents with PID remains obscure; it ranges from 5% to 20% in reports of different patient populations. Key diagnoses that must be considered in the wide differential diagnosis of such a patient include appendicitis, ectopic pregnancy, ovarian torsion/cyst, and endometriosis. Many cases go unrecognized because patients are asymptomatic or are misdiagnosed because the practitioner fails to recognize nonspecific, mild symptoms.

The majority of patients (80%) present with abdominal pain. The pain is often described as constant, dull, crampy, or aching in quality and is often bilateral. A subset of patients present with right upper quadrant pain with few or no abdominal symptoms. The majority of patients present within 7 days of their last menstrual period. Patients may complain of abnormal vaginal bleeding or vaginal discharge. Patients may complain of anorexia and nausea, but in general gastrointestinal symptoms are not primary complaints. The pelvic examination aids in identifying abnormal vaginal discharge, a friable cervix, uterine and/or adenexal tenderness or masses, and cervical motion tenderness. Important laboratory evaluations include complete blood cell count (CBC), erythrocyte sedimentation rate (ESR) or C-reactive protein (CRP), endocervical or vaginal swabs for ligase chain reaction or culture for *N. gonorrhoeae* and *C. trachomatis,* urine for β-HCG, urinalysis and culture, wet mount for *Trichomonas,* and a Gram stain on vaginal secretions looking for more than 10 WBCs per high-power field. Pelvic ultrasonography can eliminate other diagnoses as well as document the presence of PID or TOAs.

In the 2002 Guidelines for Sexually Transmitted Diseases, the Centers for Disease Control and Prevention (CDC) revised the diagnostic criteria for PID. Relaxation of these guidelines was aimed at capturing and treating as many cases as possible. Empiric treatment for PID is recommended for women at risk for sexually transmitted diseases if one of the following symptons is present and no other illness is identified: uterine/adenexal tenderness or cervical motion tenderness. Further criteria that can be used to increase specificity include presence of oral temperature greater than 38.3°C, elevated ESR, elevated CRP, abnormal cervical or vaginal mucopurulent discharge, pres-

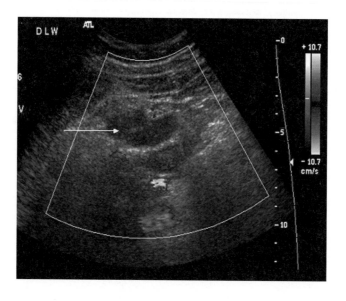

ence of white cells in vaginal secretions by microscopy, or laboratory evidence of *N. gonorrhoeae* or *C. trachomatis* infection. The absence of WBCs on the Gram stain of cervical or vaginal secretions makes the diagnosis of infection unlikely.

Broad-spectrum, empiric regimens to cover *N. gonorrhoeae, C. trachomatis,* anaerobes, gram-negative facultative bacteria, and streptococci are recommended. Prevention of sequelae is directly linked to immediate administration of appropriate antibiotics. Criteria for hospitalization include pregnancy, severe disease, unclear diagnosis, patient's inability to tolerate or follow an outpatient oral regimen, failed outpatient treatment, presence of TOA, and presence of an immunodeficiency. Both parenteral and oral regimens have been demonstrated to be effective (see table). Parenteral therapy may be discontinued 24 hours after the patient improves clinically, and oral treatment with 100 mg of doxycycline twice daily should be continued for 14 days. For those in whom a TOA has been diagnosed, most clinicians recommend at least 24 hours of inpatient treatment. Metronidazole is often included in the subsequent outpatient regimen to improve anaerobic coverage. Ofloxacin, which is effective against *N. gonorrhoeae* and *C. trachomatis,* has been shown to be effective as a single agent in two clinical trials, although its lack of anaerobic coverage remains a cause for concern.

Adolescents who are treated with oral regimens should have scheduled follow-up in 48 to 72 hours, at which time they should have substantial clinical improvement in their symptoms. If they have not improved, further evaluation may be indicated as well as admission for parenteral therapy. Patient partners in the preceding 2 months should be referred for treatment. Additionally, adolescents should be educated regarding the signs, symptoms, and consequences of sexually transmitted diseases, as well as behaviors that increase and decrease their risk for these. Consequences include recurrence of disease (12–33%), TOA, infertility (13–20% risk after one episode, increase to 55–75% after three episodes), ectopic pregnancy (6- to 10-fold risk after one episode), and chronic abdominal pain (18% after one episode).

The present patient was admitted for further treatment and scheduled for a pelvic ultrasonography, which revealed a tubo-ovarian abscess. She received intravenous cefoxitin and oral doxycyline. Her pain was successfully controlled with ketorolac.

Parental Regimens Recommended by the CDC

A. Cefotetan 2 g IV every 12 hrs *or* Cefoxitin 2 g IV every 6 hrs
plus
Doxycycline 100 mg PO or IV every 12 hrs

B. Clindamycin 900 mg IV every 8 hrs
plus
Gentamicin 2 mg/kg IV/IM loading dose, then 1.5 mg/kg every 8 hrs

---

Oral Regimens Recommended by the CDC

A. Ofloxacin 400 mg PO twice daily for 14 days
with
Metronidazole 500 mg PO twice daily for 14 days

B. Ceftriaxone 250 mg IM *or* Cefoxitin 2 g IM w/ probenecid 1 g PO
or other parenteral third-generation cephalosporin
plus
Doxycycline 100 mg PO twice daily for 14 days
with or without
Metronidazole 500 mg PO twice daily for 14 days

Clinical Pearls

1. PID is a clinical diagnosis; physicians should have a low threshold for diagnosing and empirically treating PID to prevent sequelae.

2. Scheduled follow-up, partner treatment, and education about the signs and symptoms of sexually transmitted diseases as well as prevention strategies are important components of treatment.

3. The differential diagnosis of PID must include consideration of appendicitis, ectopic pregnancy, ovarian torsion/cyst, and endometriosis.

REFERENCES

1. Centers for Disease Control and Prevention: Sexually transmitted treatment guidelines 2002. MMWR Morbid Mortal Wkly Rep; 51(RR-6):1–77, 2002.
2. Pletcher JR, Slap GB: Pelvic inflammatory disease. In Neinstein LS(ed): Adolescent Health Care: A Practical Guide, 4th ed, Philadelphia, Lippincott Williams & Wilkins, 2002, p 1161.
3. Lawson MA, Blythe MJ: Pelvic inflammatory disease in adolescents. Pediatr Clin North Am 46:767, 1999.
4. McCormack WM: Pelvic inflammatory disease. N Engl J Med; 330:115, 1994.
5. Kahn JG, Walker CK, Washington AE, et al: Diagnosing pelvic inflammatory disease: A comprehensive analysis and considerations for developing a new model. JAMA 226:2594, 1991.
6. Shafer M, Sweet RL: Pelvic inflammatory disease in adolescent females. Adolesc Med 1:545, 1990.

PATIENT 47

An 11-year-old girl with recurrent headache

An 11 year-old girl presents to the emergency department with a headache lasting for 3 hours. She characterizes her pain as diffuse and throbbing and associated with nausea and vomiting. She has no fever, neck pain, rash, or history of trauma. She describes near weekly episodes of this headache for the past 4 months.

Physical Examination: General: uncomfortable appearing. Temperature: 37.2°C; pulse: 104; respiratory rate: 22; blood pressure: 122/76 HEENT: no tenderness; pupils equal, round, and reactive to light with mild photophobia; optic discs normal. Neck: supple. Lungs: clear to auscultation. Cardiac: regular rate and rhythm without murmurs, rubs, or gallops. Abdomen: soft, nontender, nondistended. Skin: no lesions. Neurologic: cranial nerves, motor strength, reflexes normal. Sensation intact. finger-to-nose examination and gait normal; awake, alert, and oriented.

Questions: How would you proceed with this patient's evaluation in the emergency department? What is the most likely diagnosis?

Diagnosis and Treatment: This patient needs no further work-up in the ED, and her likely diagnosis is migraine headache.

Discussion: Headaches in children are common complaints, and 75% of children will have experienced at least one headache by 15 years of age. Although most of the many causes of headaches are benign, 7% to 15% are associated with causes that carry significant morbidity and mortality.

Regardless of the underlying origin, head pain is generally caused by tension, traction, or inflammation of innervated intracranial structures, which include the dura mater, major arteries at the base of the brain, and the great venous sinus and its branches. However, most intracranial structures are not pain sensitive. Frequently, head pain is caused by irritation of innervated extracranial structures, such as the skin, sinuses, mucous membranes, and teeth.

Because the causes of headaches are numerous, a helpful approach to the differential diagnosis of headache involves classifying headaches by the timing of onset. **Acute** headaches are single events without previous history of recurrent headaches; common causes include central nervous system (CNS) infections, non-CNS infections (the most common cause of pediatric headaches in the ED setting), and trauma. **Acute recurrent** headaches are those that recur but are separated by pain-free intervals, such as those associated with migraines or hypertension. **Chronic nonprogressive** headaches are those that intermittently worsen but generally do not go away completely (e.g., tension-type headaches). **Chronic progressive** headaches are headaches that gradually worsen over time and include such causes as brain tumors and idiopathic intracranial hypertension. **Mixed** headaches encompass elements of several types.

Frequently, the cause can be determined solely by history and physical examination. Key historical elements include the timing of headache onset, location of head pain, pain quality, relieving and aggravating factors, associated symptoms, and comparison with previous headaches. The physical examination should focus on the child's general appearance and vital signs. Additionally, the examiner should inspect and palpate the head, examine the eyes (including fundoscopic examination), and evaluate the ears, oropharynx, and throat. The neck should be examined for meningeal signs. A complete neurologic examination should be performed.

Generally, the role of laboratory testing is limited in the evaluation of the child with headache and should be undertaken only when clinically indicated. For example, rapid streptococcal testing may be helpful in a patient with a headache and pharyngitis. The most helpful diagnostic tests in evaluation of headache are lumbar puncture and neuroimaging. Lumbar puncture is essential in the evaluation of the patient with a suspected infection of the CNS. The clinician can also measure the opening cerebrospinal fluid (CSF) pressure for the patient with suspected idiopathic intracranial hypertension and can detect small amounts of blood in the CSF in patients with suspected subarachnoid hemorrhage. Although most children with headaches do not need acute neuroimaging, computed tomography (CT) scans or magnetic resonance imaging (MRI) scans can be helpful in selected patients. Several historical and physical findings should suggest the need for emergency studies (see table). In the ED, the most widely available imaging modality is the CT scan. CT scanning is highly sensitive in detecting lesions that cause mass effect, hydrocephalus, and hemorrhage. MRI scans are more sensitive for pituitary lesions, lesions in the posterior fossa, and inflammatory lesions. However, obtaining an emergency MRI scan is generally more difficult than obtaining an emergency CT scan. Patients undergoing MRI are more likely to require sedation and monitoring.

Indications for Neuroimaging

- Sudden onset
- Worsening in severity or frequency
- Change from baseline
- Persistent vomiting
- Headache upon awakening/awakens patient from sleep
- Worse when lying down
- Altered mental status
- Focal neurologic findings
- Age ≤3 years

Treatment for headache is directed toward treatment of the underlying cause. While there are specific interventions for some headaches (e.g., lumbar puncture for idiopathic intracranial hypertension; antibiotics for meningitis), commonly, a specific cause for a child's headache cannot be determined. Fortunately, most headaches in children respond quite well to over-the-counter analgesics.

The present patient was believed to have migraine headaches. Migraines are the most common cause of headaches in patients who are referred to pediatric neurology clinics. Although the precise mechanisms of migraine headaches are unknown, migraine symptoms result from a complex interaction of neurons and cranial vasculature.

The diagnosis of migraine headaches is made clinically, based on modified criteria from the International Headache Society (see table) As with most causes of pediatric headaches, migraines are quite responsive to acetaminophen and ibuprofen. Second-line agents include dopamine antagonists such as metoclopramide and prochlorperazine.

Additional antimigraine medications include 5-hydroxytryptamine agents. Older 5-hydroxytryptamine agents such as dihydroergotamine have been replaced by the newer triptan agents (e.g., sumatriptan).

The present patient was given ibuprofen and had complete resolution of her headache. She was referred to the pediatric neurology clinic, where her presumptive ED diagnosis of migraine headache was confirmed.

International Headache Society Diagnotic Criteria For Migraine

Migraine without aura
1. At least five attacks fulfilling criteria 2 through 4
2. Headaches last 2 to 48 hours (1 to 48 hours)
3. Headache has at least two of the following characteristics:
a. Unilateral (or bilateral, either frontal or temporal) location
b. Pulsating quality
c. Moderate to severe intensity
d. Aggravated by routine physical activity
4. During headache, at least one of the following signs occurs:
a. Nausea and/or vomiting
b. Photophobia and (and/or) phonophobia

Migraine with aura
1. At least two attacks fulfilling criterion 2
2. At least three of the following features:
a. One or more fully reversible aura symptoms indicating focal cortical and/or brainstem dysfunction
b. At least one aura symptom that develops gradually over 4 or more minutes, or two or more symptoms occur in succession
c. No aura lasts more than 60 minutes
d. Headache follows aura with a free interval of less than 1 hour

---

( ) = Proposed pediatric revisions for children under age 15

Modified from Burton LJ, Quinn B, Pratt-Cheney JL, et al: Headache etiology in a pediatric emergency department. Pediatr Emerg Care 13:1–4, 1997.

Clinical Pearls

1. Most causes of headaches in children are benign and resolve with over-the-counter analgesics.

2. Most causes of headache can be diagnosed clinically, and laboratory testing is infrequently helpful in determining a diagnosis.

3. Although most children with headache do not need neuroimaging, certain worrisome historical features or findings on physical examination should prompt an emergency CT or MRI scan.

REFERENCES
1. Goadsby PJ, Lipton RB, Ferrari MD: Migraine—Current understanding and treatment. New Engl J Med 346:257–270, 2002.
2. Bullock B, Tenenbein M: Emergency department management of pediatric migraine. Pediatr Emerg Care 16:196–201, 2000.
3. Burton LJ, Quinn B, Pratt-Cheney JL, et al: Headache etiology in a pediatric emergency department. Pediatr Emerg Care 13:1–4, 1997.
4. Winner P, Martinez W, Mate L, et al: Classification of pediatric migraine: Proposed revision to the IHS criteria. Headache 35:407–410, 1997.
5. Rothner AD: Pathophysiology of recurrent headaches in children and adolescents. Pediatr Ann 24:458–466, 1995.

Rex Mathew, MD
Anthony J. Dean, MD

PATIENT 48

A 23-year-old woman with abdominal pain and jaundice

A 23-year-old woman with a history of hereditary spherocytosis and gallstones presents to the emergency department reporting 2 weeks of crampy abdominal pain. It radiates to the back, is worse over the past 2 days, and is accompanied by nausea and vomiting. The patient is otherwise healthy and has no known allergies.

Physical Examination: Temperature 37°C; pulse 91; respiratory rate 34; blood pressure 116/57. General appearance: uncomfortable. HEENT: icteric, dry mucous membranes. Chest: clear to auscultation. Cardiac: regular rate and rhythm. Abdomen: nondistended, normal bowel sounds, right upper quadrant (RUQ) and midepigastric tenderness to palpation with guarding. No rebound or splenomegaly. Back: no flank tenderness. Extremities: no edema. Neuromuscular: normal.

Laboratory Findings: CBC: WBC 11,300/μL, hemoglobin 11.3 g/dl, platelets 201,000/μL. Blood chemistries: normal. Liver function studies: total bilirubin 17.5 (normal 0–1.2) mg/dL, conjugated bilirubin 12.8 mg/dL (normal 0–0.1), unconjugated bilirubin 2.0 mg/dL (normal 0–1.0), alkaline phosphatase 315 U/L (normal 35–125), aspartate aminotransferase 234 U/L (normal 14–36), alanine aminotransferase 522 U/L (normal 9–52). Pancreatic enzymes: amylase 2172 U/L (normal 0–140), lipase 24,762 U/L (normal 0–300). Emergency medicine bedside ultrasonography (EMBU): multiple gallstones, normal gall bladder (GB) wall-thickness, and a stone in the common bile duct (CBD) with associated dilatation of the intra- and extrahepatic bile ducts suggesting complete CBD obstruction (see figures).

Questions: What is the most likely cause of the patient's abdominal pain? What other life-threatening diagnoses must be considered in this patient?

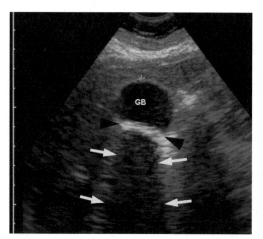
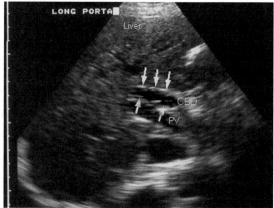

Diagnosis and Treatment: Acute pancreatitis associated with complete biliary obstruction secondary to choledocholithiasis is almost certainly the cause of the patient's symptoms in the context of markedly elevated pancreatic enzymes and the EMBU findings. With the jaundice and RUQ pain and tenderness, the patient has two of the three components of Charcot's triad (the third is fever). Although both of these findings, as well as the elevated white blood cell count, can be explained by the leading diagnosis, the high bilirubin and sonographic findings in the liver suggest that cholestasis is long-standing, so the potentially lethal coexistent complication of ascending cholangitis is of concern. In a patient with hemolytic anemia and splenomegaly, splenic rupture could also be considered, but is unlikely in the context of stable vital signs and hemogram and is ruled out by the absence of free fluid on EMBU. The differential diagnosis includes perforated peptic ulcer, other perforated viscus, acute cholecystitis, bowel obstruction, abdominal aortic aneurysm, pneumonia, myocardial infarction, diabetic ketoacidosis, and renal colic.

Initial therapy should include pain control, intravenous hydration, and bowel rest. The use of nasogastric suction is controversial. Cholecystectomy and common bile duct exploration are definitive therapy. If a contraindication to surgery exists, endoscopic retrograde cholangiopancreatography with removal of the obstructing gallstone, or temporizing stent, would be indicated. In view of the possibility of ascending cholangitis, broad-spectrum antibiotics covering bowel flora should be given empirically. Appropriate choices would include any of the following: ampicillin/ sulbactam, ticarcillin/cluvulanate, a third-generation cephalosporin with clindamycin or metronidazole or ampicillin, gentamycin, and clindamycin.

Discussion: Gallstones and alcoholism are the two most common causes of acute pancreatitis, with gallstones being more common in women and alcoholism more common in men. In the United States, 80% of gallstones are of the cholesterol variety, with the remainder either pure pigment stones or a combination of the two. Risk factors for cholesterol stone formation include female gender, pregnancy, estrogen replacement, obesity, fasting, weight loss, certain cholesterol-lowering drugs, chronic intestinal loss (e.g., Crohn's disease or ileal resection), age, and genetics (e.g., certain native American groups in the Southwest).

Pigment stones are formed by precipitates of bilirubin and calcium. Most pigment stones occur in states of increased heme turnover and/or conditions associated with increased secretion of unconjugated bilirubin (e.g., cirrhosis, chronic alcohol abuse, hemolytic disease, hypersplenism, or ineffective erythropoiesis).

Gallstone pancreatitis usually manifests as a steady pain in the midepigastrium or RUQ and occasionally with radiation to the back. The event may have been preceded by episodes of biliary colic or postprandial RUQ pain. Physical examination findings may include fever and tachycardia. Dullness to percussion of the chest may suggest the presence of a pleural effusion. In 1% of cases, ecchymosis of the flank (Grey-Turner sign) or the periumbilical region (Cullen's sign) occurs, but these signs may also be seen in other diseases involving retroperitoneal or intraperitoneal hemorrhage, respectively. Laboratory markers include elevated amylase (usually greater than three times the upper limit of normal) or lipase. Elevations of bilirubin and liver function test findings may also occur and suggest a biliary origin. An elevation in alanine aminotransferase of greater than three times normal in the setting of pancreatitis has a positive predictive value of 95% for gallstones as the cause.

Although 90% of patients recover without complications, acute pancreatitis can be lethal and is associated with a large number of complications. Those of most concern in the emergency setting include hypocalcemia, hyperglycemia, hypotension, acute renal failure, shock, disseminated intravascular coagulation, and necrosis of local abdominal organs. Patients at risk for poor outcome are identified using the Ranson criteria (see table). In addition, obesity has been shown to be a major risk factor for severe pancreatitis. Patients with fewer than three Ranson criteria have a 1% mortality rate; with three or four criteria, there is a 16% mortality rate; with five or six criteria, the mortality rate is 40%. Patients with more than six criteria have a 100% mortality rate.

Ranson's Criteria

At Admission or Diagnosis	During Initial 48 Hours
Age > 55 years	Hematocrit fell >10%
Blood glucose > 200 mg/dl	BUN increase >8 mg/dL
WBC count >16,000/μl	Arterial Po_2 <60 mm Hg
Serum LDH >700 IU%	Base deficit >4 mEq/L
AST > 250 SF units % (56 units/dl)	Estimated fluid sequestration >6 L

Transabdominal ultrasonography or computed tomography of the abdomen can be performed to confirm the diagnosis. Ultrasonography is highly sensitive in detecting gallstones in the gallbladder and frequently can provide images of the biliary tract, including obstructing gallstones, often seen at the ampulla of Vater. Assessment of the gall bladder walls and pericholecystic spaces confirms or refutes the presence of acute cholecystitis. Ultrasonography also provides information about the liver, pancreas, and spleen in patients presenting with undifferentiated abdominal pain. A diffusely enlarged, hypoechoic pancreas is the classic ultrasonographic finding in acute pancreatitis. A dilated pancreatic duct is often seen in patients with disease of a biliary origin.

The primary focus of EMBU evaluation of the RUQ is in the diagnosis of gallstones. With experience, however, it is not difficult for the emergency physician to identify the common bile duct and examine the liver for signs of intrahepatic cholestasis. The normal common bile duct is considered to be smaller than 3 mm, although there are many reports of larger CBDs not associated with pathologic conditions. Some authors allow 1 mm per decade of age. A CBD of greater than 9 mm is universally accepted as abnormally enlarged. As with all tests in emergency medicine, the EMBU is interpreted in the context of the patient's entire clinical picture. In the present setting with a high pretest probability of biliary obstruction, the CBD of 12 mm is clearly abnormal. In-

trahepatic bile ducts are not sonographically visible in healthy persons. With obstruction, the bile passages appear as reduplication of the portal venous system, leading to sonographic findings that have been variously described as "too many tubes," the "railroad sign," and the "shot gun sign." Sonographic signs of intrahepatic cholestasis develop gradually, usually over a period of 24 hours or more. Bacterial colonization proximal to the CBD obstruction may occur, leading to ascending cholangitis. Both CBD dilatation and intrahepatic cholestasis were identified in the present patient, allowing the emergency physician to fulfill his primary responsibility of identifying potentially lethal conditions—in this case, ascending cholangitis. As a result, antibiotics were added to the usual therapy for pancreatitis, and early urgent consultation was obtained, allowing for expedited definitive care.

Hemolytic anemia causing cell breakdown and bile-pigment stone formation is the most likely cause of gallstones in the present patient. The early formation of bile-pigment stones is the most common complication in cases of hereditary spherocytosis, occurring in about 50% patients. Splenectomy in patients with mild to moderate hemolysis is recommended to prevent these complications. In this patient, endoscopic retrograde cholangiopancreatography was performed, revealing a black, pigmented stone in the common bile duct that was removed. She subsequently had outpatient cholecystectomy and splenectomy.

Clinical Pearls

1. The emergency physician must strive to identify the minority of patients with pancreatitis who are at risk for life-threatening complications.

2. The clinical presentation of acute pancreatitis mimics that of many other conditions, which must be ruled out before the diagnosis is made.

3. Bedside ultrasonography performed by the treating physician, while limited in focus, may provide information that allows for expedited care of patients with critical illnesses.

REFERENCES
1. Bank S, Indaram A: Causes of acute and recurrent pancreatitis: Clinical considerations and clues to diagnosis. Gasrtroenterol Clin North Am 28:571–589, 1999.
2. del Giudice EM, et al: Coinheritance of Gilbert syndrome increases the risk for developing gallstones in patient with hereditary spherocytosis. Blood 94:2259–2262, 1999.
3. Mergener K, Baillie J: Endoscopic treatment for acute biliary pancreatitis: Clinical considerations and clues to diagnosis. Gasrtroenterol Clin North Am 28:601–613, 1999.
4. Tenner S, Dubner H, Steinberg W: Predicting gallstone pancreatitis with laboratory parameter: A meta analysis. Am J Gastroenterol 89:1863–1866, 1994.

Allyson Kreshak, MD
Stephanie Abbuhl, MD

PATIENT 49

A 57-year-old woman with fever, malaise, and weight loss

A 57-year-old woman who has had human immunodeficiency virus (HIV) disease for several years presents with fever, malaise, and weight loss over a 2-week period. She denies any hemoptysis, chest pain, dyspnea, abdominal pain, or other symptoms. She is not taking any medications for her HIV disease and has no other medical problems.

Physical Examination: Temperature: 36.7°C; pulse 106; respiratory rate 22; blood pressure 110/70; pulse oximetry 95%. General: ill-appearing, in mild distress. HEENT: pale conjunctiva. Pulmonary: clear to auscultation bilaterally. Cardiac: regular tachycardia. Abdomen: normal. Extremities: no clubbing, cyanosis, or edema. Neurologic: normal. Skin: normal

Laboratory Findings: CBC: WBC 3.9, hemoglobin 6.7 g/dl, no change compared to CBC 1 month ago. Blood chemistries: normal. Urinalysis: normal. ECG: sinus tachycardia. Chest x-ray (see figure): cavitation in left upper lobe with bilateral infiltrates.

Questions: What is the likely cause of a pulmonary cavitary lesion in an HIV-positive patient with symptoms of fever, malaise, and weight loss? What practical measures should be performed while the patient is in the emergency department?

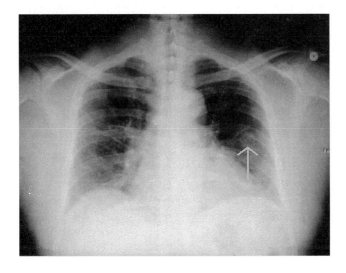

Diagnosis and Treatment: The possible causes of a cavitary lesion in an HIV patient include *My-cobacterium tuberculosis* (MTB) infection, *Pneumocystis carinii* infection, bacterial infections, and fungal infections. Making a presumptive clinical diagnosis depends on the consideration of a number of factors, including the patient's symptoms, details about the past and present history, the appearance of the chest radiograph, CD4 count, and physical examination findings. A recent CD4 count can be helpful, for example, in that TB frequently occurs in patients with counts between 200 and 500 cells/μl, whereas PCP and fungal infections do not occur until immunosuppression is more severe and the counts are less than 200/μl. Although a definitive diagnosis can rarely be made in the ED, emergency physicians should maintain a high index of suspicion for MTB infection so that immediate isolation can be instituted to prevent transmission to other patients and health care workers.

Discussion: MTB is transmitted by the inhalation of droplet nuclei (particles ≤ 5 μm) produced by coughing and sneezing from patients with active disease. The small size of the droplets allow their suspension in air for long periods of time. The ED is a high-risk area for the transmission of tuberculosis, and infection control measures should be instituted as soon as it is appreciated that TB is a possibility. The ideal form of isolation for a potential TB patient is in a negative pressure room with a minimum of six air exchanges per hour and venting of the air from the room directly outside. Other measures include the use of ultraviolet lamps for germicidal irradiation. Many EDs do not have these facilities, however, and if nothing else, the health care workers involved in the care of a patient with suspected TB should wear tight-fitting "N-95" masks, otherwise known as high-efficient particulate filter masks (not the standard surgical mask). These are capable of filtering out particles in the 1 to 5 μm range and do not leak significant air around the edges.

Once infected droplets are inhaled, they are taken up by respiratory macrophages and multiply. The infection then spreads to local lymph nodes and becomes disseminated. After 4 weeks of infection, the host's immune system clears most of the mycobacteria from the infected tissues. Uncleared mycobacteria are contained within a granuloma designed to protect the body from further invasion of the organism, and some patients may demonstrate a Ghon or Ranke complex (calcified primary focus and calcified primary focus with calcified hilar lymph node, respectively). This stage of infection is usually asymptomatic. In other patients, a chest radiograph at this time may show pleural effusions, pulmonary infiltrates, and/or ipsilateral adenopathy. If the host is immunocompromised, infection may result in active tuberculosis. Otherwise, approximately 10% of persons infected develop active disease later in life. Most cases of tuberculosis are reactivation from infection at a previous time. Populations at risk for primary infection and reactivation include immunocompromised (especially HIV-positive) patients, immigrants, low-income inner city minorities, prisoners, and people residing in homeless shelters or other group living situations.

Symptoms of tuberculosis may be systemic or organ specific. Systemic symptoms include low-grade fever, fatigue, malaise, anorexia, and night sweats. Organ-specific symptoms often involve the lung and include hemoptysis, pleuritic chest pain, shortness of breath, and cough. However, extrapulmonary symptoms may be present and are found with increased frequency among more severely immunocompromised patients. Symptoms may begin insidiously and be present for weeks or months prior to diagnosis. On physical examination, these patients often appear chronically ill and malnourished. Chest radiographs of reactivation tuberculosis commonly show upper lobe infiltrates with cavitation, but atypical radiographic patterns may occur in up to 30% of cases, especially in HIV-positive patients. In patients with advanced HIV disease and low CD4 counts, TB often presents as a diffuse interstitial pneumonia mimicking *P. carinii* infection.

Nontuberculous mycobacterial (NTM) infections are acquired from environmental sources and are increasing in prevalence, especially among HIV-positive patients. Symptoms of NTM infections are variable and nonspecific and usually manifest as a slowly progressive pulmonary infection that resembles tuberculosis. Dissemination is rare, except in immunocompromised patients. Chest radiographs may show infiltrates with or without nodules, cavitation, or multiple nodules.

Evaluation of patients in whom tuberculosis or NTM infection is suspected includes complete blood cell count, electrolytes, chest radiograph, and HIV test, since HIV is an important risk factor for the development of tuberculosis. Tuberculin skin testing should be performed, but up to 60% of patients with acquired immunodeficiency syndrome and up to 30% of those without HIV infection have a negative PPD test result even when they are infected. Sputum samples or bronchial washings should be sent for smear and culture. Acid-fast bacilli–positive smears serve as the initial confirmation of suspicion of MTB or NTM infection. Definitive diagnosis requires identification of the organism from culture or DNA analysis.

Hospitalization is necessary for patients in whom the diagnosis is uncertain, if the patient is unlikely to be compliant with medication, or if the patient is hypoxic, has significant hemoptysis, or is otherwise systemically ill. Empiric therapy should be started with one of three treatment options (see table) combining isoniazid, rifampin, and pyrazinamide with the addition of either ethambutol or streptomycin, based on the prevalence of geographic-specific patterns of resistance to isoniazid. If local resistance to isoniazid is 4% or greater (most of the United States), then four-drug therapy is recommended, including either ethambutol or streptomycin. If local resistance to isoniazid is less than 4%, then ethambutol or streptomycin may be excluded from treatment. Treatment should be modified once patient sensitivities are reported. Drug therapy for HIV-positive patients involves any of these three treatment options, except that an alternative to rifampin is necessary in patients concurrently receiving antiretroviral therapy. Public health department notification is imperative. Additionally, treatment should be coordinated through health care providers who will monitor treatment and any medication side effects. High-risk patients with positive tuberculin skin tests but without active disease should be treated for latent tuberculosis with isoniazid.

The present patient was placed in respiratory isolation and sputum samples were sent to the laboratory. Initial smears revealed AFB-positive sputum, and the patient was treated with combination therapy. During her hospital course, infection with *Mycobacterium tuberculosis* was confirmed by DNA amplification. She was ultimately discharged and continued on multidrug therapy in coordination with the public health department.

Initial Treatment Options for Suspected Tuberculosis

Option One	Isoniazid, rifampin, pyrazinamide, and ethambutol or streptomycin daily for 8 weeks, then isoniazid and rifampin two to three times weekly for 16 weeks, if strains are susceptible to isoniazid and rifampin.
Option Two	Isoniazid, rifampin, pyrazinamide, and ethambutol or streptomycin for 2 weeks, then these same medications twice weekly for 6 weeks, then isoniazid and rifampin twice weekly for 16 weeks, if strains are susceptible to isoniazid and rifampin.
Option Three	Isoniazid, rifampin, pyrazinamide, and ethambutol or streptomycin three times weekly for 6 months.

Clinical Pearls

1. A high index of suspicion is necessary to detect mycobacterial infections. MTB and NTM infections should be suspected in all patients with respiratory or extrapulmonary symptoms, especially if the patient is from a high-risk population. Patients who are immunocompromised may present with "atypical" findings. Diagnosis is a collective assessment of clinical, radiographic, and microbiologic criteria.

2. The protection of other patients and health care personnel is of critical importance in the initial management of patients with possible TB. Suspected patients should be placed in a respiratory isolation room, and health care workers should wear a tight fitting N-95 mask to reduce exposure.

3. Because of multidrug resistance, initial empiric treatment with combination therapy should be initiated if smears are AFB positive. Treatment should be altered based on subsequent drug susceptibilities. High-risk patients with latent tuberculosis infection should be treated with isoniazid.

4. Public health department notification is imperative to facilitate appropriate treatment of the patient and to help maintain tuberculosis-control programs.

REFERENCES

1. American Thoracic Society and The Centers for Disease Control and Prevention: Diagnostic standards and classification of tuberculosis in adults and children. Am J Respir Crit Care Med 161:1376–1395, 2000.
2. Horsburgh RC, Feldman S, Ridzon R: Practice guidelines for the treatment of tuberculosis. Clin Infect Dis 31:633–639, 2000.
3. Centers for Disease Control and Prevention: Prevention and treatment of tuberculosis among patients infected with human immunodeficiency virus: Principles of therapy and revised recommendations. MMWR Morbid Mortal Wkly Rep 47: RR-20, 1998.
4. American Thoracic Society: Diagnosis and treatment of disease caused by nontuberculous mycobacteria. Am J Respir Crit Care Med 156:S1–S25, 1997.
5. Centers for Disease Control and Prevention: Initial therapy for tuberculosis in the era of multidrug resistance: Recommendations of the Advisory Council for the Elimination of Tuberculosis. MMWR Morbid Mortal Wkly Rep 42:RR-7, 1993.

Kevin C. Osterhoudt, MD

PATIENT 50

A 14-week-old boy with crankiness and poor feeding

A 14-week-old baby boy is evaluated in the emergency department for "being cranky" and "acting sick." He was born at full term via uncomplicated vaginal delivery and had been well until 5 days prior. Stooling has changed from four per day to only one per day, but today it is normal in consistency. Over the past few days, the baby has seemed "congested," and has developed a mild "gaggy" cough. For the past 24 hours he has been cranky with a "whining" cry, has not slept much, and has lost interest in nursing. The number of wet diapers is reduced. The baby has not had a fever and is consoled when carried by his mother.

Physical Examination: Temperature 37.1°C.; pulse 152; respiratory rate 38. General: alert, low-volume cry, expressionless face with occasional weak social smile. HEENT: anterior fontanelle flat, tympanic membranes normal, decreased tears, increased salivary pool. Chest: normal. Cardiovascular: normal. Abdomen: distended, hyperactive bowel sounds, flatulence, no masses, no organomegaly. Genitourinary: normal. Extremities: well perfused. Skin: normal. Neuromuscular: cranial nerve function intact, poor suck, intact gag, mild hypotonia, deep-tendon reflexes present.

Laboratory Findings: Hemogram: WBC 10,700/μl, hemoglobin 12.6 g/dl, platelets 377,000/μl. Serum chemistries: Na 141 mEq/L, K 4.8 mEq/L, CO_2 20 mEq/L, creatinine 0.5 mg/dl. Urinalysis: specific gravity 1.020, no leukocytes or blood. Abdominal obstruction radiographs: dilated gas-filled intestine with air present from stomach to rectum.

Question: Beyond general supportive care, what specific pharmacologic therapy might be helpful to this baby as an inpatient?

Treatment: Botulism immune globulin

Discussion: Consideration of a whining baby with poor feeding behaviors, cough, and congestion might suggest a simple viral syndrome as the cause for this baby's illness. However, careful notation of the baby's affect, poor suck, distended abdomen, and hypotonia portend a more significant malady. Sepsis is to be considered, but the baby is afebrile and can be consoled by the mother. Urinary tract infection is unlikely based on a normal urinalysis result. Crankiness and abdominal distension merit thought of intussusception, and the history of diminished stooling might suggest Hirschprung's disease. However, poor suck, pooling of saliva, an expressionless face, a weak cry, and hypotonia suggest that this baby's symptomatology is derived from weakness (see table). The differential diagnosis can be narrowed significantly with a good medical history and physical examination and, perhaps, with directed laboratory investigation.

Serial physical examinations note the loss of previously attained motor control of the head, a diminished gag reflex, and bilateral ptosis of the eyelids. The history of constipation and the findings of generalized weakness and cranial neuropathies in a previously healthy infant strongly suggest the diagnosis of infant botulism (see table).

Infant botulism typically occurs in children younger than 6 months and involves intestinal colonization by ingested *Clostridium botulinum* spores. With spore germination, *botulinum* neurotoxin is absorbed into the blood stream, where it inhibits acetylcholine release at the presynaptic membranes of the neuromuscular junctions, and ganglionic and postganglionic synapses. Movements that require frequent neuromuscular transmission, such as sucking, peristalsis, and eye opening, are frequently more overtly affected.

The "gold standard" for the diagnosis of infant botulism is identification of *C. botulinum* organisms or toxin in the feces. Most infants can be appropriately managed based on clinical diagnosis, however. Electromyography can provide diagnostic support. Clinical management should focus on support of hydration and nutrition, maintenance of ventilation and oxygenation, and prevention of secondary infections (especially aspiration pneumonia). Currently, the California Department of Health Infant Botulism Treatment and Prevention Program [*www.infantbot.org*] produces a human-derived botulism immune globulin (BIG), which may be administered to infants through a Treatment Investigational New Drug protocol with the U.S. Food and Drug Administration. The average hospitalization of untreated infants may exceed 5 weeks. Preliminary use of BIG suggests that it can drastically reduce inpatient hospitalization by more than 50% and lower treatment costs.

In the present patient, the infant's weakness was recognized in the emergency department, and

Differential Diagnosis of Acute Floppiness During Infancy

Cortical Dysfunction
    Hypoxic/ischemic encephalopathy
    Intracranial hemorrhage
    Leukodystrophies
Anterior Horn Cell Dysfunction
    Spinal muscular atrophy
    Type II glycogen storage disease
    Poliomyelitis
Peripheral Nerve Dysfunction
    Guillain-Barré syndrome
    Metal poisoning
Neuromuscular Junction Dysfunction
    Infant botulism
    Myasthenia gravis
    Tick paralysis
Muscle Dysfunction
    Myotonic dystrophy
    Inflammatory myopathy
Systemic Illness
    Sepsis
    Meningitis/encephalitis
    Urinary tract infection
    Hypoglycemia
    Acidemia
    Electrolyte abnormality
    Cardiac failure
    Hypothyroidism
    Intussusception
    Poisoning

Common Symptoms and Signs of Infant Botulism

Symptoms	Signs
Constipation	Hypotonia
Poor feeding	Facial weakness
Weak cry	Diminished gag reflex
Drooling	Ptosis
Irritability	Sluggishly reactive
Loss of develop-	pupils
mental motor	Hyporeflexia
milestones	

the child was admitted to an intensive care unit. An electromyogram demonstrated brief, small-amplitude, abundant motor unit potentials and the "staircase phenomenon" and supported the admission diagnosis of infant botulism. A nasoduodenal tube was used for nutritional support, and respiratory function was monitored through measurement of negative inspiratory pressures. BIG was administered, bulbar weakness was resolved within 1 week, and oral feeding was resumed within 2 weeks of diagnosis. The baby recovered uneventfully.

Clinical Pearls

1. Muscular weakness can be subtle in infants and may be manifest by weak cry, loss of head control, or failure to bring hands to the midline.

2. Constipation, and the new onset of generalized weakness and cranial neuropathies, strongly suggests the diagnosis of botulism among infants under the age of 6 months.

3. Aminoglycoside antibiotics can potentiate neuromuscular weakness and should be avoided in suspected cases of infant botulism.

4. Although expensive, BIG is a beneficial and cost-effective active treatment for infant botulism.

REFERENCES

1. Davis DH, Priestley MA: A BIG treatment for a small infant with constipation and weakness. Pediatr Case Rev; 2:133–140, 2002.
2. Arnon SS: Infant botulism. In Feigen RD, Cherry JD (eds): Textbook of Pediatric Infectious Diseases. Philadelphia, WB Saunders, 1998, pp 1570–1577.

PATIENT 51

A 79-year-old woman with dyspnea

A 79-year-old woman with unknown past medical history presents to the emergency department via ambulance after several hours of progressive dyspnea at home. Paramedics report an initial room air oxygen saturation of 66% and attribute the patient's symptoms to congestive heart failure. En route, the patient received sublingual nitroglycerin (0.4 mg) and 80 mg IV furosemide without improvement. She arrives markedly dyspneic, unable to speak more than an occasional single word. She denies chest pain, productive cough, or fever.

Physical Examination: Temperature 37.1°C; pulse 120; respiratory rate 34; blood pressure 185/82; pulse oximetry 97% on 50% Venturi mask. General appearance: severe respiratory distress, diaphoretic, lethargic but arousable and cooperative. HEENT: normal. Neck: no increased jugular venous pressure. Chest: symmetrically decreased breath sounds, scant bibasilar rales, scattered wheezes, and rhonchi. Cardiac: tachycardiac, regular rhythm, without gallops or murmurs. Abdomen: normal. Extremities: no edema. Skin: no lesions. Neuromuscular: mild somnolence, no focal deficits.

Laboratory Findings: ABG (50% Venturi mask): pH 7.13, $Paco_2$ 77 mm Hg, Pao_2 107 mm Hg; calculated bicarbonate 26 mEq/L. ECG: sinus tachycardia, rate 120, left ventricular hypertrophy with repolarization abnormality (strain), no acute ST segment changes. Portable chest radiograph: lung hyperinflation and slight flattening of the diaphragm.

Questions: What is the most likely cause of this patient's respiratory distress? What intervention(s) should be considered prior to intubating this patient?

Diagnosis and Treatment: The patient demonstrates acute hypercapneic respiratory failure with relative hypoxemia, most likely due to an exacerbation of chronic obstructive pulmonary disease (COPD). In addition to inhaled beta-agonists and intravenous corticosteroids, this patient would likely benefit from an immediate trial of noninvasive positive pressure ventilation before endotracheal intubation and mechanical ventilation are attempted.

Discussion: Acute respiratory failure can be defined as any rapid decline in effective oxygenation, ventilation, or both. Impaired oxygenation results in hypoxemic failure, whereas impaired ventilation produces hypercapnea. Mixed presentations are frequent. Common causes of acute respiratory failure include asthma, COPD, pneumonia, pulmonary edema, neuromuscular disease, massive pulmonary embolism, and pulmonary hypertension. Although all of the above plus precipitant myocardial ischemia must be considered in the present patient, the physical findings and chest radiograph most strongly suggest COPD. The paramedics' assertion of congestive heart failure seems unlikely.

Regardless of the specific cause of respiratory failure, the "gold standard" of emergency respiratory support is endotracheal intubation (ETI) and mechanical ventilation. However, ETI is associated with a number of significant hazards and complications, especially in the setting of COPD. A misplaced tube can have severe, potentially fatal consequences. Successful intubations carry risk of vocal cord injury, pulmonary barotrauma, and nosocomial pneumonia. Ventilation of patients with COPD is complicated and can be associated with decreased cardiac output and hypotension.

Alternatives should be considered to avoid these risks. Noninvasive ventilation (NIV), defined as ventilatory support given to a spontaneously breathing patient without the use of an endotracheal airway is one such alternative. In practice, NIV usually takes the form of positive-pressure ventilation administered via nasal mask or full-face mask (see figure). Airway pressure can be held constant throughout the respiratory cycle or higher during inspiration (bilevel ventilation). Volume-controlled modes can also be used.

NIV can provide rapid correction of acid-base and gas exchange abnormalities, with greater patient comfort, decreased need for sedation, and preservation of normal airway defense mechanisms against infection. However, NIV requires an alert, cooperative patient without excessive se-

cretions. Risks of NIV are few and include facial skin necrosis (mostly over the bridge of the nose), aerophagia, and vomiting with aspiration (especially when a full face mask is used). When considering ETI versus NIV, the clinician must weigh the risks inherent in ETI against its major advantage of providing a definitive, secure airway. Contraindications to the use of NIV are listed in the table.

Contraindications to Noninvasive Positive-Pressure Ventilation for Acute Respiratory Failure

Uncooperative patients or patients with profound obtundation, coma, or altered mental status
Hemodynamic instability, active cardiac ischemia, serious arrhythmias, or upper gastrointestinal bleeding
Excessive oral or pulmonary secretions requiring frequent suctioning
Laryngeal edema or other need for a definitive, secure airway
Significant facial trauma

For acute respiratory failure due to COPD exacerbation, there is demonstrated benefit of NIV in reducing the need for intubation, the risk of nosocomial infection, and overall hospital mortality. Although less compelling than the COPD data, there is mounting evidence to support the use of NIV in selected patients with acute respiratory failure due to pulmonary edema and asthma. Data regarding the use of NIV for other specific causes is currently lacking.

The present patient was placed on bilevel ventilation via full-face mask and titrated to settings of 15 cm H_2O inspiratory pressure over 5 cm H_2O expiratory pressure. Within minutes, her mental status improved, respiratory rate slowed, and dyspnea lessened. A repeat ABG measurement after 30 minutes showed pH 7.32, $Paco_2$ 56 mm Hg, Pao_2 145 mm Hg. The patient was admitted to the intensive care unit but never required intubation. She was discharged home in good condition 5 days later.

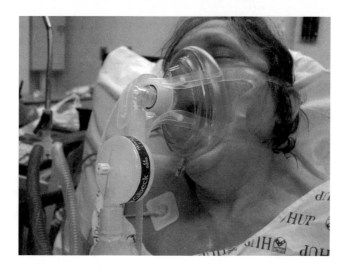

Clinical Pearls

1. NIV is not a universal substitute for endotracheal intubation, but in appropriately selected patients with acute respiratory failure, it can provide equivalent results with fewer complications.

2. A prompt empirical trial of NIV is warranted for all appropriate patients, since improvement is usually rapid and there is no evidence to suggest that a delay in intubation for those who fail to respond to NIV results in worse outcomes.

3. NIV may also be useful for patients with potentially treatable respiratory failure who are not candidates for immediate intubation because of advanced directives or terminal illness, or while awaiting clarification of individual or family preferences.

REFERENCES

1. Widger HN, Hoffmann P, Mazzolini D, et al: Pressure support noninvasive positive pressure ventilation treatment of acute cardiogenic pulmonary edema. Am J Emerg Med 19:179–181, 2001.
2. Poponick JM, Renston JP, Bennett RP, Emerman CL: Use of a ventilatory support system (BiPAP) for acute respiratory failure in the emergency department. Chest 116:166–171, 1999.
3. Hotchkiss JR, Marini JJ: Noninvasive ventilation: An emerging supportive technique for the emergency department. Ann Emerg Med 32:470–479, 1998.
4. Antonelli M, Conti G, Rocco M, et al: A comparison of noninvasive positive-pressure ventilation and conventional mechanical ventilation in patients with acute respiratory failure. N Engl J Med 339:429–435, 1998.
5. Keenan SP, Brake D: An evidence-based approach to noninvasive ventilation in acute respiratory failure. Crit Care Clin 14:359–372, 1998.

Purvi Shah, MD
Jill M. Baren, MD, FACEP, FAAP

PATIENT 52

A 24-year-old man with a swollen right hand

A 24-year-old man presents to the emergency department with fever and a painful swollen right hand. The patient was seen in the same ED 24 hours prior to the current visit for a small laceration on the dorsum of the right hand; the wound was determined not to need sutures. He states the cut occurred "at a bar when opening a bottle."

Physical Examination: Temperature 39.0°C, heart rate 106, respiratory rate 16, blood pressure 116/74. General: well appearing, no distress. Extremities: right hand with 3 mm abrasion over the fourth metacarpophalangeal (MCP) joint on the dorsum of hand with surrounding warmth and erythema (see figure). Small amount of purulent material expressed and marked tenderness with palpation of this joint. Limited range of motion on active and passive extension of the third and fourth fingers secondary to pain. Neurologic: sensation intact to light touch and two-point discrimination over the entire right hand and all fingers.

Laboratory Findings: WBC 16,000/μl, hemoglobin 14.6 g/dl, platelets 265,000/μl. Right hand plain radiograph: no fracture, no air in soft tissue, no evidence of osteomyelitis, no foreign body.

Questions: What is the most likely diagnosis? Why was this not picked up on the initial ED visit?

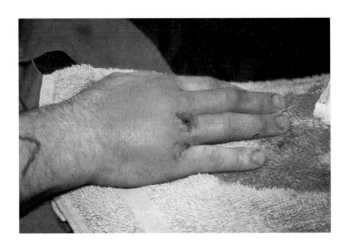

Diagnosis: Clenched-fist injury/human bite wound with subsequent septic arthritis and tenosynovitis. The injury was most likely missed during the initial encounter because the laceration was inappropriately treated as a minor wound without adequate assessment, exploration, and prophylactic antibiotic therapy.

Discussion: Clenched-fist human bite wounds are puncture wounds that occur at the third to fifth metacarpal joints on the dorsum of the hand. Affected patients are usually males, ages 18 to 34 years, who have been involved in an altercation with another individual but are reluctant to provide this information. Lacerations are typically 3 to 5 mm in length and initially may present as a benign abrasion or superficial laceration. Penetration of the tooth may violate soft tissue, extensor tendon and sheath, and possibly the MCP joint capsule. This occurs during a blow to an opponent's mouth with the assailant's fist in a clenched position (full flexion at the MCP joints). When painful contact with a tooth occurs, the assailant draws back in pain, immediately relaxing the fist and extending the fingers at the MCP joints. The soft tissues and the extensor tendons migrate proximally, potentially trapping a bacterial innoculum in the joint. Infection in this area is accelerated for two reasons. First, the joint and extensor tendon are avascular and have a decreased capacity to fight infection. Second, human saliva contains a highly concentrated amount of pathogenic organisms, reaching levels as high as 1×10^8 organisms/ml. Organisms most likely to cause infection, from most to least common, include *Staphylococcus aureus, Streptococcus* spp., *Corynebacterium* spp., and *Eikenella corrodens*. Anaerobic bacteria can also be isolated from more than 50% of wounds.

A patient may present early before any clinical manifestations of infection begin. The patient will have a harmless-appearing superficial laceration and abrasions accompanied by mild erythema. More commonly, however, the patient will ignore such a "benign-looking" insult and present several days later when signs and symptoms of infection are evident. Swelling, erythema, pain, limited range of motion, fever, and lymphadenopathy are the most common complaints. Cellulitis, tenosynovitis, and septic arthritis are common complications.

A diagnosis of soft tissue injury from a clenched-fist mechanism becomes apparent by history if explored properly, but the diagnosis is usually evident even when the patient denies a history of an altercation. Plain radiographs should be obtained to look for fractures, foreign bodies, and early signs of osteomyelitis. Surgical debridement and subsequent culture of specimen may reveal infection by pathogens present in human saliva. Bone biopsy may be necessary if bony infection is present.

All lacerations to the dorsum of the hand should be assumed to be a clenched-fist injury until proven otherwise. ED management may include appropriate exploration of deep structures as well as copious irrigation with normal saline. Puncture wounds are exceedingly difficult to irrigate, so wound care must be supplemented with appropriate broad-spectrum antibiotic prophylaxis. Amoxicillin/clavulanate, or trimethoprim sulfa/clindamycin in penicillin-allergic patients, are the best choices in patients who present early without current infection. Once a wound becomes infected, intravenous ampicillin/sulbactam, cefoxitin, or ticaracillin/clavulanate are appropriate agents, with the combination of clindamycin and a fluoroquinolone for penicillin-allergic patients. Duration of therapy depends on clinical presentation, however a general rule of thumb is 3 to 7 days for infection prophylaxis and 10 to 14 days for cellulitis and tenosynovitis.

Tetanus immunization should be updated, although transmission through oral flora is unlikely. Lastly, surgical consultation should be obtained regarding wound closure. The present patient presented after inadequate treatment of his clenched-fist human bite wound. The patient developed a septic arthritis of the third MCP joint, cellulitis, and tenosynovitis from invasion of his extensor tendon compartment. The wound was irrigated and debrided. The patient was admitted for intravenous antibiotic therapy and released 5 days later with resolving infection.

Clinical Pearls

1. Any laceration to the dorsum of the hand should be treated as a potential clenched-fist wound and appropriately irrigated, explored, and treated.

2. Most patients with clenched-fist injuries present late in the infectious course because the wound is initially ignored and as such is already infected.

3. Treatment regimens in penicillin-allergic patients can be ineffective against *Eikenella* infections. Extremely close follow-up should be arranged if the decision is made to treat these patients at home.

REFERENCES

1. Gonzales MH, Papierski P, Hall RF: Osteomyeltis of the hand after a human bite. J Hand Surg 18:520–522, 1993.
2. Kelly LP, Cunney RJ, Coleville J: The management of human bite injuries of the hand. Injury 27:481–484, 1996.
3. Chadaev AP, Jukhtin VI, Butkevich, Emkuzhev VM: Treatment of infected clench-fist human bite wounds in the area of metacarpophalangeal joints. J Hand Surg Am 21:299–303, 1996.
4. Pressutti J: Bite wounds. Postgrad Med 101:243–254, 1997.
5. Perron AD, Miller MD, Brady WJ: Orthopedic pitfalls in the ED: Fight bite. Am J Emer Med 20:114–117, 2002.
6. Baddour LM: Soft tissue infections due to human bites. Up To Date. *www.UpToDate.com:* Accessed July 21, 2002.

Diane P. Calello, MD
Kevin C. Osterhoudt, MD

PATIENT 53

A 3-year-old girl with a snakebite

A 3-year-old girl is brought to the hospital after being bitten by a snake while walking through the woods with her father behind her Pennsylvania home about 2 hours earlier. She was bitten on her left ankle once and immediately felt pain at the site of the bite. She now reports severe pain and swelling of the affected leg. She sustained no other injuries. She has no significant medical history or allergies.

Her father, a seasoned hiker, managed to disable and capture the snake and has brought it in for inspection. He has also placed a compression bandage around the patient's left leg.

Physical Examination:　Temperature 37.2°C; pulse 130; respiratory rate 40; blood pressure 90/55. General appearance: anxious, pale child who is alert and oriented. Extremities: two fang marks on the dorsum of the foot, with surrounding edema (see figure); extremely tender from the wound to just above the ankle; pulses equal in both extremities. Remainder of examination: normal.

Examination of the now-dead snake reveals a two-foot long snake with a copper-colored triangular head, elliptical pupils, and a single row of caudal plates on its undersurface (see figure).

Initial Laboratory Findings:　CBC (including platelet count), PT/PTT, fibrinogen, and D-dimer: normal.

ED Course:　The patient is placed on cardiac and blood pressure monitors, and the compression bandage is removed. The left lower extremity is immobilized and kept at a level below her heart. Despite administration of narcotics, she complains of worsening pain throughout her leg. She reports being nauseated and has three episodes of emesis. On repeat examination, she has an elevated pulse of 150 beats/min. Edema and ecchymosis have progressed to involve more than half of her left lower extremity, extending to well above the knee. Pulses are still equal in both extremities, and sensation is intact. Repeat laboratory findingsare significant for PT 14.0 (normal range 11.7–13.2), PTT normal, and D-dimer 0.6 (normal range 0.1–0.6).

Questions:　What is the diagnosis? What should the treatment plan be?

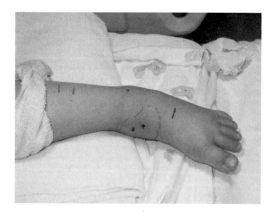 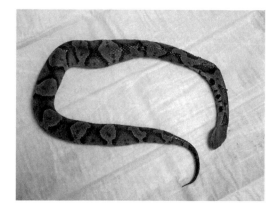

Diagnosis and Treatment: Copperhead envenomation. Given the patient's age, progression of local symptoms, and development of systemic manifestations, she is admitted to the intensive care unit and treated with crotaline antivenom.

Discussion: At least 50,000 snakebites occur in the United States each year, and at least 6000 of these are from venomous snakes. Children, along with snake handlers, collectors, and intoxicated men are the most likely victims. Snakebites can occur at any time but usually happen from May to October (when snakes are not in hibernation), between the hours of 2 and 6 PM. Bites are most often sustained on the extremities, during deliberate handling of the snake. Although bites from snakes indigenous to the United States are seldom fatal, they can have serious systemic manifestations, and fatalities, although rare, do occur.

There are approximately 30 species of venomous snakes native to this country, and most are Viperidae (subfamily Crotalinae), also known as pit vipers. Named for the heat-sensing pit behind their nostrils, these include rattlesnakes (*Crotalus*), copperheads (*Agkistrodon contortix*), and water moccasins (*Agkistrodon piscivorus,* or cottonmouths). Up to 60% of envenomations in this country are from rattlesnakes, and most lethal snakebites are inflicted by the eastern or western diamondback rattlesnake. The other group of venomous snakes found in the United States is the Elapidae, or coral snakes.

Following a bite, it is helpful to identify the offending snake. Emergency physicians should familiarize themselves with the species native to their region. In the case of snake handlers and collectors, the victim may be able to provide this information. Fortunately, in this case, the snake was brought in for inspection. Special care must be taken when inspecting snakes, even if they are dead and even decapitated, as envenomation can still occur.

Pit vipers, in contrast to their nonvenomous counterparts, have a triangular head, vertically elliptical pupils, visible long fangs (when the mouth is open), and a single (instead of double) row of caudal plates. Rattlesnakes can be up to 2 m long, and some have distinctive patterns of scales, as in the symmetrical diamond pattern of a diamondback; a "rattle" may be heard prior to attack. The water moccasin is indigenous to the Southeast and Mississippi valley and has a white mouth and buccal mucosa, thus the name "cottonmouth." The copperhead is very commonly found in the Eastern United States, is smaller, has a copper-tinged head, and is responsible for approximately 30% of venomous snakebites.

Coral snakes, in comparison, have round pupils and shorter fangs, causing them often to bite their victims repeatedly. Their distinctive black, red, and yellow bands aid in identification but may be confused with those of the nonvenomous king snake. In coral snakes, the red and yellow bands touch, whereas in the king snake the red and yellow bands are separated by a black band ("Red on yellow kills a fellow; red on black, venom lack").

Pathophysiology: Pit viper venom is a heterogeneous composition of enzymes and polypeptides that have a vast array of hematotoxic, neurotoxic, nephrotoxic, and necrotizing effects. Most pit viper venom causes endothelial injury and increased capillary permeability, leading to edema and tissue necrosis. The Mojave rattlesnake in particular has a potent neurotoxin that can cause cranial nerve dysfunction and respiratory paralysis. The South American rattlesnake's venom has potent opioid effects, leading to analgesia at the wound that can mask impending systemic effects.

Envenomation results in both local and systemic effects, owing to the fact that venom is initially deposited into the tissue surrounding the bite and subsequently distributed throughout the circulation. The quantity of venom injected varies with the species and temperament of snake, the geographic location, and the time of year. In fact, up to 20% of pit viper bites are "dry," with no envenomation at all. Intuitively, the more venom that is injected, the more extensive the envenomation will be. In addition, children and the elderly are at much greater risk for severe manifestations. The site of the bite may also influence the amount of toxicity; face, head and neck wounds result in particularly extensive involvement, because high vascularity hastens systemic distribution of venom. Rattlesnake envenomation is the most severe, followed by water moccasins; copperhead envenomation is usually mild, with few systemic effects.

Clinical Presentation: Even if the snake cannot be positively identified, the characteristic effects of its venom should be. Within seconds to minutes after a pit viper bite, the victim will feel pain, often severe, at the site. Over the next 30 to 60 minutes, edema, erythema, and ecchymosis develop around the bite, as microvascular injury worsens. Serous or hemorrhagic blebs often arise, sometimes accompanied by signs of lymphangitis. Patients may complain of tingling or paresthesias of the affected extremity. As vascular permeability increases, direct tissue necrosis can ensue, with both local myonecrosis and generalized se-

Local: pain, edema, ecchymosis, petechiae, hemorrhagic/serous blebs, myonecrosis
Neurologic: perioral paresthesias, taste abnormalities, tingling/numbness in affected area, altered mental status, coma, fasciculations, cranial nerve palsies, respiratory paralysis
Renal: acute renal failure
Gastrointestinal: nausea, vomiting, diarrhea, abdominal pain, hematemesis, hematochezia
Respiratory: acute respiratory distress syndrome, pleural effusions, pulmonary edema
Cardiovascular: tachycardia, hypotension, cardiovascular collapse/cardiac arrest
Heme: thrombocytopenia, hypofibrinogenemia, hypoprothrombinemia, hemolysis, fibrinolysis

---

vere rhabdomyolysis. An exception to this dramatic local presentation is a bite from the Mojave and South American rattlesnakes, which cause deceptively mild local effects.

Systemic effects develop minutes to hours after local toxicity, as the venom reaches the general circulation slowly through subcutaneous lymphatic channels. Fortunately, direct intravascular injection of venom, often fatal, is rare. Systemic manifestations range from mild to severe (see table) and involve multiple organ systems. Mild effects (tachycardia, tachypnea, nausea, vomiting, pallor, diaphoresis, and altered mental status) are often indistinguishable from the anxiety and terror most patients experience after a snakebite. Increased capillary permeability leads to pulmonary edema, hypovolemia, acute renal failure, decreased end-organ perfusion, and shock. Neurotoxins can have a wide range of effects, from a metallic taste and perioral paresthesias to fasciculations, weakness, cranial nerve dysfunction, and respiratory paralysis. Pit viper venom can also cause renal failure via myoglobinuria, hemoglobinuria, and cardiovascular collapse, as well as through direct nephrotoxic effects.

The effect of crotaline venom on coagulation and platelet count causes a broad derangement of hematologic parameters. The prothrombin time (PT), activated partial thromboplastin time (PTT), fibrin split products, and D-dimer can be markedly elevated, and the fibrinogen level and platelet count markedly decreased. As a result, after a pit viper bite, patients may develop a consumptive coagulopathy very similar to disseminated intravascular coagulation, with a risk of both life-threatening bleeding and clot formation.

Prehospital Management: For the prehospital setting, many unnecessary practices have been promulgated in both the lay and medical literature. Cryotherapy and, in most settings, tourniquet placement have been shown to have little to no benefit in ameliorating pit viper envenomation and may delay time to definitive hospital care and antivenom administration. Incision and mechanical

suction (mouth suction should never be performed) removes a variable amount of venom, must be performed within 30 minutes of the attack, may increase tissue ischemia and infection, and is indicated only, if ever, in the deteriorating patient with severe rattlesnake envenomation. The most important goal of prehospital care is to transport the patient to the emergency department as expeditiously as possible. Constrictive clothing, watches, and jewelry should be removed. In addition, the affected body part should be immobilized at or below the level of the heart, and activity, which may hasten the distribution of venom through the general circulation, should be avoided.

In circumstances in which severe envenomation has most definitely occurred and/or the patient is hours away from medical care, the placement of a loose compression band proximal to the site of the bite may be effective in slowing systemic absorption of venom. It is crucial that this is not an arteriovenous tourniquet, which can worsen tissue ischemia, but a wide (2–4 cm), loose, constricting band intended to decrease lymphatic flow. No prospective data exist on the benefits of this practice, and it may worsen local tissue damage as the venom pools in the affected extremity. Also, sudden worsening of systemic symptoms after compression band removal has been reported, so once in place, the band should be removed gradually and, if applicable, only after antivenom administration.

In-Hospital Management: Patients without any signs of envenomation, in whom a bite from a venomous snake cannot be ruled out, should be observed for at least 8 hours for the possibility of a delayed reaction. After a copperhead bite, if the patient is asymptomatic or shows only local manifestations with no progression, he or she may be released after 4 to 6 hours. If the bite is from a Mojave rattlesnake, coral snake, or non-native species of snake, observation for 24 hours is recommended.

In the symptomatic patient, after the principles of basic life support are established, a focused history and physical examination should be performed, with special attention to the patient's tetanus immunization status, history of prior snakebites or snake exposure, and history of contact with horses or horse serum products (see crotaline antivenom, below). Circumferential measurements of the affected area proximal and distal to the bite should be obtained, and the advancing edge of edema should be marked; these should be re-evaluated every 20 minutes for progression.

Initial laboratory evaluation should include a complete blood cell count (CBC), electrolytes, blood urea nitrogen (BUN), creatinine, urinalysis, PT/PTT, fibrinogen, and fibrin split products or D-dimer assay. These should be repeated every 4 to 6 hours as abnormalities evolve. Additional studies to consider initially include a creatine kinase level, blood typing and screening, chest radiographs, and electrocardiogram.

Antivenom: The decision to administer antivenom to a snakebite victim should be individualized based on the patient's age, the species of the snake, and the severity of clinical presentation. In general, antivenom should be considered in any patient who demonstrates systemic toxicity and progression of local injury or whose condition becomes unstable at any time.

There are two types of antivenom available for the treatment of crotaline snakebite in the United States, both of which are in somewhat short supply. ACP (Antivenin Crotalidae Polyvalent, Wyeth-Ayerst) is an equine product containing crotaline-specific IgG obtained from the sera of hyperimmunized horses exposed to four species of Viperidae. It is effective against all species of pit vipers, although some reports suggest it may have limited efficacy against copperheads and the timber rattlesnake. Owing to its imperfect purification process, a number of other immunogenic proteins, such as albumin, globulins, and nonspecific IgM, are also found in this antivenom. As a result, there is a significant risk of acute reactions, such as urticaria and anaphylaxis (23–56%) and an even greater incidence of serum-sickness reactions 7 to 10 days later (75–86%).

Another antivenom has recently emerged that seems to have a more favorable side-effect profile. Crotalidae Polyvalent Immune Fab (CroFab, FabAV, Protherics and Savage Laboratories) is obtained by immunizing flocks of sheep to one of four crotaline venoms. However, the immune sera obtained are then digested with papain to produce Fab and Fc antibody fragments; the immunogenic Fc fragments are discarded, leaving the more specific Fab fragments in the antivenom. In addition, the concentration of other extraneous proteins is much lower. It is not surprising, then, that preliminary data suggest a much lower rate of acute (14%) and delayed (16%) reactions with FabAv.

Clearly the risks of adverse reactions are significant with either product, and for that reason antivenom should without exception be administered in an intensive care setting. Skin testing with horse sera (for ACP) and pretreatment with antihistamines may be of some value. Suggested initial doses and dosage schedules vary; these decisions should be made in consultation with a local poison center and toxicologist. An important issue to bear in mind, however, is that recurrence of symptoms does occur after initial administration of antivenom, and repeated doses are often necessary, especially with the newer FabAV product.

The present patient, although she initially demonstrated mild local symptoms, developed progression of local toxicity (increased swelling, ecchymosis, and pain) as well as early signs of coagulopathy. Although copperhead bite victims rarely require antivenom, her young age and therefore increased risk for severe envenomation warranted this treatment early in her course. After a negative anti-horse-serum skin test, pretreatment with diphenhydramine was given, and five vials of ACP were infused over 90 minutes. She experienced no acute reaction. Her hematologic parameters normalized, and she experienced no further progression of local symptoms. She was discharged home 2 days later.

Clinical Pearls

1. The pit vipers, or Crotalinae, consist of rattlesnakes, copperhead, and cottonmouths and are responsible for more than 90% of snakebites in the United States.

2. First-aid measures such as incision and suction, cryotherapy, and tourniquet placement have little value and may actually harm crotaline snakebite victims.

3. Copperhead snakebite, while usually associated with mild symptoms, may be more severe in children and may require antivenom therapy.

4. There are two antivenoms available against crotaline snakebites. Both are in short supply, with significant side effects, and the decision to use them should be based on the age of the patient, the species of the snake involved, and the severity of envenomation.

REFERENCES

1. Gold BS, Dart RC, Barish RA: Bites of venomous snakes. N Engl J Med 347:347–356, 2002.
2. Roberts JR, Otten EJ: Snakes and other reptiles. In Goldfrank LR, Flomenbaum NE, Lewin NA, et al (eds): Goldfrank's Toxicologic Emergencies, 7th ed. New York, McGraw-Hill, 2002.
3. Dart RC, McNally J: Efficacy, safety, and use of snake antivenoms in the United States. Ann Emerg Med 37:181–188, 2001.
4. Dart RC, Seifert SA, Boyer LV, et al: A randomized multicenter trial of crotalinae polyvalent immune Fab (ovine) antivenom for the treatment for crotaline snakebite in the United States. Arch Intern Med 161:2030–2036, 2001.
5 Hodge D, Tecklenburg FW: Bites and Stings. In Fleisher GR, Ludwig S (eds): Textbook of Pediatric Emergency Medicine, 4th ed. Philadelphia, Lippincott Williams & Wilkins, 2000.
6. Dart RC, Seifert SA, Carroll L, et al: Affinity-purified, mixed monospecific crotalid antivenom ovine Fab for the treatment of crotalid venom poisoning. Ann Emerg Med 30:33–39, 1997.
7. Dart RC, Hurlbut KM, Garcia R, Boren J: Validation of a severity score for the assessment of crotalid snakebite. Ann Emerg Med 27:321–326, 1996.

Nancy N. Sun, MD
Suzanne Shepherd, MD, DTM&H

PATIENT 54

A 50-year-old man with altered mental status

A 50-year-old man is brought to the emergency department by a friend after he was found disoriented, vomiting, incontinent of urine, and wandering around his apartment with a slow, uncoordinated gait. His past medical history is significant for poorly controlled hypertension, for which he takes clonidine, felodipine, atenolol, and furosemide.

Physical Examination: Temperature 36.2°C; pulse 73; respirations 28; blood pressure 290/152. Skin: no lesions. HEENT: normal. Pupils 4 mm, round, reactive to light and accommodation. Patient unable to cooperate with fundoscopic examination. Gag reflex intact. Chest: clear to auscultation. Cardiac: regular rate and rhythm without gallops or murmurs. Abdomen: normal. Extremities: no edema. Neuromuscular: awake and oriented to person only, murmurs incomprehensibly, responds to voice, spontaneously moves all extremities, withdraws to pain, but does not follow commands. Normal muscle strength and reflexes. Shuffling but steady gait noted.

Laboratory Findings: CBC: normal. Blood chemistries: Normal anion gap. Elevated BUN 44 (normal < 20), creatinine 3.8 (normal <1.5, patient's baseline 2.0), glucose 97. Liver function tests: normal. Cardiac enzymes: normal. ABG: normal. Urinalysis: moderate protein and blood. Urine toxicology screen positive for cocaine. ECG (see figure next page): 1-mm ST segment depressions in lead II, III, AVF. Chest radiograph: no active disease.

Questions: How would you manage this patient's blood pressure? How would you manage his cardiac ischemia?

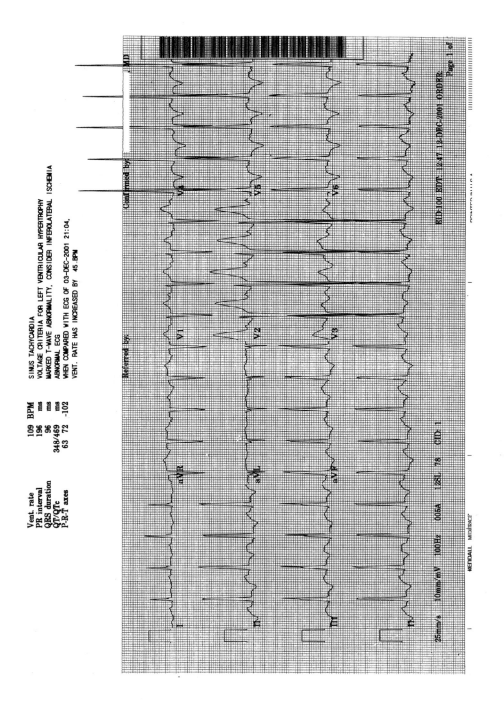

Diagnosis and Treatment: Hypertensive emergency/malignant hypertension with evidence of end-organ damage. Hypertensive encephalopathy, cardiac ischemia, and renal insufficiency are all present in this patient. For treatment options, see table.

Discussion: Hypertensive encephalopathy and evaluation for an acute hypertensive intracranial hemorrhage is a true medical emergency. Blood pressure will need to be reduced emergently to reduce the likelihood of death and further end-organ damage. The goal is reduction of mean arterial pressure by 20% to 25% over 1 hour, and lowering diastolic pressure to 100 to 110 mm Hg. More rapid reduction can worsen end-organ damage. If an elderly patient has been hypertensive for many years, normal cerebral autoregulation mechanisms may be lost, and reduction should take place over several hours. True hypertensive emergencies require parenteral agents for management and immediate titration of effects. A centrally acting oral agent such as clonidine should be avoided. Use of diuretic agents should also be avoided unless it is necessary to treat fluid overload states such as congestive heart failure. The agent of choice for most hypertensive emergencies is intravenous nitro-

prusside, a fast-acting vasodilator with a short duration of action. This agent is relatively contraindicated in pregnancy.

There are several causes for the present patient's extreme hypertension: baseline essential hypertension and renal insufficiency, acute cocaine intoxication, and possible clonidine withdrawal due to noncompliance. His cardiac ischemia is most likely secondary to increased left ventricular wall stress and myocardial oxygen demand in the setting of severe hypertension. Reduction of blood pressure in the setting of cardiac ischemia is best achieved with intravenous labetalol and/or intravenous nitroglycerin/nitroprusside. Ischemia will likely be reversed with a decrease in blood pressure, and therefore typical agents used to treat ischemia, such as heparin, may not be indicated for this patient because of the risk of hemorrhage. In the setting of renal end-oran damage, a relatively newer agent, fenoldopam, has shown good results. Fenoldopam, a dopamine agonist, has been found to improves natriuresis, diuresis, and creatinine clearance.

The present patient's blood pressure was refractory to management and required intravenous infusions of nitroprusside, nicardipine, and phentolamine to lower blood pressure to 190/120. Use of intravenous labetalol was attempted but aborted after the patient developed bronchospasm. An arterial line was established for monitoring purposes. A subsequent magnetic resonance imaging scan of the brain was notable for multiple thalamic infarcts. Further injury to the kidneys and heart were averted.

Treatment Options in Hypertensive Emergencies

CAUSE	TREATMENT DRUG
Stroke/acute cocaine intoxication	Labetalol
Other neurologic (not including stroke)	Nitroprusside or labetalol
Cardiac	Nitroglycerin or nitroprusside and labetalol
Renal	Fenoldopam
Pregnancy	Hydralazine
Catecholamine excess	Phentolamine

Clinical Pearls

1. Careful reduction of blood pressure should be the goal of treatment in hypertensive emergencies, with the recognition that rapid decreases can result in greater morbidity.

2. There is no single agent appropriate in every case of hypertensive emergency with end-organ damage. Each clinical situation must be examined independently before pharmacologic choices are made.

3. In the setting of hypertensive emergency and cardiac ischemia, usual anti-ischemic agents may not be necessary if blood pressure control is achieved rapidly.

REFERENCES
1. Gray R, Mathews J: Hypertension. In Rosen P, et al (eds): Emergency Medicine: Concepts and Clinical Practice, 5th ed. St. Louis, Mosby-Year Book, 2002.
2. Elliott WJ: Hypertensive emergencies. Crit Care Clin 17:435–451, 2001.
3. Vaughan CJ, Delanty N: Hypertensive emergencies. Lancet 356:411–417, 2000.

Todd Severson, MD
Anthony J. Dean, MD

PATIENT 55

A 60-year-old man with weakness

A 60-year-old man with past medical history of hypertension, myocardial infarction 2 years ago (status-post angioplasty with stent placement), and mild congestive heart failure, presents to the emergency department complaining of progressive generalized weakness for the past 24 hours. The patient's wife reports that he has not been feeling well for several days, and tonight was too weak to feed himself. His speech seemed slurred earlier, but it is normal now. The patient denies chest pain, shortness of breath, fevers, or other symptoms.

Physical Examination: Temperature 37°C; pulse 74; respiratory rate 16; blood pressure 100/64; pulse oximetry 98% on 2 L nasal cannula oxygen. General appearance: lethargic but interactive, answers appropriately. HEENT: normal. Neck: no increased jugular vein pressure. Chest: lungs clear to auscultation. Cardiac: distant heart sounds, regular rate and rhythm, no murmurs, gallops, or rubs. Abdomen: normal. Rectal: normal tone, brown stool, guaiac negative. Extremities: no edema. Skin: no lesions. Neuromuscular: profound proximal muscle weakness of all four extremities with strength 3/5, milder distal extremity weakness 4/5, symmetric 1+ reflexes, cranial nerves intact, normal speech, sensation grossly intact.

Laboratory Findings: Fingerstick glucose: 113. Initial ECG (Fig. 1): normal sinus rhythm, rate 74, anteroseptal Q waves and right bundle-branch block. When compared to the patient's baseline ECG, the only significant changes are lengthening of the PR interval and less prominent P waves. While awaiting blood test results, the nurse notes a change on the cardiac monitor. A repeat ECG is obtained (Fig. 2).

Questions: What is the cause of this patient's weakness? What immediate interventions are necessary?

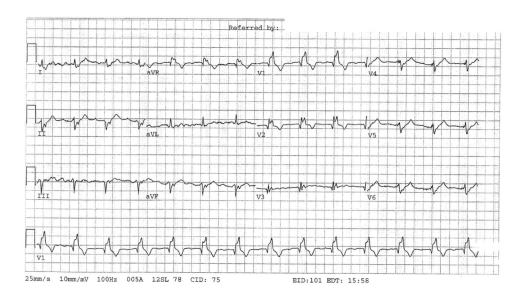

25mm/s   10mm/mV   100Hz   005A   12SL 78   CID: 75   EID:101 EDT: 15:58

FIGURE 1

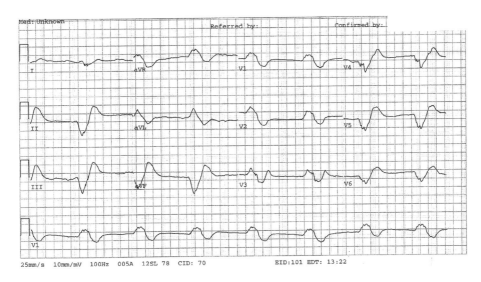

Med: Unknown   Referred by: Confirmed by:

25mm/s   10mm/mV   100Hz   005A   12SL 78   CID: 70   EID:101 EDT: 13:22

FIGURE 2

Diagnosis and Treatment: Figure 2 shows a wide complex ventricular escape rhythm with a nearly "sine wave" pattern, consistent with profound hyperkalemia. The patient received immediate treatment with 9.2 mEq of intravenous calcium gluconate (20 ml of 10% solution) and 100 mEq of intravenous sodium bicarbonate, resulting in rapid, appreciable narrowing of the QRS complexes on the cardiac monitor.

Discussion: Hyperkalemia is a potentially life-threatening metabolic abnormality. Elevated potassium has a direct effect on cardiac conduction tissue, which may result in serious arrhythmias, including ventricular fibrillation, complete heart block, and asystole. Other symptoms of hyperkalemia include muscular weakness, areflexia, paresthesias, nausea, and vomiting. Hyperkalemia may be classified as mild (K+ 5.5–6.0 mmol/L), moderate (K+ 6.1–7.0 mmol/L), or severe (K+ > 7.0 mmol/L). While the severity of clinical manifestations generally correlates with the degree of potassium elevation, symptom thresholds may vary widely among individual patients, depending in part on the rapidity of the increase. Renal failure, both acute and chronic, is the most common cause of hyperkalemia. However, a number of other conditions can result in elevated potassium, including adrenal insufficiency, diabetic ketoacidosis, rhabdomyolysis, acute digoxin toxicity, and use of medications affecting kidney function (such as nonsteroidal anti-inflammatory drugs [NSAIDs], angiotensin-converting enzyme inhibitors, beta-blockers, and potassium-sparing diuretics).

Diagnosis of hyperkalemia is confirmed by definitive serum measurements; however, given the inherent delays involved in blood sampling and laboratory analysis, early diagnosis and treatment of hyperkalemia are often dependent on recognition of its characteristic electrocardiographic manifestations. The most common (and most frequently recognized) ECG abnormality of hyperkalemia is tall, "peaked" T waves in the precordial leads. Other changes with mild to moderate hyperkalemia include prolongation of the PR interval and P-wave flattening. At severe elevations, the QRS complex widens, ultimately blending with the T wave to produce a "sine wave" pattern that can rapidly deteriorate into ventricular fibrillation or asystole. Importantly, contrary to common opinion, the ECG is not perfectly reliable for determining hyperkalemia. Classic manifestations may be absent, and atypical changes may also occur.

In the present patient, the initial ECG does not demonstrate classically peaked T waves. Because of this, the existing P wave and PR segment changes were not immediately recognized as hyperkalemia. Initial patient care became focused on sorting through the differential diagnosis: sepsis, stroke, myocardial infarction, neuromuscular disease, metabolic derangements, drugs, or toxins. Laboratory results were delayed, and as a result, the correct diagnosis of hyperkalemia was not made until potentially life-threatening QRS widening occurred.

Treatment of symptomatic hyperkalemia must be rapid and aggressive. The three phases of treatment are: (1) stabilization of cardiac membrane tissue, (2) redistribution of potassium from the extracellular to the intracellular space, and (3) elimination of excess potassium from the body. Stabilization is achieved initially with intravenous calcium (chloride or gluconate). Sodium bicarbonate helps stabilize membranes and also shifts potassium intracellularly. Combined administration of insulin and dextrose, as well as use of inhaled beta-agonists, can further shift potassium into cells. Potassium excretion can be achieved by use of loop diuretics and/or cation exchange resin (sodium polystyrene, Kayexalate). Emergency hemodialysis may also be required to correct severe or persistent hyperkalemia, but because of the delays inherent in arranging this procedure, symptomatic patients must be stabilized initially with the pharmacologic steps outlined above.

After administration of calcium and bicarbonate, the present patient received 10 units of regular insulin IV along with 25 g IV dextrose. In addition, he received 0.5 ml nebulized albuterol, 50 g oral sodium polystyrene sulfonate (Kayexalate), and 40 mg IV furosemide. Subsequent laboratory results demonstrated acute renal failure with a serum creatinine level of 9.4 mg/dl (prior baseline was 1.5 mg/dl). The initial potassium level was 8.5 mmol/L. The patient was admitted to the ICU for further management and consideration of hemodialysis. His acute renal failure was believed to be due to a combination of dehydration and excessive NSAID use after a preceding viral illness. The patient recovered well and was discharged to home in good condition 7 days later.

Clinical Pearls

1. Recognition of characteristic electrocardiographic abnormalities is often crucial to the early diagnosis of hyperkalemia; however, the ECG is not perfectly reliable in this regard. "Classic" ECG changes are not always present, and atypical manifestations can occur.

2. The three phases of emergency treatment for symptomatic hyperkalemia are membrane stabilization, redistribution from the extracellular to the intracellular space, and excretion. Rapid, aggressive intervention is essential.

3. In cases of hyperkalemia due to acute digoxin toxicity, calcium administration is relatively contraindicated and should be used with caution, as it may enhance the toxic effects of cardiac glycosides.

REFERENCES

1. Mattu A, Brady WJ, Robinson DA: Electrocardiographic manifestations of hyperkalemia. Am J Emerg Med 18:721–729, 2000.
2. Ahee P, Crowe AV: The management of hyperkalemia in the emergency department. J Accid Emerg Med 17:188–191, 2000.
3. Thadhani R, Pascual M, Bonventre JV: Acute renal failure. N Engl J Med 334:1448–1459, 1996.

PATIENT 56

An 8-year-old girl with fever and a neck mass

The mother of a previously healthy 8-year-old girl brings her to the emergency department because of persistent fevers and a left-sided neck mass. The child was initially evaluated at an outside hospital 6 days prior for fevers to 40°C and a painful swelling of the left side of her neck. A rapid strep test at the time was negative and the child was started on amoxicillin/clavulanate for presumed bacterial lymphadenitis. The day prior to coming to the emergency department, the child developed bilateral "red eyes" and a rash involving the trunk, palms, and soles. She continues to have fever daily, occasionally reports chills, and has had several loose stools each day but no vomiting. She denies having a sore throat. Her oral intake has been poor. She was born in the United States and has had no recent travel. There are no pets at home and no known tick exposure.

Physical Examination: Vital signs: temperature 39.2°C orally; pulse 112; respiratory rate 22; blood pressure 102/65; pulse oxymetry 100% on room air. General: ill appearing but in no distress. HEENT: bilateral conjunctival injection sparing the limbus without exudate, pearly tympanic membranes bilaterally, no nasal discharge, dry mucous membranes, oropharynx erythematous without exudates, uvula midline, "strawberry tongue," no cracked lips. Neck: supple without meningismus, left-sided neck mass that is 4 cm by 4 cm, moderately tender, mobile, with no overlying erythema or fluctuance, no other lymphadenopathy. Chest: clear to auscultation without stridor. Cardiac: regular rate and rhythm without murmur, rubs, or gallop, 2-second capillary refill. Abdomen: normal bowel sounds, soft, not distended, tender in the right upper quadrant with a palpable mass 5 cm in diameter, rectal is guiac negative. Skin: erythematous maculopapular rash prominent in the axilla and inguinal region, erythroderma of the palms and soles, no peeling of the digits, and no petechiae.

Laboratory Findings: CBC: WBC 18,000/μl with 75% PMNs and 8% bands, hemoglobin 11.7 g/dl, and platelets 243,000/μl. Electrolytes: within normal limits with the exception of a phosphorus of 2.0 mg/dl (normal range 2.5–4.5 mg/dl). Albumin 2.3 g/dl (normal 3.5–5.0 g/dl), total bilirubin 6.3 mg/dl, direct bilirubin 5.2 mg/dl (normal range <0.4 mg/dl and <1.3 mg/dl, respectively), transaminases within normal limits, GGT 163 U/L (normal range<50 U/L). ESR: 111 mm/hr (normal <20 mm/hr). Urine dipstick: pH 7.0, SG 1.025, large leukocytes, negative nitrites, moderate ketones, positive for bilirubin, and no blood, glucose, or protein. Urine microscopy: WBC >50/hpf, RBC 0/hpf, bacteria negative. ECG: see figure. Chest x-ray: no infiltrate, no mediastinal mass, normal heart size.

ED Course: The child was given a 20 ml/kg normal saline bolus. An ultrasonogram of the abdomen was performed, revealing a distended, fluid-filled gallbladder without stones, consistent with hydrops. Cardiology was consulted, given the ECG findings of RV conduction delay and inverted/flattened T-waves in inferolateral leads. The patient was admitted to the general inpatient floor for definitive therapy.

Questions: What is the diagnosis? What are the potential complications?

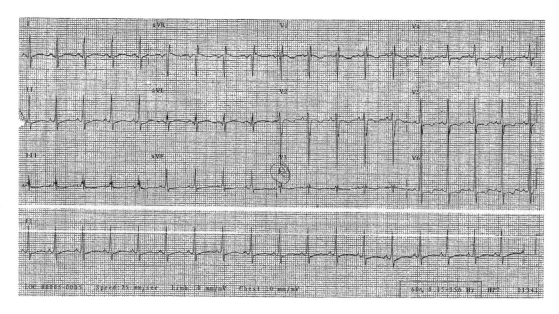

Diagnosis: Kawasaki disease (mucocutaneous lymph node syndrome). The most serious complication is coronary artery aneurysms and acute myocardial infarction.

Discussion: In 1962, Dr. Tomisaku Kawasaki first described what later came to be called the *mucocutaneous lymph node syndrome*, and now the disease that bears his name. Kawasaki disease (KD) is a clinical diagnosis requiring four of the five CDC disease-defining criteria. The child must have fever for at least 5 days, have no other explanation for the illness, and possess at least four of the following:

1. Bilateral conjunctival injection. It is often prominent and nonexudative and spares the corneal-scleral junction (i.e., the limbus).

2. Oral mucous membrane involvement. This may include generalized oropharyngeal erythema, red/cracked lips, or a "strawberry tongue."

3. Polymorphous rash. Any type of rash may be associated with KD, but it is often most prominent in the diaper region in smaller children and intertrigenous areas of older children.

4. Peripheral extremity changes. This may include either hand/foot swelling or palmer/plantar erythema. Late in the disease, there may be desquamation of the fingers and toes.

5. Cervical lymphadenopathy. Often unilateral and isolated to one node, this is the least commonly associated finding in KD.

Up to 10% of cases of KD are "atypical," having fever and cardiac abnormalities that are highly suggestive of the disease but with fewer than four of the above criteria.

KD is a systemic vasculitis that may affect any organ system. Hypothesized causes have included carpet cleaner use, living near standing bodies of water, and infectious agents. Recent studies have implicated bacterial superantigens. This remains controversial, and evidence exists that both supports and refutes the theory. There are several risk factors associated with developing KD. Males are affected more commonly than females, with a ratio of 1.5:1. It is more common in toddler-aged children, with approximately 85% of cases occurring in children less than 5 years old. Regional epidemics have been reported and peaks occur in the spring and winter. Being of Asian ancestry is a major risk factor, although the disease has been reported in nearly every ethnic group. Current estimates of the incidence of KD in the United States range from 4 to 15 per 100,000 children under 5 years old. In contrast, the incidence in Japan is 30 times greater, with similar rates seen in Japanese Americans.

Although the diagnosis of KD is based on the presence of the aforementioned clinical criteria, several commonly associated symptoms and laboratory abnormalities may provide additional supportive evidence. Most affected children are quite irritable, and up to one third have aseptic meningitis. Common gastrointestinal complaints include mild abdominal pain, vomiting, loose stools, and right upper quadrant tenderness. The last symptom may be due to hydrops of the gallbladder, an infrequent but clinically significant complication that can lead to direct hyperbilirubinemia or even surgical exploration. Arthritis, particularly of the small joints, is common in the first week of illness. Nonspecific markers of inflammation such as C-reactive protein or the erythroycte sedimentation rate are often markedly elevated; if normal, they might suggest an alternate diagnosis. There maybe a mild to moderate peripheral leukocytosis and a normochromic, normocytic anemia. The serum albumin and phosphorus levels can be low but rarely require intervention. There is often an associated sterile pyuria. Initial ECG findings may include evidence of pericarditis, myocarditis, or ST-segment changes. In the second week of the disease, the platelet count may exceed 1 million/mm^3 and the fingers and toes may begin to peel.

Approximately 20% of untreated children with KD develop cardiac complications, including pericarditis, myocarditis, coronary artery aneurysms, acute myocardial infarction, or sudden death. Currently, KD is the most common cause of acquired heart disease in children in developed countries. The larger the coronary artery aneurysms are at presentation, the less likely they are to regress and the more likely they are to form stenotic lesions. There may be endothelial dysfunction even in children without detectable coronary artery lesions.

The initial treatment for KD is intravenous immunoglobulin (IVIG), 2 g/kg administered over 10 hours and high-dose aspirin therapy (>80 mg/kg/day). When administered within 10 days of the onset of fever, IVIG has been shown to decrease the incidence of coronary artery abnormalities by 10-fold. Although most centers continue to use high-dose aspirin therapy initially, recent evidence suggests that it may be unnecessary when using the 2 g/kg IVIG protocol. Treatment with steroids remains controversial and limited to children with recrudescent disease who have failed repeated doses of IVIG.

In the present patient, the presence of all five diagnostic criteria in association with prolonged fever confirms the diagnosis of KD. In addition, many of the commonly associated laboratory findings are present. Her ECG is worrisome for the fact that she already has evidence of cardiac involvement. She was begun on an infusion of IVIG and high-dose aspirin. Echocardiography revealed mild mitral regurgitation and a low-normal left ventricular shortening fraction of 28%, consistent with myocarditis. No coronary artery aneurysms were noted. She defervesced and clinically improved within 24 hours of beginning treatment. She was discharged from the hospital on low-dose aspirin therapy (4 mg/kg/day) with the duration of treatment pending follow-up echocardiography results. An echocardiogram 6 weeks later showed normal cardiac function, no evidence of mitral regurgitation, and normal coronary arteries.

Clinical Pearls

1. Early diagnosis and treatment of Kawasaki disease is important to reduce the risk of cardiac sequelae.

2. The clinician must maintain a high index of suspicion, as not all of the diagnostic criteria for KD may be present at the same time, making a detailed review of the patient's history imperative.

3. The vasculitis may affect multiple organ systems, including the cardiovascular system, central nervous system, gastrointestinal tract, skin, and joints.

4. Close follow-up of these children is imperative to reduce the risk of long-term cardiac sequelae.

REFERENCES

1. Burns JC, Kushner HI, Bastian JF, et al: Kawasaki disease: A brief history. Pediatrics 106:e27, 2000.
2. Meissner HC, Leung DY: Superantigens, conventional antigens and the etiology of Kawasaki syndrome. Pediatr Infect Dis J 19:91–94, 2000.
3. Curtis N, Levin M: Kawasaki disease thirty years on. Curr Opin Pediatr 10:24–33, 1998.
4. Durongpisitkul K, Gururaj VJ, Park JM, Martin CF: The prevention of coronary artery aneurysm in Kawasaki disease: a meta-analysis on the efficacy of aspirin and immunoglobulin treatment. Pediatrics 96:1057–1061, 1995.

Marilyn Howarth, MD

PATIENT 57

A 35-year-old woman with acute onset of dyspnea

A 35-year-old female day care worker was transported by ambulance to the emergency department after becoming short of breath immediately after eating salad (no dressing) at a restaurant with her family. The EMTs reported that she was breathing fairly comfortably when they arrived. They noted her medical alert bracelet indicating that she had latex allergy. They immediately removed the latex gloves that they were wearing, but very soon after, the woman became much more short of breath.

Physical Examination: Vital signs: temperature 37°C, pulse 120, respiratory rate 38 and labored, blood pressure 148/84. Skin: diffuse urticaria. HEENT: angioedema of the lips and oropharynx. Chest: labored breathing with use of accessory muscles of respiration, diffuse wheezing. Cardiac: tachycardia with no murmurs. Abdomen: normal. Extremities: no cyanosis, clubbing, or edema. Neurologic: alert, oriented, and anxious.

Laboratory Findings: CBC: normal. Blood chemistries: normal. Electrocardiogram: sinus tachycardia at 120. Chest x-ray: normal. ABG (room air): pH 7.47, $PaCO_2$ 30 mm Hg, PaO_2 120 mm Hg, calculated bicarbonate 22 mEq/L.

Questions: What should be done to treat this severe allergic reaction (anaphylaxis)? Why is it important to attempt to identify the cause of the allergy early in the care?

Diagnosis and Treatment: Anaphylaxis due to type I latex allergy. Initial treatment should be supportive with epinephrine, intravenous fluids, diphenhydramine, and oxygen. If unsuccessful, airway obstruction must be considered and endotracheal intubation may be required. It is equally important to identify and remove all latex-containing materials from the patient's health care environment.

Discussion: Anaphylaxis is a life-threatening systemic allergic reaction to an antigen in a previously sensitized patient. The classic signs are respiratory distress, with or without vascular collapse usually preceded by urticaria and/or angioedema. Angioedema and urticaria are caused by the release of endogenous histamine. Vascular collapse likely involves histamine and prostaglandin (PGD_2). Natural rubber latex is a complex mixture of hundreds of proteins and lipids extracted from the sap of a tree. At least 10 proteins found in natural rubber latex have been found to be antigenic, but it remains unclear whether patients with type I latex allergy react to one or more of these proteins or others yet to be identified. Few type I latex allergic patients have anaphylaxis, but those who do are at risk for recurrence.

Latex is found in more than 40,000 commercial products. However, only 1 to 2% of the general population is allergic to latex. The exact mechanism of sensitization has not been elucidated. Epidemiologic studies have identified several risk factors for the development of latex allergy: atopy, history of repeated urogenital procedures as a child, spina bifida, and work that requires frequent latex glove use. Prevalence rates range from 15% in atopic patients, to 18% in some groups of health care workers, to 60% in patients with spina bifida. Avoiding all latex is virtually impossible. Avoiding direct contact with latex, in particular gloves, tourniquets, balloons, and other products with a similar elastic consistency has been shown to decrease symptoms in sensitized patients.

Soon after eating salad that had been prepared by a food handler wearing latex gloves, the present patient became acutely short of breath and noted generalized pruritis. The patient's husband administered epinephrine and she began to feel better. By this time, the restaurant owner had called the ambulance. This patient had type I latex allergy noted on her medical alert bracelet and she and her husband both informed the EMTs of her allergy immediately. However, the EMTs only carried latex gloves and were wearing them when they arrived. They immediately removed the gloves but the patient's bronchospasm worsened dramatically. Removal of latex gloves liberates latex protein into the air. Since the EMTs were in close proximity to the patient when they removed the gloves and then continued to care for her without washing remaining latex proteins from their hands, the patient was likely exposed via inhalation to latex airborne particles from the gloves.

In the emergency department, a latex-free crash cart was immediately employed in the resuscitative effort. The hospital's purchasing department had previously been asked to identify latex-free products that would be required for resuscitation. The Food and Drug Administration requires labeling of latex-containing medical equipment that comes into direct contact with patients. All hospitals are required to have policies describing methods for providing safe medical care to latex-allergic patients.

Not everyone with skin reactions to gloves has true latex allergy. The management of reactions associated with latex glove use is described in the table.

Management of Reactions to Latex

CONDITION	PRESENTATION	MANAGEMENT
Irritant contact dermatitis (irritation not allergic)	Fissuring and cracking of skin in areas of glove contact	Cotton glove liners
Allergic contact dermatitis (delayed hypersensitivity reaction to glove additives not latex)	Erythematous, itchy rash	Change gloves to avoid additive of concern Patch testing is helpful
Latex allergy (immediate hypersensitivity reaction to latex proteins)	Contact urticaria, dermatitis, rhinitis, conjunctivitis, angioedema, asthma, anaphylaxis	No latex direct contact Avoid proximity to latex aeroallergen Carry injectable epinephrine

Clinical Pearls

1. Latex is ubiquitous in the home and hospital environment. The care of patients with type I latex allergy must exclude medical equipment containing latex so that systemic allergic reactions are not exacerbated.

2. Latex-free resuscitation and other patient care items should be identified and easily located to avoid delays in care.

3. Latex exposure can occur not only by direct contact but also by inhalation of aerosolized particles and ingestion of particles left by food handling. Considering latex as a potential offending allergen in systemic reactions depends on an understanding of these possible routes of exposure.

4. Health care workers are not the only at-risk profession for latex allergy. Day care workers who uses gloves to change many diapers each day may develop latex allergy from glove use.

REFERENCES

1. Food and Drug Administration: Latex-containing Devices: User Labeling. 21CFR Part 801 [Docket No. 96N-0119].
2. Hamilton RG, Abmli D, Brown RH: Impact of personal avoidance practices on health care workers sensitized to natural rubber latex. J Clin Immun 105:839–841, 2000.
3. Liss GM, Sussman G: Latex sensitization: Occupational versus general population prevalence rates. Am J Ind Med 35: 196–200, 1999.
4. Hunt LW, Boone-Orke JL, Fransway AF, et al: A medical-center-wide, multidisciplinary approach to the problem of natural rubber latex allergy. J Occup Environ Med 38:765–770, 1996.

Paul Ko, MD
Jill M. Baren, MD, FACEP, FAAP

PATIENT 58

A 19-year-old man with facial trauma after a fall from a bicycle

A 19-year-old man with no significant past medical history presents to the emergency department after hitting a parked truck while riding his bicycle without a helmet. He landed on his face without loss of consciousness. He was ambulatory at the scene and walked home without any difficulty. He presents 10 hours later reporting jaw pain and inability to close his mouth completely. He denies any nausea, vomiting, headache, neck pain, or difficulty breathing. Except for his jaw, he had no pain.

Physical Examination: Vital signs: temperature 36°C; heart rate 60; respiratory rate 18; blood pressure 119/69; room air pulse oximetry 100%. General: no apparent distress. Head: 2-cm hematoma over right parietal/occipital scalp, no crepitus or bony deformity. Superficial abrasions over left forehead. Eyes: PERRLA, EOMI, no orbital bony deformity palpable. Face: maxillary and nasal bone stable; mandible has point tenderness over left parasymphyseal area with edema over entire left mandible; able to close mouth, but unable to bite down completely; mild trismus; intraoral: teeth stable and intact, ecchymosis of left mucosal vestibule; bilateral anterior open bite (malocclusion). Neck: no cervical spine tenderness.

Laboratory Findings: Mandible x-ray: see figure.

Questions: What do these clinical findings make you suspect in this patient? What associated injuries should be excluded?

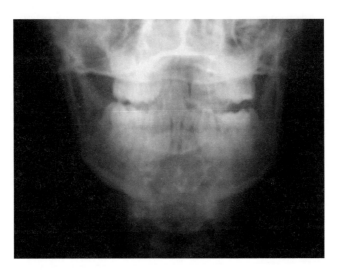

Diagnosis: Mandible fracture

Discussion: The hallmarks of a mandibular fracture are jaw pain, tenderness, ecchymosis of the floor of the mouth, and malocclusion. Malocclusion is defined as the inability to close the mouth completely with the teeth meeting comfortably. Other associated findings include deviation of the chin, inability to open the mouth fully, fractured teeth, gingival lacerations, and crepitus on jaw motion.

The mandible is the third most commonly fractured facial bone, following nasal and zygomatic fractures. Common causes are motor vehicle crashes, assault, and falls. The amount of impact expressed in force of gravity required to fracture the angle of the mandible is approximately 70 g. General knowledge of mandibular anatomy is important in understanding the pathogenesis of fracture.

The mandible has a horseshoe-shaped partial ring anatomy. It is divided into six anatomical parts: condyle, coronoid process, ramus, angle, body, and symphysis. Because of its ring-shaped structure, more than 50% of mandibular fractures result in fractures in more than one location and fractures can occur distant from the area of direct impact. The most commonly fractured sites are the body (21%), angle (20%), condyle (36%), and symphysis (14%). The condyles are the growth centers of the bone and their fracture in children can retard future growth of the mandible and result in facial asymmetry.

Radiographic studies for the evaluation of mandibular trauma include anteroposterior views, right and left oblique lateral views, and special views such as a Towne view (better visualization of the condyles and angles), Waters projection (mandibular symphysis), and Cadwell's view (posteroanterior view). When available, a dental panoramic view of the mandible can provide a nearly complete view of the whole mandible.This is not always available in many emergency departments, however, and it requires the patient to be able to sit still for a longer period of time. A computed tomographic (CT) scan is rarely indicated and is mainly used when a condylar fracture is suspected but not visualized on plain radiographs.

The plain radiograph of the present patient shows a left parasymphyseal fracture of the mandible and right angle fracture (see figure). This is consistent with the idea that the mandible is a ring-shaped structure and that most impacts will result in multiple fractures. This radiographic finding is also consistent with the patient's examination findings and symptoms.

Before obtaining a consultation for mandibular fracture, other concurrent injuries also need to be ruled out. Because of the high impact force involved, other facial fractures, cervical spine fractures, and possible head trauma need to be evaluated. Facial fractures in children should alert the examining physician to ask about social and family situations to rule out nonaccidental trauma as a possible cause of the injury.

Medical management includes analgesia, a soft diet, and antibiotic coverage with penicillin for open fractures. Surgical intervention is done either with closed reduction and fixation with Ivy loops (24-gauge wiring between the teeth for maxillomandibular fixation) or with placement of arch wires for intermaxillary fixation. Open reduction is indicated in displaced fractures of the angle, body, or parasymphyseal regions or with multiple fractures. There are various approaches to open reduction with internal fixation (ORIF) that involve the insertion of plates and screws. In this patient, an ORIF approach was undertaken because of the multiple locations of his fractures.

The major complications associated with mandible fractures are abscess formation, osteomyelitis, and permanent malunion or malocclusion. In general, the healing and prognosis from mandible fractures is quite good, with studies showing greater than 99% bone healing in most cases.

Clinical Pearls

1. In patients with suspected facial trauma, always test for malocclusion and inability to open or close mouth as indications of a mandible fracture.

2. The anatomical shape of the mandible causes injury distant to the area of initial impact and causes the majority of injuries to result in multiple fractures.

3. Assess for head trauma and cervical spine trauma in all patients with mandible fractures.

REFERENCES

1. Lazow SK: The mandible fracture: A treatment protocol. J Craniomaxillofac Trauma 2:24–30, 1996.
2. Redman H, Purdy P, Miller G, Rollins N: Emergency Radiology. Philadelphia, W.B. Saunders, 1993, pp 105–113.
3. Schwartz G, Cayten CG, Mangelsen MA, et al: Principles and Practice of Emergency Medicine, 3rd ed. Philadelphia, Lea & Febiger, 1992, pp 1013–1015.
4. Schwartz DT, Reisdorff EJ: Emergency Radiology. New York, Mcgraw-Hill, 2000, pp 379–381.
5. Marx JA, Hockberger RS, Walls RM: Rosen's Emergency Medicine: Concepts and Clinical Practice, 5th ed. St Louis, Mosby, 2002, pp 322–327.
6. Barrera JE, Batuello SG: Mandibular body fracture. Accessed July, 2002 at http://www.emedicine.com/ent/topic415.htm.

PATIENT 59

An 11-year-old boy with vomiting and lethargy

An 11-year-old boy is brought to the emergency department with a chief complaint of lethargy and weakness. His mother reports that for the past few days he has had progressive fatigue, vomiting, and dizziness. She also reports that on the morning of the ED visit he was difficult to arouse from bed and has been very lethargic. She denies fever, diarrhea, or respiratory symptoms. On further questioning, the mother states that she has noticed changes in his facial complexion, with the appearance of darkly pigmented spots on his face that were not there previous to the onset of the illness.

Physical Examination: Temperature 39.2°C.; pulse 142; respiratory rate 22; blood pressure 78/42. General: somnolent, sluggishly responsive. HEENT: mucous membranes tacky, dry cracked lips. Chest: clear to auscultation bilaterally. Cardiovascular: normal S1 and S2, no murmur. Abdomen: soft, nontender, no organomegaly. Genitourinary: normal male genitalia. Extremities: cool, pulses thready. Skin: cool and dry; tan coloration with multiple dark brown macules on face (see figure). Neurologic: cranial nerves intact, strength 5/5 in all groups, DTRs 2+.

Laboratory Findings: WBC 24,600/μl, hemoglobin 14.7 g/dl, platelets 424,000/μl. Na 123 mEq/L (normal 133–146 mEq/L), K 6.7 mEq/L (normal 3.4–4.7 mEq/L), Cl 89 mEq/L (normal 98–107 mEq/L), CO_2 7 mEq/L (normal 20–28 mEq/L), BUN 34 mg/dl (normal 5–18 mg/dl), Cr 1.4 mg/dl (normal 0.3–0.7 mg/dl), glucose <20 mg/dl (normal 60–100 mg/dl). Venous blood gas: pH 7.19, $PaCO_2$ 30.7 mm Hg, PaO_2 53 mm Hg, HCO_3 12 mEq/L, base excess −14. Cortisol 1.4 μg/dl (normal 10–25 μg/dl).

Questions: In addition to intravenous access, fluid resuscitation, and dextrose administration, what medication should be included in this child's initial management?

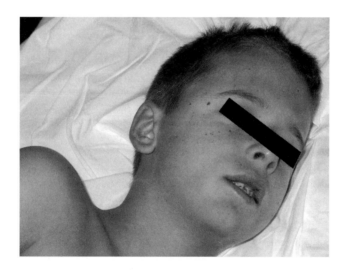

Answer: Intravenous hydrocortisone

Discussion: The combination of hypotension, shock, and hyperpigmentation accompanied by hyponatremia, hypoglycemia, and hyperkalemia are hallmark findings of acute adrenal insufficiency. The present patient was eventually given the diagnosis of new-onset Addison disease.

Addison disease is defined as destruction of the adrenal cortex with resultant adrenocortical hormone synthetic deficiency. In childhood, this is most commonly the result of an autoimmune process. Early in the disease, the predominant clinical effect is that of isolated cortisol deficiency, with mineralocorticoid deficiency and salt wasting occurring later. The term *Addison disease* is reserved for the primary failure of adrenocortical hormone synthesis, but acute adrenal insufficiency can result from many congenital and acquired causes in children, with congenital adrenal hyperplasia being most common in infancy, and autoimmune adrenalitis being most common in older children and adolescents. Two syndromes, termed *autoimmune polyglandular syndromes* (APS), occur children with Addison disease and are marked by the concurrence of mucocutaneous candidiasis and hypoparathyroidism (type I) and autoimmune thyroid disease or insulin-dependent diabetes (type II).

The clinical features of adrenal insufficiency are nonspecific and can mimic many other conditions, including infectious, gastrointestinal, neuromuscular, and psychiatric conditions. Fatigue, malaise, and weakness are common. Vomiting, weight loss, poor weight gain in young children, muscular weakness, and dehydration can also occur. Hyperpigmentation is sometimes seen in children with long-standing adrenal insufficiency. The pigmentation changes may be first apparent on the face and hands and are typically most intense around the genitalia, umbilicus, axillae, nipples, and joints. Scars, freckles, and mucous membranes can also become hyperpigmented. The pathophysiology of the skin changes is unclear, although the cleavage of pro-opiomelanocortin (POMC), the precursor to adrenocorticotropic hormone(ACTH), results in the release of melanocyte-stimulating hormone (MSH) as a by product that could account for increased pigmentation.

Diagnosis of adrenal insufficiency requires a high degree of suspicion, because the disorder is so nonspecific in its clinical manifestations. Additionally, clinically significant adrenal insufficiency has been demonstrated to be common in critical disease states other than those primarily involving the adrenal glands, including sepsis and burns. One study in adults by Rivers et al. found that 14% of adults presenting to an ED with hypotension and shock had significant hypocortisolemia; however, there was no significant difference in survival between these patients and other enrolled patients in similar clinical states whose cortisol levels were normal. Laboratory findings consistent with salt wasting (hyponatremia, hyperkalemia) and hypoglycemia should alert the clinician to the diagnosis. Definitively diagnosing adrenal insufficiency requires tests of serum cortisol and ACTH before the institution of therapy. Assessing the endogenous response to ACTH through a stimulation assay is the confirmatory method of choice.In an emergency setting, however, results of these assays are unlikely to be quickly available, and therapy should be empirically instituted on the basis of sufficient clinical suspicion alone.

The cornerstone of therapy for acute adrenal insufficiency is steroid replacement. The normal physiologic production of cortisol in children has been cited by different authors to be between 7.5 and 15 mg/m^2/day, and it has been recommended that replacement doses for acute adrenal insufficiency be administered at between two and five times the physiologic dose. For children, a bolus dose of 2 mg/kg of hydrocortisone IV push improves hemodynamics within minutes, and often normalizes hemodynamics within several hours. One study by De Vroede et al. preliminarily showed that rectal administration of hydrocortisone may be an effective alternative when intravenous administration is difficult. Electrolyte disturbances that accompany adrenal insufficiency most often normalize without specific therapy; isotonic intravenous fluids and dextrose should be administered in normal resuscitative doses. Maintenance steroid replacement following the first dose should be given in doses of 50 mg/m^2/day, divided, every 6 to 8 hours. Children with primary adrenal insufficiency require lifelong corticosteroid replacement and should be cared for by an endocrinologist.

The present patient received isotonic intravenous fluid and dextrose boluses. Cortisol and ACTH levels were drawn in the ED and 2 mg/kg of hydrocortisone was given via intravenous push. The patient's hemodynamic instability normalized with 6 to 8 hours; he was admitted to the pediatric intensive care unit but never required vasopressor drug infusion. His electrolytes gradually corrected and he was transitioned to an oral corticosteroid replacement regimen before being discharged to home on hospital day 5.

Clinical Pearls

1. Adrenal insufficiency can be a primary or secondary disorder.
2. In addition to signs of shock and hypoperfusion, skin hyperpigmentation can be a sign of adrenal insufficiency.
3. Laboratory hallmarks include hypoglycemia, hyponatremia, and hyperkalemia.

REFERENCES

1. Annane D: Corticosteroids for septic shock. Crit Care Med 29:S117–S120, 2001.
2. Ten S, New M, Maclaren N: Addison's disease 2001. J Clin Endocrinol Metab 86:2909–2922, 2001.
3. Rivers EP, et al: Adrenal dysfunction in hemodynamically unstable patients in the emergency department. Acad Emerg Med 6:626–630, 1999.
4. De Vroede M, Beukering R, Spit M, Jansen M: Rectal hydrocortisone during stress in patients with adrenal insufficiency. Arch Dis Child 78:544–547, 1998.
5. DiGeorge AM, Levine LS: Disorders of the adrenal glands. In Behrman RE, Kliegman RM, Arvin AM, eds: Nelson Textbook of Pediatrics. Philadelphia, W.B. Saunders, 1996.
6. Kohane DS, Tobin TR, Kohane IS: Endocrine, mineral, and metabolic disease in pediatric intensive care. In Rogers MC, ed: Textbook of Pediatric Intensive Care. Baltimore, Williams & Wilkins, 1996.
7. Sheridan RL, Ryan CM, Tompkins RG: Acute adrenal insufficiency in the burn intensive care unit. Burns 19:63–66, 1993.
8. New MI: Replacement doses of glucocorticoids. J Pediatr 119:161, 1991.
9. Nickels DA, Moore DC: Serum cortisol responses in febrile children. Pediatr Infect Dis J 8:16–20, 1989.

Anthony J. Dean, M.D.

PATIENT 60

A healthy 24-year-old woman with syncope and unexplained hypotension

A 24-year-old woman is brought to the emergency department by ambulance after fainting at home. The patient has been experiencing pelvic pain for several hours and she fainted on the way to the bathroom. On scene, they found a patient who was awake, alert and oriented, but diaphoretic with a blood pressure of 60/P. On arrival in the ED, the patient continues to report mild suprapubic pain with discomfort in her right upper quadrant. Family witnesses describe a brief loss of consciousness, with complete loss of postural tone, and absence of tonic/clonic movements or incontinence. The patient recovered consciousness in 30 to 60 seconds. She denies irregular, heavy, or missed menses (last normal menstrual period 2 weeks ago). She has no history of gynecologic problems, including sexually transmitted disease, tubal ligation, or previous pregnancy. She has no urinary or gastrointestinal symptoms. She denies fever, chills, dyspnea, chest pain, or palpitations. She has no history of seizures, cardiac disease, or previous syncope.

Physical Examination: Vital signs: temperature 37.6°C, heart rate 75, respiratory rate 16, blood pressure 103/59. The patient is orthostatic without pallor or diaphoresis. HEENT: moist mucous membranes. Neck, chest, and lung normal. Abdomen: normal bowel sounds with mild suprapubic tenderness without guarding, rebound, or masses. Negative psoas and obturator signs. No cervical discharge, no cervical motion tenderness. Rectal examination normal, heme-negative stool.

Laboratory Findings: Room air pulse oximetry 99%. Urine HCG negative. Hemogram normal with hemoglobin 12.1 g/dl. Serum chemistry normal with anion gap 15. Blood glucose 115. Amylase, lipase, liver function tests all normal. ECG normal. Confirmatory serum HCG negative. Emergency medicine bedside ultrasonography (EMBU) of the abdomen, aorta and heart: large amount of free fluid in the pelvis and a small amount in the hepatorenal space (see figures—*left*, transverse suprapubic view of left adnexal area shows uterus [UT] and bowel loops [B] surrounded by free fluid [FF], which appears dark; *right*, sagittal section shows liver overlying kidney and infrahepatic space and hepatorenal space [Morison's pouch, *arrows*] filled with free fluid.)

Questions: What are the likely causes of syncope in this patient? Does the normal hemoglobin level rule out acute hemorrhage? How is the differential diagnosis modified by the EMBU?

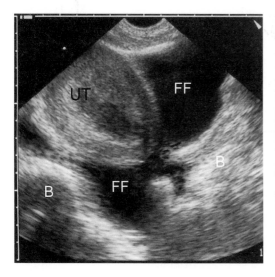
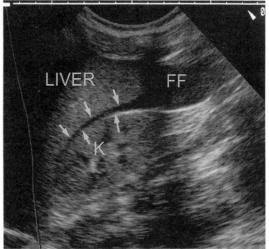

Diagnosis and Treatment: The patient is placed on a monitor and provided with an intravenous line. Since she is symptomatically orthostatic and has no history or clinical findings to suggest heart disease, she is given 2 L of normal saline wide open. The EMBU identification of large quantities of intra-abdominal free fluid in a patient without any active clinical reason for ascites suggests intra-abdominal hemorrhage, thus explaining her syncope and persistent hypotension. Pelvic discomfort suggests hemorrhage from a ruptured ovarian cyst, but to rule out occult hemorrhage from another site, a computed tomographic (CT) scan of the abdomen and pelvis with contrast is obtained and shows normal abdominal organs and vasculature with large amount of clot and fluid in the pelvis and some free fluid around the liver. Repeat hemoglobin is 8.6 g/dl.

Discussion: Syncope is the presenting symptom in 1 to 2 % of all patients visiting the ED. Its causes range from benign to lethal. The emergency physician must determine, with limited time and resources, where on this spectrum an individual patient belongs. The definition of syncope is a transient, completely reversible loss of consciousness. The physiologic mechanism allowing for rapid loss and then recovery of consciousness is transient interruption of global cerebral perfusion. It is therefore useful to categorize the causes of syncope according to various forms of circulatory impairment (see table).

Cerebrovascular ischemia is an extremely rare cause of syncope. A brief, reversible period of occlusion of all sources of cerebral circulation, or of the entire reticular activating system, is extremely unlikely without residual neurologic deficit. For this reason, CT scan of the head is not indicated in the evaluation of nontraumatic syncope unless subarachnoid hemorrhage is suspected. It should be noted that while medications are listed among the "other" causes of syncope, medications and drugs are often responsible for syncope by circulatory, cardiac, or autonomic mechanisms. Cardiac and antihypertensive medications, widely used in patients at risk for malignant causes of syncope, should be carefully investigated. Syncope must be distinguished from hypoglycemia (usually gradual onset and resolution; loss of postural tone occurs rarely) and seizures (often clonic movements or tics, with gradual resolution). This is usually possible with a careful history. If it is not, it will be necessary to evaluate the patient for both disorders.

The cause of syncope can be determined in the ED in about 50% of cases (further work-up and testing improves this number only marginally).In more than 75% of cases in which a cause is identified, however, the diagnosis can be made on the basis of the history and physical examination alone. Therefore, diagnostic testing should be directed by the clinical evaluation. Prospective

---

Causes of Syncope, Classified by Cause of Circulatory Impairment

Circulatory
Impaired venous return
  Intravascular volume depletion
  Tricuspid or mitral stenosis
  Mechanical obstruction (e.g., myxoma)
  Situational (e.g., post-tussive, post-micturition)
Impaired pulmonary outflow
  Pulmonary embolus
  Pulmonary hypertension
Impaired aortic outflow
  Aortic stenosis
  Hypertrophic cardiomyopathy
Impaired arterial circulation
  Aortic dissection
  Subclavian (or other) steal

Cardiac
Dysrhythmias
  Slow: sick sinus syndrome, heart blocks, pacemaker problems
  Fast: ventricular tachycardia, supraventricular tachycardia, Wolff-Parkinson-White syndrome
Ischemia
Congenital heart disease

Autonomic Dysfunction
Vasovagal syncope
Postural syncope
Carotid hypersensitivity

Other
Hyperventilation
Medications and drugs
Migraine
Cerebrovascular ischemia
Psychiatric

studies have shown that syncope is unlikely to have a malignant cause in patients who are younger than 45 years of age, have no history of dysrhythmia or congestive heart failure, and have an electrocardiogram (ECG) that is normal or with nonspecific ST-T wave abnormalities. For this reason, an ECG is obtained in almost all cases.

The present patient is young and healthy, with no past medical history and a normal examination. This makes cardiac causes unlikely. The event occurred while she was standing, so postural causes are possible, although in young patients these usually happen after prolonged standing. Vasovagal syncope is associated with emotional stress or pain. A primary autonomic derangement would not cohere with the patient's persistent orthostasis. Considering the list of circulatory causes, the patient does have signs of hypovolemia, and all other causes, except for atrial myxoma, can be excluded based on the clinical picture. With respect to the evaluation of this patient's syncope, therefore, the ECG, pregnancy test, and complete blood cell count are most likely to be helpful. However, due to her continued abdominal pain and unexplained hypotension, a wider battery of tests was performed.

Prior to the performance of the EMBU, the patient continued to have unexplained abdominal pain, with no clear cause for her hypotension or syncope. In the absence of other causes, the unexplained intravascular volume depletion is most likely the result of occult hemorrhage. The three sites where this can occur are the gastrointestinal tract, peritoneal space, and pleural spaces. Massive gastrointestinal hemorrhage has been ruled out by the normal rectal examination findings. With recent advances in technology, the EMBU has made it possible to rule in or exclude the other two. In addition, EMBU will be able to assess for a significant atrial myxoma, which was not definitively ruled out on clinical evaluation.

Unexplained hypotension is not uncommonly encountered in the emergency department. Like pulseless electrical activity and syncope, with which it shares many etiologies, its causes are often life-threatening and time sensitive. Many of the causes of these three syndromes can be rapidly identified using bedside ultrasonography to evaluate the heart, abdominal aorta, and peritoneal cavity (see table at right). These diagnoses can be made within minutes by the treating physician without the need to remove the patient from the resuscitation area. In addition to the rapidity with which diagnosis is possible, this arrangement allows a single physician to perform a test, where previously two separate consultations (one to cardiology for the transthoracic examination, and one to radiology for the abdominal examination), with attendant expenditure of time and resources, were necessary. With the accumulation of experience in bedside ultrasonography, applications of this technology are evolving to help answer the unique clinical challenges in emergency medicine.

In the present patient, due to the high risk of ectopic pregnancy, a serum quantitative β-HCG was checked. It was negative. After a total of 4 L IV normal saline solution, her hypotension and orthostatic hypotension resolved. The large volume of free fluid in the pelvis, in the absence of other apparent pathology, suggested the diagnosis of ruptured ovarian cyst. Of note, the initially normal serum hemoglobin did not rule out significant hemorrhage; in fact, it is characteristic of it. Since whole blood is being lost, the composition of the blood remaining in the intravascular compartment is unchanged. Conversely, the subsequent fall in hemoglobin does not necessarily imply continued hemorrhage since repletion of the intravascular compartment with crystalloid solution causes dilution of the blood, reflected in lower hemoglobin and hematocrit levels.

The consultant gynecologist thought that there was no indication for emergency laparotomy or laparoscopy if the patient's condition stabilized with conservative management. The patient was admitted to the gynecology service for observation, where her hemoglobin dropped as low as 7.1, although she remained symptomatically stable. After 2 days without symptoms and with stable hemoglobin levels, the patient was discharged on iron supplements with the presumptive diagnosis of hemorrhage from a ruptured ovarian cyst.

Causes of Unexplained Hypotension Identifiable by Emergency Medicine Bedside Ultrasonography

---

Transsthoracic EMBU
   Pericardial tamponade
   Pulmonary embolus*†
   Intravascular volume depletion*
   Proximal aortic dissection*†
   Massive hemothorax or pleural effusion
EMBU of the aorta
   Abdominal aortic aneurysm*
   Distal aortic dissection*†
Evaluation of the peritoneal cavity
   Intraperitoneal hemorrhage*

Note: all also cause pulseless electrical activity.

* Indicates conditions that can also cause syncope.

† Indicates diagnoses that can be ruled in, but cannot reliably be ruled out with EMBU.

Clinical Pearls

1. The primary goal of the emergency physician treating syncope is to identify potentially lethal causes.

2. The majority of potentially lethal causes of syncope are cardiac in origin.

3. Patients who are young, with a normal ECG, and without heart disease, usually have benign causes of syncope and can be discharged if a plausible cause can be identified clinically.

4. Several causes of syncope, as well as unexplained hypotension and PEA can be identified by using bedside ultrasonography.

REFERENCES

1. Hendrickson RG, Dean AJ, Costantino TG: A novel use of ultrasound in pulseless electrical activity: The diagnosis of an acute abdominal aortic aneurysm rupture. J Emerg Med 21:141–144, 2001.
2. Rose JS, Bair AE, Mandavia D, Kinser DJ: The UHP ultrasound protocol: A novel ultrasound approach to the empiric evaluation of the undifferentiated hypotensive patient. Am J Emerg Med 19:299–302, 2001.
3. Kapoor WN: Syncope. N Engl J Med 343:1856–1862, 2000.
4. Linzer M, Yang EH, Estes NA 3rd, et al: Diagnosing syncope. Part 1: Value of history, physical examination, and electrocardiography. Clinical Efficacy Assessment Project of the American College of Physicians. Ann Intern Med 126:989–996, 1997.
5. Martin TP, Hanusa BH, Kapoor WN: Risk stratification of patients with syncope. Ann Emerg Med 29:459–466, 1997.

PATIENT 61

An 18-year-old woman with headache and diplopia

An 18-year-old obese woman presents to the emergency department with a 2-week complaint of headache, nausea with intermittent vomiting, occasional double vision, and a ringing in her ears. She denies any other symptoms.

Physical Examination: Temperature 37°C; blood pressure 116/65; pulse 94; respiratory rate 20; weight 114 kg. General: She is sitting in the room with the lights off, leaning forward and holding her head. Skin: no petechiae. HEENT: normacephalic, no tenderness to palpation, pupils equal and reactive to light, extraocular muscles intact, right subconjunctival hemorrhage, fundi pale (see figure), tympanic membranes intact and clear, mucus membranes moist. Neck: no nuchal rigidity. Chest: clear to auscultation. Cardiac: regular rate with no murmurs. Abdomen: normal. Extremities: normal. Neurologic: Alert and oriented × 4; no cranial nerve deficits; no visual field deficit; no motor or sensory deficits; gait steady.

Laboratory Findings: CBC: normal. Blood chemistries: normal. Erythrocyte sedimentation rate: normal. Computed tomography (CT) of the head: negative for intracranial bleed, mass effect, or midline shift. Lumbar puncture: opening pressure 220 cm H_2O, cerebrospinal fluid (CSF) clear and colorless with no red blood cells or white blood cells, protein 29, glucose 52.

Questions: What is the cause for the patients' elevated opening pressure on the lumbar puncture? What is the most appropriate initial therapy?

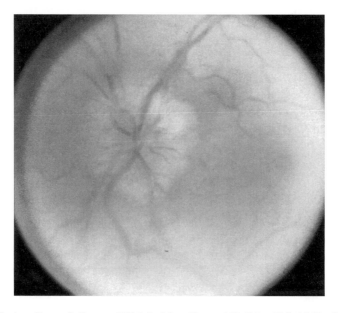

From Mandell GL: Infectious disease. In Braunwald E (ed): Atlas of Internal Medicine. Philadelphia, Current Medicine, 1999; with permission.

Diagnosis: Idiopathic intracranial hypertension, also commonly referred to as *pseudotumor cerebri*. Initial therapy is acetazolomide, which lowers cerebrospinal pressure by decreasing overall total body fluid. However, weight loss remains the cornerstone of therapy.

Discussion: Idiopathic intracranial hypertension (IIH) is a condition of elevated CSF pressure in the absence of a mass in the brain. The cause is not known, and other causes of elevated CSF pressure must be excluded before this diagnosis can be made. If untreated, IIH can cause visual loss and even blindness in about 5% of patients. It is commonly found in overweight females of childbearing age, but it may also occur in men and children. The symptoms often start or worsen during a period of weight gain. Common signs and symptoms include headache (94%), transient visual obscurations or blurring (68%), pulse synchronous tinnitus or "whooshing noise" in the ear (58%), pain behind the eye (44%), double vision (38%), visual loss (30%), and pain with eye movement (22%).

Headache is the usual symptom for which patients seek medical attention. The headaches of the IIH patient are usually severe, daily, retro-ocular, and worse with eye movements and throbbing. They are different from previous headaches, may awaken the patient, and can last for hours. Nausea and vomiting are common. Visual obscurations are described as episodes of transient blurred vision lasting less than 30 seconds with full recovery. The attacks may involve one or both eyes. Pulsatile intracranial noises or pulse-synchronous tinnitus is common and often unilateral. Compression of the jugular vein on the side of sound may abolish it.

Evaluation of patients with suspected IIH involves a thorough history and physical examination, including a fundoscopic examination to look for edema of the optic disc (papilledema). If present, neuroimaging should be performed to exclude other causes of elevated CSF pressure. If imaging does not reveal the cause, the CSF pressure is measured by a lumbar puncture. Levels greater than 180 cm H_2O are considered elevated. Opening pressure must be measured in the lateral decubitus position with the legs relaxed. Pressures recorded in the sitting or prone (i.e., under fluoroscopy) position may be artificially elevated. Laboratory studies on the CSF must be normal.

Treatment for patients with IIH can be divided into medical and surgical. The cornerstone of medical treatment is weight loss, but effect does not correspond to the total number of pounds lost. Losing 1 pound every week or two for several months and then maintaining the weight loss is effective for some patients. The loss of fluid accompanying weight loss may be the significant factor, but this is unproven. Loss of fluid can also be obtained using diuretics; acetazolamide is the one most commonly prescribed, and furosemide is also used. These are relatively safe but produce benign tingling in the fingers and toes in most patients. Corticosteroids rapidly decrease intracranial pressure, but their side effects of weight gain and fluid retention preclude their use in the acute setting. They may be employed for the treatment of patients with visual loss in conjunction with a surgical procedure. Two surgical treatments are currently in use for cases refractory to medical therapy: optic nerve sheath fenestration and lumbar shunting.

The present patient was treated with a 3-day course of acetazolamide and started on a weight loss program by her physician. Her symptoms improved and she was weaned off diuretics.

Clinical Pearls

1. The diagnosis of IIH can be made only after all other causes of increased CSF pressure are excluded.

2. Papilledema is the hallmark finding of IIH, but because it is difficult to ascertain in the ED, consider this diagnosis in *all* headache patients, especially those who are female, obese, and of childbearing age.

3. CSF opening pressure should be measured with the patient in the lateral decubitus position with the legs relaxed. Measurement in the sitting or prone positions results in artificially elevated pressure.

REFERENCES
1. Digre KB: Idiopathic intracranial hypertension headache. Curr Pain Headache Rep 6:217–225, 2002.
2. Kosmorsky G: Pseudotumor cerebri. Neurosurg Clin North Am 12:775–797, 2001.
3. Friedman DI: Papilledema and pseudotumor cerebri. Ophthalmol Clin North Am 14:129–147, 2001.
4. Movsas TZ, Liu GT, Galetta SL, et al: Current neuro-ophthalmic therapies. Neurol Clin 19:145–172, 2001.
5. Jones JS, Nevai J, Freeman MP, et al: Emergency department presentation of idiopathic intracranial hypertension. Am J Emerg Med 17:517–521, 1999.

PATIENT 62

A 13-month-old girl with left arm pain after a fall

A previously healthy 13-month-old girl is brought to the emergency department by her parents with concerns about left arm pain. They report that the child seemed to have pain in her left arm when she was picked up by both her hands to swing her earlier that day. The child has a history of falling down four steps onto outstretched arms on a tile floor the day prior to presentation. She did not sustain any head trauma or other injury, according to the parents. She was able to play using the left arm without difficulty following the fall and continues to use the arm. She has had no fever or other trauma.

Physical Examination: Vital signs: temperature 37.1°C rectally; pulse 100; respiratory rate 28; blood pressure 94/48. General: well-nourished and well-developed child, interactive, moving both arms without difficulty. Chest: clear, equal breath sounds. Cardiac: regular rate without murmur. Extremities: minimal edema at left wrist with some tenderness over distal forearm; 2+ left radial pulse, brisk capillary refill. Skin: no lesions.

Laboratory Findings: Left forearm x-ray: see figures.

Question: What is the diagnosis?

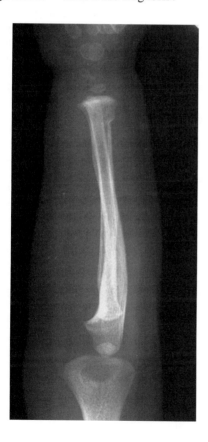
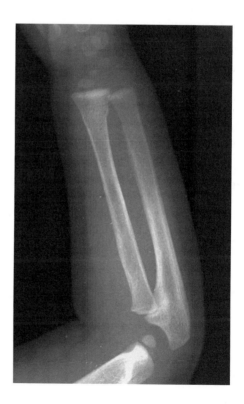

Diagnosis: Torus, or buckle, fracture of the distal radius

Discussion: A buckle, or torus, fracture is one of several fracture patterns commonly seen in and limited to pediatric patients. This fracture results from a compressive failure at the metaphyseal/diaphyseal junction or in the metaphysis. On radiographs, it appears as a buckling of the cortex at the fracture site. Buckle fractures are considered to be stable fractures, especially when unilateral cortical disruption occurs. If bilateral cortical injury is visible on radiographs, the fracture has the potential for displacement.

Torus fractures occur commonly in younger children and may result from a relatively minor, low-impact injury. Children with these fractures may present with pain and swelling at the affected area. They may not present immediately following the inciting trauma, as these fractures are stable and protected by an intact periosteum, leading to less pain and limitation of use. Torus fractures are diagnosed by plain radiographs of the affected area. They are sometimes subtle and visible on only one view. The fracture presented is visible on both the anteroposterior and lateral views. Simple torus fractures generally heal without complications.

Emergency management of these fractures includes ruling out any other injury that may have occurred with the trauma that caused the fracture as well as performing a complete neurovascular examination of the affected limb. The fracture should be immobilized in a splint or cast (a short-arm splint or cast may be used in the case of a simple torus fracture), and standard fracture care, including rest, ice, and elevation, is recommended. The patient with a simple buckle fracture may be referred to an orthopedist for follow-up.

When evaluating pediatric patients for orthopedic injuries, it is important to remember that there are several anatomic differences between adults and children that lead to different injury types. Relative to adults, the bones in children are more porous, have a thick and more active periosteum, contain cartilaginous physes or growth plates, and may undergo remodeling after an injury. The greater porosity and the presence of active growth plates, which are not as strong as the accompanying ligaments, lead to more frequent fractures when a child experiences trauma. Conversely, the occurrence of sprains and joint dislocations are relatively uncommon in the growing child.

Some of the other fracture patterns unique to children include bowing, greenstick, and physeal fractures. Bowing fractures occur when a longitudinal force is applied to a long bone, leading to plastic deformation of the bone without fracture of the cortex. This fracture type has limited remodeling capacity. A greenstick fracture is an incomplete fracture in which the periosteum and cortex remain intact on the side that is compressed. Finally, physeal or growth plate fractures are unique to growing children. One of the most common systems for classifying these fractures is with the Salter-Harris system, which divides these injuries into five types. In general, the higher the number type of physeal fracture, the greater the chance for problems with healing and normal growth.

Clinical Pearls

1. There are a number of anatomic differences between pediatric and adult bones which result in a number of fracture types, including torus, physeal, and bowing, that are unique to children.

2. Buckle, or torus, fractures are stable fractures caused by compression failure at the diaphyseal/metaphyseal junction.

3. Torus fractures may be difficult to see on radiographs. A high index of suspicion is often necessary to make this diagnosis.

4. Routine fracture care, including immobilization, ice, elevation, and orthopedic follow-up, constitute the emergency management of torus fractures.

REFERENCES

1. Waters PM: Distal radius and ulna fractures. In Beaty JH, Kasser JR (eds): Rockwood and Wilkins' Fractures in Children, 5th ed. Philadelphia, Lippincott Williams & Wilkins, 2001, pp. 408–413.
2. Bachman D, Santora S: Orthopedic trauma. In Fleisher GR, Ludwig S (eds): Textbook of Pediatric Emergency Medicine, 4th ed. Philadelphia, Lippincott Williams & Wilkins, 2000, pp. 1435–1441, 1455–1457.
3. England SP, Sundberg S: Management of common pediatric fractures. Pediatr Clin North Am 43:991–1012, 1996.
4. Dicke TE, Nunley JA: Distal forearm fractures in children: Complications and surgical indications. Orthop Clin North Am 24:333–340, 1993.

Y. Veronica Pei, MD, MEd
Jill M. Baren, MD, FACEP, FAAP

PATIENT 63

A 45-year-old man with confusion and acute renal failure

A 45-year-old man with history of substance abuse, hepatitis C, and cirrhosis was brought to the emergency department by his wife for right forearm pain after a fall onto his right side 2 days ago. He was initially evaluated at an outside hospital and was found to have a right upper extremity muscle hematoma and an elevated creatinine level of 3.2 mg/dl. He was discharged to follow-up with his primary physician. He then noted worsening of right arm pain associated with paresthesias and right hip pain, severely limiting his activity. His wife also reports worsening of his baseline confusion and memory deficit. Review of systems is significant for decreased urine output and intermittent nausea and vomiting.

Physical Examination: Vital signs: temperature 36.6°C; pulse 80; respiratory rate 16; blood pressure 133/66. Skin: warm and dry; multiple abrasions on right upper extremity. HEENT: normal. Chest: normal. Cardiac: regular rate and rhythm; normal heart sounds without murmurs. Abdomen: mild right costovetebral angle tenderness. Extremities: mild swelling of right forearm; no tense compartments; tender to palpation and pain with passive extension of the right wrist; reflexes equal bilaterally; +2 pulses bilaterally. Neuromuscular: alert and oriented to person, place, and time but difficulty recalling events of past few days; cranial nerves intact; motor: 3/5 right wrist and finger extensors; sensation intact.

Laboratory Findings: CBC: normal, except platelets 45,000/μl (normal 150,000–400,000/μl). Blood chemistries: sodium 131 mmol/L (normal 133–143 mmol/L), potassium 4.7 mmol/L (normal 3.5–5.5 mmol/L), chloride 97 mmol/L (normal 97–107 mmol/L), CO_2 16 mmol/L (normal 22–30 mmol/L), urea nitrogen 106 mg/dl (normal 10–20 mg/dl), creatinine 7.6 mg/dl (normal 0.8–1.3 mg/dl), glucose 230 mg/dl (normal 70–110 mg/dl), calcium 7.7 mg/dl (normal 8.5–10.5 mg/dl), anion gap 18. Liver function tests: total bilirubin 3.3 mg/dl (normal 0–1.2 mg/dl), alkaline phosphatase 137 U/L (normal 35–125 U/L), aspartate aminotransferase 1395 U/L (normal 17–59 U/L), alanine aminotransferase 1807 U/L (normal 21–72 U/L), albumin 2.4 g/dl (normal 3.5–5.8 g/dl). Creatine kinase 18,680 U/L (normal 60–400 U/L), CK-MB 50.9 ng/ml (normal 0–7.5 ng/ml). Ammonia: 74 μmol/L (normal 9–33 μmol/L). Coagulation studies: INR 2.2, APTT 30.2 sec (normal 22–33.3 sec). Urinalysis: yellow urine, moderate blood, trace protein, 100 glucose, negative leukocyte esterase and nitrates. Urine microscopy: 0 RBCs per hpf, 0 WBCs per hpf.

Question: Given that this patient's last serum creatinine level was 0.8 mg/dl 5 months ago, what is the most likely cause of his new-onset renal failure?

Diagnosis and Treatment: Acute renal failure secondary to rhabdomyolysis. Therapy includes aggressive intravenous fluids and urine alkalinization.

Discussion: *Rhabdomyolysis* refers to the process of muscle cell breakdown resulting in the release of intracellular contents into the circulation. It does not represent one specific syndrome but rather is a pathologic process that is associated with many serious complications.

Common causes of rhabdomyolysis include trauma, exercise, seizures, infections, substance abuse, and medications (see table). Regardless of the initial insult, the end result is the loss of function of the muscle cell membrane leading to disruption of the Na^+, K^+, and Ca^{2+} gradients across the cell membrane. This leads to an increase in intracellular calcium, which promotes intracellular proteolytic enzyme activity, resulting in eventual cell death and release of intracellular contents.

Patients should be asked about a history of recent trauma, excessive exertion, toxic ingestions or exposures, medications, use of illicit drugs, and known history or family history of muscle dysfunction or disease. Clinically, the patient may report localized or diffuse muscle weakness, myalgia, and/or swelling as well as systemic symptoms such as malaise, confusion, nausea, emesis, and tea-colored urine. Physical examination may reveal tenderness to palpation of affected muscle groups, local swelling, or overlying skin discoloration with or without associated sensory and/or motor deficits. Absence of characteristic findings does not rule out rhabdomyolysis.

The presentation of rhabdomyolysis is variable and includes features of early and late complications. Acute renal failure (ARF), electrolyte abnormalities, disseminated intravascular coagulation, and compartment syndrome are some of the most common complications. The mechanisms of renal injury are believed to be related to (1) myoglobin-induced renal vasoconstriction resulting in decreased glomerular filtration rate and renal blood flow; (2) direct cytotoxic effect of hemoprotein on the renal tubular cells secondary to the formation of free radicals of oxidants; and (3) renal tubular obstruction by the formation of myoglobin—renal tubular protein (Tamm—Horsfall protein) casts. The degree of creatine kinase (CK) elevation is poorly correlated with the severity of ARF, so even mild elevations must be taken seriously. Metabolic abnormalities are secondary to the release of intracellular contents and include hypocalcemia, hyperkalemia, hyperphosphatemia, and hypoalbuminemia. Disseminated intravascular coagulation may develop as a result of massive tissue necrosis and the release of thromboplastin. Compartment syndrome may be an early or late complication. Damaged muscles cause capillary leakage into the interstitial space, resulting in increased compartment pressure and ischemia. Consultation with an orthopedic surgeon is necessary if compartment syndrome is suspected.

Causes of Rhabdomyolysis

PHYSICAL CAUSES	NONPHYSICAL CAUSES
Excessive muscle use: exercise, seizure, delirium tremens	Metabolic disorders: hyponatremia, hypernatremia, hypokalemia, hypophosphatemia, DKA, thyroid storm
Trauma: crush injury, electric shock, burns	Drugs/toxins: HMG-CoA reductase inhibitors, diuretics, steroids, cocaine, zidovudine, alcohol, ecstasy, PCP/amphetamine, carbon monoxide, cyanide, ethylene glycol, snake venom.
Ischemic: vascular injury, prolonged immobilization, direct compression, compartment syndrome	Infections: toxic shock syndrome, septic shock, tularemia, infection with *Streptococcus, Salmonella, Legionella,* or *Staphylococcus,* human immunodeficiency virus, Epstein-Barr virus, cytomegalovirus, coxsackie virus, influenza, malaria
Hyperthermia: neuroleptic malignant syndrome, malignant hyperthermia, heat stroke	Immune mediated: polymyositis, dermatomyositis
	Ischemic: sickle cell anemia, vasculitis, shock, thromboembolism
	Hereditary: any enzyme deficiency in the pathway of ATP generation, most commonly carnitine palmitotransferase deficiency
	Idiopathic

The most reliable diagnostic marker for rhabdomyolysis is the measurement of serum CK. It is measurable immediately after muscle injury and is not rapidly cleared. In contrast, myoglobin has a very short half-life in serum (1–3 hours) and thus is not a useful marker. Urinalysis is a good initial screening tool, although positive blood on dipstick does not differentiate between myoglobin, hemoglobin, and RBCs. Urine microscopy and serum CK levels are additional tests that aid in the diagnosis (see table).

The goal of treatment is the prevention of ARF. Aggressive intravenous fluid therapy to achieve a urine output of 1–2 ml/kg/hour corrects intravascular depletion. Acidic urine pH greatly favors the formation of myoglobin (Tamm—Horsfall) protein casts which cause renal tubular obstruction. Therefore, urine alkalinization to a pH of 6.5 or greater is another treatment goal. Mannitol has been used as an osmotic diuretic to prevent renal tubular obstruction through increased urine flow.

In cases of oliguric ARF, hemodialysis may be necessary. Electrolyte abnormalities should be corrected to prevent life-threatening arrhythmias.

In the present patient, the recent trauma was the inciting event for the development of rhabdomyolysis and subsequent ARF. Muscle hematoma, worsening confusion, and elevated creatinine were consistent with the diagnosis. There was clinical suspicion for right forearm compartment, syndrome, although that was later ruled out. The laboratory studies revealed common metabolic abnormalities associated with rhabdomyolysis, including elevated anion gap, hypocalcemia, hyperphosphatemia, and hypoalbuminemia. The elevated CK level of 18,680 U/L and moderate blood on urine dipstick without significant RBCs on microscopy were most consistent with the diagnosis of rhabdomyolysis. The patient received aggressive hydration and bicarbonate therapy, with significant improvement in his creatinine level on discharge from the hospital.

Characteristics of Urine Under Different Conditions

CHARACTERISTIC	RHABDOMYOLYSIS	HEMOLYSIS	HEMATURIA
Urine color	Tea-colored	Red-colored	Tea-colored
Blood on dipstick	+	+	+
RBC on urine microscopy	0–few	0–few	Many
Elevated serum CK	+	−	−

Clinical Pearls

1.   Rhabdomyolysis is a pathologic process, not a specific disease; a broad differential diagnosis is associated and a comprehensive work-up is indicated to determine the cause.
2.   The extent of CK elevation is poorly correlated with severity of ARF.

REFERENCES
1. Visweswaran P, Guntupalli J: Rhabdomyolysis. Crit Care Clin 15:415–428, 1999.
2. Vanholder R, Sever MS, Erek E, et al: Rhabdomyolysis. J Am Soc Nephrol 11:1553–1561, 2000.
3. Sauret JM, Marinides G, Wang GK: Rhabdomyolysis. Am Fam Physician 65:907–912, 2002.

Cynthia Jacobstein, MD

PATIENT 64

A 6-week-old boy with apnea and cyanosis

A 6-week-old boy is brought to the emergency department with the history that he stopped breathing and turned blue. The event occurred 1 hour after his last feed. He seemed to be trying to breathe. His parents report that he seemed a little stiff, but that his eyes remained open throughout the event. No formula came from his mouth or nose. His face was blue around the nose and lips. His parents estimate that the event lasted 20 to 30 seconds and say it resolved with a small amount of gentle stimulation, followed by the infant falling to sleep. There is no history of fever or upper respiratory infection symptoms. He has been feeding, urinating, and stooling normally. The infant was born at term following an uncomplicated pregnancy, labor, and delivery and went home from the hospital with his mother. He has been growing well and has had only routine well-child visits to his pediatrician.

Physical Examination: Vital signs: temperature 37.3°C rectally; pulse 140; respiratory rate 40; blood pressure 85/45; oxygen saturation in room air 99%. General: well-nourished, well-developed infant, alert and active. HEENT: head atraumatic, anterior fontanelle soft and flat, red reflex visible bilaterally, tympanic membranes clear, moist mucous membranes with no lesions in the oropharynx. Chest: clear, equal breath sounds bilaterally with no increased work of breathing. Cardiac: Regular rate and rhythm without murmur or gallop. Abdomen: Soft, nondistended, nontender with no organomegaly or mass, normoactive bowel sounds. Skin: No rashes. Extremities: Pink and warm. Neurologic: Alert, cries with examination but is consoled easily with pacifier, good tone.

Laboratory Findings: No laboratory tests performed initially in the emergency department.

Questions: What is the initial impression? What are the next steps in the management of this patient?

Diagnosis and Management: Apparent life-threatening event (ALTE). The patient was admitted to the inpatient pediatric ward for observation and pH polysomnography study.

Discussion: The formal definition of an ALTE comes from a National Institutes of Health Consensus Conference on Infantile Apnea held in 1986. An ALTE is "an episode that is frightening to the observer and that is characterized by some combination of apnea (central or occasionally obstructive), color change (usually cyanotic or pallid but occasionally erythematous or plethoric), marked change in muscle tone (usually marked limpness), choking, or gagging."

An ALTE may be the result of a wide range of underlying conditions, potentially involving almost any organ system, and thus may be considered a presenting symptom rather than a final diagnosis. The table lists many of the possible causes. No definitive cause is found in approximately 50% of cases.

Possible Causes of ALTE

Infectious	**Central Nervous System**
Respiratory	Seizure
syncytial virus	Mass/lesion
Pertussis	Central hypoventilation
Pneumonia	**Metabolic**
Sepsis	Hypoglycemia
Meningitis/	Inborn error of
encephalitis	metabolism
Cardiac	**Hematologic**
Dysrhythmia	Anemia, especially in
Structural heart	preterm infant
disease	**Abuse/Münchausen**
Gastrointestinal	**by proxy**
Gastroesophageal	**Idiopathic**
reflux	
Dysfunctional	
swallowing	

It is the job of the emergency physician to evaluate the episode and decide whether it represents a true ALTE or normal infant physiology. If the episode is believed to be truly pathologic, the physician's role then includes beginning the diagnostic evaluation and therapeutic interventions as indicated. The history is one of the most important diagnostic tools in the evaluation of the infant who presents with an ALTE. It should be complete and include as many details of the event as the person who witnessed it is able to provide. A thorough physical examination is also essential.

The diagnostic work-up in the ED should always be individualized to the specific patient's presentation. There is no routine set of tests that must always be performed. Tests to consider include those that would diagnose the conditions listed in the differential diagnosis table, based on the individual presentation. If there are any indications of an infectious origin, such as hyper- or hypothermia, tachycardia, or lethargy, then a full sepsis evaluation is warranted in the ED. A chest x-ray or electrocardiogram (ECG) may be utilized as an initial work-up if any cardiac abnormality is indicated on physical examination (murmur, poor growth, tachycardia) or on history (sweating or tiring with feeds). Admission to the hospital for observation and monitoring should be considered for all events that seem to represent something other than normal infant physiology.

The current patient had a worrisome, yet nonspecific, history but completely normal physical examination findings on presentation to the emergency department. He was admitted to the hospital for observation, and pH polysomnography was performed. The patient was found to have gastroesophageal reflux without documented episodes of apnea or cyanosis. He was treated with ranitidine and metoclopramide and discharged home.

Clinical Pearls

1. An ALTE encompasses a large and heterogeneous group of diagnoses and should be considered as a presenting symptom rather than a diagnosis.

2. A thorough history and physical examination are key to determining whether an event is truly an ALTE and abnormal or rather a normal physiologic event, such as choking.

3. The emergency department evaluation of the infant with an ALTE should be focused on the details of each individual patient, rather than the performance of a long list of tests for all possible causes of ALTE.

4. Admission of the patient for observation and further focused evaluation is warranted for any event that is believed to represent a true ALTE.

REFERENCES

1. Palfrey S: Overcoming ALTEphobia: A rational approach to "spells" in infants. Contemp Pediatr 16:132–157, 1999.
2. Brooks JG: Apparent life-threatening events. Pediatr in Rev 17:257–259, 1996.
3. National Institutes of Health Consensus Development Conference on Infantile Apnea and Home Monitoring: Consensus statement. Pediatrics 79:292–299, 1987.

Allison R. Silver, MD

PATIENT 65

A 55 year-old woman with chest pain and shortness of breath

A 53-year-old Spanish-speaking woman presents to the emergency department accompanied by her nephew. Obtaining the history is difficult because of extreme respiratory distress and the language barrier. She is able to report that she has chest pain radiating down her left arm. Her son arrives and explains that the patient has non-insulin-dependent diabetes and hypertension. She has been reporting dyspnea, heat intolerance, diarrhea, and diaphoresis for 4 days. She recently spent 6 months in the Dominican Republic, where she was started on a new medication for similar symptoms. She had run out of this medication approximately 2 weeks earlier.

Physical Examination: Vital signs: temperature 37°C; heart rate 190; blood pressure 110/72; respiratory rate 50. General: extreme respiratory distress with central cyanosis, cough with pink frothy sputum, vomiting. HEENT: normal. Chest: diffuse crackles. Cardiac: tachycardiac. Abdomen: normal. Extremities: normal.

Laboratory Findings: CBC: WBC 15,100/μl, otherwise normal. Chemistries: glucose 274 mg/dl, otherwise normal. U/A: glucose $+++$, otherwise negative. Urine drug screen: negative. ABG (100% O_2): pH 7.29, PCO_2 49 mmHg, PO_2 106 mmHg, HCO_3 24 mEq/L. ECG: rapid atrial fibrillation (see figure). Chest x-ray: pulmonary edema and congestive heart failure (see figure).

Questions: What diagnosis can explain all of the patient's symptoms? What blood test could one order to help confirm the diagnosis? What may have been the medication that she ran out of?

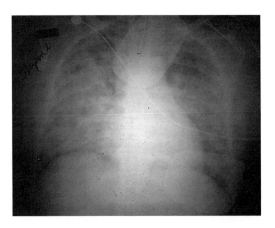

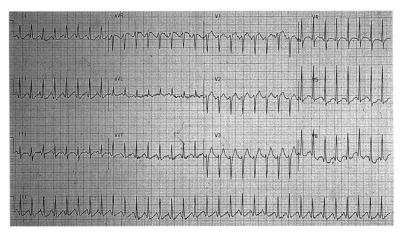

Diagnosis: The patient receives adenosine 6 mg and then 12 mg IV with no response. She is cardioverted at 50, 100, and 200 Joules with no change in her cardiac rhythm. She is endotracheally intubated. Subsequently, her son returns to the emergency department with an empty box that had contained the medication she was given in the Dominican Republic. The hospital pharmacist was consulted to help translate the name of the medication from Spanish and concludes that it was propylthiouracil (PTU). Treatment is begun for the presumed diagnosis of thyroid storm and a confirmatory thyroid-stimulating hormone (TSH) level is ordered. The result is 0.00 mIU/ml.

Discussion: A patient is considered thyrotoxic when he or she exhibits clinical, physiologic, and biochemical findings resulting from tissue exposure to excess thyroid hormone. Thyroid storm is a rare but life-threatening syndrome characterized by exaggerated manifestations of thyrotoxicosis. It is generally precipitated by illness or surgery, or, in the case of the present patient, noncompliance with medications. It is a purely clinical diagnosis requiring a high degree of suspicion, and it has a mortality rate of approximately 30% for hospitalized patients.

The thyroid gland is made up of follicles containing a peptide called *thyroglobulin,* which is iodinated and broken down to form L-thyroxine (T_4) and L-thyronine (T_3), the biologically active compound. Production is mediated by the hypothalamus' release of thyroid-releasing hormone (TRH), which in turn stimulates release of TSH from the anterior pituitary. Much of the body's T_3 is made in peripheral tissues by conversion from T_4.

Thyrotoxicity carries a wide range of symptoms, including fatigue, heat intolerance, weight loss, change in bowel habits, and cardiovascular symptoms, as seen in this patient. Ninety-five percent of patients have some type of tachycardia. Many of the signs and symptoms are attributable to stimulation of the adrenergic system.

It is helpful to view the treatment of this condition as multifaceted strategy:

1. Block hormone synthesis: This is generally the first step. There are two classes of thioamide antithyroid drugs represented by the drugs propylthiouracil (PTU) and methimazole. They both interfere with the iodination of thyroglobulin.

2. Inhibit hormone release: There are various forms of inorganic iodide (Lugol's solution, SSKI, sodium iodide, radiographic contrast dyes, amiodarone), all of which stop thyroglobulin proteolysis.

3. Blocking conversion of T_4 to T_3: Several modalities are available, including radiographic iodine, amiodarone, corticosteroids, propanolol, and PTU. Dexamethasone or hydrocortisone is usually used for this purpose.

4. Lessen adrenergic effects: Historically, this was done by the drugs reserpine and guanethidine; beta-blockade is now favored. Propanolol is the most widely studied drug and is administered in small doses until symptoms abate. Esmolol is also being used more, as it is quickly titratable.

5. Remove excess circulating hormone: Considered if conventional therapy fails. Options include plasmapheresis, dialysis, exchange transfusion, and more.

6. Supportive care: The "ABC's," with close attention to temperature control, fluid resuscitation with central venous monitoring if necessary, dextrose repletion, and treatment of associated congestive heart failure (CHF).

7. Treat precipitating illness: This is not always obvious and requires full investigation.

8. Definitive care: Ultimately, when a patient is stable, options include radioactive iodine or surgical ablation of the gland.

Patients such as the present patient require admission to an intensive care unit setting. Clinical improvement is expected within 1 to 2 hours after administration of antiadrenergic agents, with decrease in T_3 and T_4 levels as soon as 24 hours. Full recovery takes about 1 week.

The present patient received 200 mg PTU via nasogastric tube, 10 mg dexamethasone IV, and an esmolol infusion. One hour later she was given 10 drops of Lugol's iodine solution. She was discharged to home 10 days later on methimazole and propanolol. She returned to the ED a few days later with a supraventricular tachycardia after losing her prescription for propanolol. Two months later, she underwent I^{131} ablation and is now doing well, maintained on thyroid hormone replacement therapy.

Clinical Pearls

1. Iodides given to block hormone release must be given at least 1 hour after the antithyroid medications to prevent a paradoxical *increase* in the production of hormone that would occur as iodides are used as substrate for hormone synthesis.

2. The empiric administration of glucocorticoids is just that, *empiric*. It is on the basis of a theorized relative adrenal insufficiency that has never been proven, but steroids also have an important role in blocking conversion of T_4 to T_3.

3. Do not be afraid to use β-blockers in thyrotoxic patients with CHF. CHF in a patient with thyroid storm is often rate-related or secondary to atrial fibrillation, and blockade is therefore very helpful.

REFERENCES

1. Manifold CA: Hyperthyroidism, thyroid storm and Graves disease. eMedicine.com, 2000. Accessed April 2003.
2. Cooper DS: Treatment of thyrotoxicosis. In Werner and Ingbar's The Thyroid, 7th ed. Philadelphia, Lippincott, 1996, pp 713–724.
3. Wartofsky L: Thyrotoxic Storm. Werner and Ingbar's The Thyroid, 7th ed. Philadelphia, Lippincott, 1996, pp 701–707.
4. Tietgens ST, Leinung MC: Thyroid storm. Med Clin North Am 79:170–184, 1995.
5. Burch HB, Wartofsky L: Life threatening thyrotoxicosis: Thyroid storm. Endocrinol Metab Clin North Am 22:263–277, 1993.
6. Brunette DD, Rothong C: Emergency department management of thyrotoxic crisis with esmolol. Am J Emerg Med 9: 232–234, 1991.

Eron Friedlaender, MD
Kathy Shaw, MD, MSCE

PATIENT 66

A 2-year-old girl with fever and rash

A previously healthy 2-year-old girl is brought to the emergency department with several hours of headache and a nonpruritic, progressive rash. She has had 24 hours of fever associated with several episodes of nonbloody, nonbilious vomiting and diarrhea. Her immunizations are up to date and her only medication is intermittent doses of acetaminophen. Recent sick exposures included multiple classmates in day care diagnosed with acute viral gastroenteritis.

Physical Examination: Vital signs: temperature 39.1°C rectally; pulse 180; respiratory rate 40; blood pressure 113/55. General: ill-appearing, lethargic. HEENT: no photophobia, dry mucous membranes. Neck: supple, negative Kernig's sign, and negative Brudzinski's sign. Chest: clear to auscultation. Cardiac: tachycardiac with regular rhythm, no murmur or gallop. Abdomen: soft, nontender, nondistended. Extremities: cool hands and feet, 3 to 4-second capillary refill. Neurologic: pupils 3 mm bilaterally and equally reactive, responds to voice with eye opening, moves all extremities spontaneously and symmetrically. Skin: showers of petechiae and purpura scattered over trunk and extremities (see figure).

Laboratory Findings: WBC 18,500/μl with 17% bands, 72% neutrophils; hemoglobin 12.3 g/dl, platelets 412,000/μl. Sodium 131 mEq/L. Prothrombin time 15.3 seconds (normal 11.7–13.2 seconds), partial thromboplastin time 36.8 seconds (normal 26.0–38.0 seconds), fibrinogen 700 mg/dl (normal 172–471 mg/dl), D-dimer 3.96 UGFEU/ml (normal 0.1–0.6 UGFEU/ml). Cerebrospinal fluid: WBC 1850, RBC 62, protein 137 mg/dl, glucose 121 mg/dl; Gram stain, many WBCs, rare diplococci.

ED Course: Two large-bore peripheral intravenous catheters were placed. The patient was then given 60 ml/kg normal saline and meningitic doses of vancomycin and ceftriaxone. A dopamine infusion was prepared to be ready at the bedside.

Question: What is the most likely diagnosis?

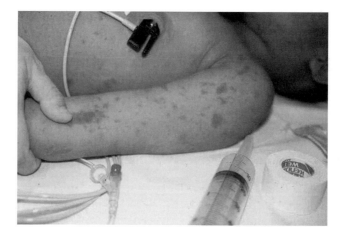

Diagnosis: Meningococcal meningitis with meningococcemia

Discussion: *Neisseria meningitidis* is an encapsulated, gram-negative, aerobic diplococcus responsible for a wide spectrum of disease states, ranging greatly in severity but including irreversible, rapidly progressive multisystem organ failure. Immediate recognition of patients with invasive meningococcal infection allows for initiation of aggressive antibiotic therapy and supportive care designed to moderate the potentially devastating sequelae of this invasive bacterial disease.

The incidence of meningococcal disease in the United States is approximately 1.1 cases per 100,000 people per year. Rates of infection peak in the winter and early spring months. The disease disproportionately affects the young, with 46% of cases in children 2 years of age or younger. Thirteen serotypes of *N. meningitidis* are responsible for producing disease. The majority of meningococcal disease in this country results from infection with strains from groups B, C, and Y, whereas serotypes A and C predominate worldwide.

Meningococcal disease is spread through the aerosolization of infected respiratory droplets. The organisms invade through the microvilli of the mucosal cells in the nasopharynx, thereby gaining access to the blood stream and allowing for the dissemination of bacteria throughout the host. Clinical findings generally occur within 2 weeks of contact with the bacteria. Increased susceptibility to the development of meningococcemia occurs with exposure to tobacco smoke and coincident viral upper respiratory tract infections as a result of disruption of the integrity of the nasal mucosa. Individuals with an altered complement-mediated immune system are also at greater risk for contracting infection with *N. meningitidis*. Finally, an association between meningococcal disease and both black race and low socioeconomic status has been described and attributed to their association with urban crowding and increased chances of contact with someone harboring the organism.

Meningococcal sepsis has a dramatic clinical presentation, including the abrupt onset of high fever; myalgias; a petechial, purpuric, or urticarial rash; hemodynamic instability with myocardial dysfunction; and evidence of multisystem organ failure, including adrenal insuffiency, oliguria, and disseminated intravascular coagulation. Meningeal infection with *N. meningitidis* results from the hematogenous spread of bacteria in approximately 50% of patients with meningococcemia. These individuals report headache, stiff neck, vomiting, and photophobia and may possibly display an altered mental status. Less invasive clinical syndromes associated with meningococcal infection include pneumonia, epiglottitis, otitis media, conjunctivitis, urethritis, salpingitis, septic arthritis, and pericarditis.

The initial diagnosis of meningococcal disease rests on clinical suspicion, and empiric therapy should be initiated without delay. Confirmation of infection requires bacteriologic isolation of *N. meningitidis* from blood or cerebrospinal, pericardial, pleural, or synovial fluids. Supportive evidence of meningeal disease includes cerebrospinal fluid with either gram-negative diplococci, a leukocytosis of predominantly polymorphonuclear cells, a low glucose level, or an elevated protein count. Gram stains of scrapings from petechial lesions may also reveal intracellular organisms suggestive of meningococcal infection. Counterimmunoelectrophoresis, latex agglutination, and coagglutination studies of cerebrospinal fluid are available but are of limited utility, as they each demonstrate high false-negative rates in practice. Blood and urine antigen tests are similarly unreliable.

Early antibiotic administration in suspected cases of meningococcal disease substantially reduces morbidity and mortality. Specifically, penicillin, ceftriaxone, and cefotaxime are appropriate first-line agents. Chloramphenicol is an alternative treatment for penicillin-allergic patients. Droplet precautions are recommended during the first 24 hours of antibiotic therapy. Supportive care is often required to assist patients experiencing hemodynamic collapse, neurologic impairment, metabolic derangements, or coagulopathy. Chemoprophylaxis with rifampin, ciprofloxacin, or ceftriaxone is indicated for all individuals in either the household or day care who are in contact with the index case for at least 8 hours a day, or medical personnel exposed to the patient's oral secretions. Preventative therapy should be received within 24 hours of diagnosis of meningococcal disease. A quadrivalent polysaccharide vaccine is available that protects against serogroups A, C, Y, and W-135 by inducing bactericidal antibody production. Immunoprophylaxis with this vaccine is used during epidemics or in high-risk populations, including individuals with asplenia or terminal complement or properdin deficiencies, military recruits, college students, and people traveling to epidemic regions. Clinical efficacy rates of 85% or higher have been documented in individuals older than 5 years of age. Routine childhood immunization is not recommended given the vaccine's limited immunogenicity and brief duration of efficacy in infants and young children.

Mortality rates from invasive meningococcal disease range from 5 to 20%. Death usually results from overwhelming shock causing irreversible multisystem organ failure. Adverse outcome is associated with the following characteristics upon admission to the hospital: poor perfusion, rash, hypothermia or hyperthermia, abnormal platelet count, abnormal peripheral leukocyte and differential counts, and prolonged prothrombin and partial thromboplastin time. Sequelae of infection for survivors most commonly includes sensorineural hearing loss, vasculitis, arthritis, iritis, episcleritis, myocarditis, and subdural effusion.

The present patient was infected with *Neisseria meningitides* type C. She required aggressive fluid resuscitation, and remained in the intensive care unit for several days, where she was treated with vancomycin and cefotaxime. Antibiotics were changed to penicillin once sensitivities were available. Her mental status returned to baseline and she was discharged to home with no long-term complications.

Clinical Pearls

1. Confirmed or suspected cases of meningococcal disease should be reported to a regional public health department.
2. Antibiotic therapy should not be delayed for confirmatory laboratory evidence of meningococcal disease.
3. Chemoprophylaxis is recommended for all household and day care contacts of an index case as well as anyone exposed to oral secretions from a infected individual.
4. Infection may lead to rapidly progressive multisystem organ failure.

REFERENCES

1. Nguyen T, Malley R, Inkelis S, et al: Comparison of prediction models for adverse outcome in pediatric meningococcal disease using artificial neural network and logistic regression analyses. J Clin Epi 55:687–695, 2002.
2. Rosenstein N, Perkins B, Stephens D, et al: Meningococcal disease. N Engl J Med 344:1378–1388, 2001.
3. Rosenstein N, Perkins B, Stephens D, et al: The changing epidemiology of meningococcal disease in the United States, 1992–1996. J Infect Dis 180:1894–1901, 1999.
4. Rosenstein N, Levine O, Taylor J, et al: Efficacy of meningococcal vaccine and barriers to vaccination. JAMA 279:435–439, 1998.
5. Kirsch E, Barton R, Kitchen L, et al: Pathophysiology, treatment and outcome of meningococcemia: A review and recent experience. Pediatr Infect Dis J 15:967–979, 1996.
6. Apicella M: Neisseria meningitidis. In Mandell G, Bennett J, Dolin R, eds: Principles and Practice of Infectious Diseases. New York, Churchill Livingstone, 1995, pp 1896–1909.
7. Riedo F, Plikaytis B, Broome C: Epidemiology and prevention of meningococcal disease. Pediatr Infect Dis J 14: 643–657, 1995.
8. Periappuram M, Taylor R, Keane C: Rapid detection of meningococci from petechiae in acute meningococcal infection. J Infection 31:201–203, 1995.
9. Baker C, Edwards M: Meningococcal infections. In Oski F, ed. Principles and Practice of Pediatrics. Philadelphia, J. B. Lippincott, 1994, pp 1199–1203.
10. Edwards M, Baker C: Complications and sequelae of meningococcal infections in children. J Pediatr 99:540– 545, 1981.

M. Bradley Falk, MD
Jill M. Baren, MD, FACEP, FAAP

PATIENT 67

A 28-year-old man with facial swelling

A 28-year-old man presents to the emergency department with facial swelling that began 20 minutes earlier. He denies dyspnea, wheezing, or hoarseness. He reports minimal pruritis involving his chest and arms and swelling of his lips and tongue (see figure). Symptoms began shortly after dinner (he unintentionally ingested fish) and have been progressively more severe. In the past he has had similar but less severe reactions to seafood. He denies any new detergents, soaps, colognes, clothes, or pet contact.

Physical Examination: Vital signs: temperature 36.6°C; heart rate 100; respiratory rate 18; blood pressure 135/85; room air pulse oximetry 98%. HEENT: Marked edema of lips and tongue (anterior); airway patent; no obvious oropharyngeal or uvular edema; no stridor; tolerating his secretions; voice with normal character. Neck: supple, nontender. Chest: clear to auscultation bilaterally. Cardiac: regular rate and rhythm, no murmurs, rubs, or gallops. Abdomen: normal. Extremeties: no rash or other edema. Nasopharyngeal laryngoscopy: minimal base of tongue edema extending into the valecula; no laryngeal edema; vocal cords have good mobility.

Laboratory Findings: CBC: normal. Chemistries: normal.

Questions: Before obtaining a detailed history, what needs to be assessed on *any* patient with the above constellation of symptoms? What is one immediate medication that you can administer even without intravenous access?

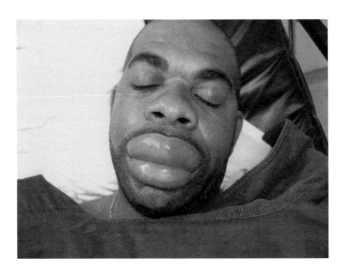

Diagnosis: Angioedema. The swelling of his lips and tongue is extremely worrisome because it signifies potential airway compromise. The patency and protection of the patient's airway is assessed before anything else. If the patient exhibits any sign of airway compromise, proceed with intubation for airway protection. Epinephrine is immediately available and often necessary in this setting. This patient should receive 0.3 mg of subcutaneous epinephrine (0.5 ml of 1:10,000 epinephrine). An important caveat to consider when using epinephrine is that patients with coronary artery disease may develop ischemia as a result of epinephrine's adrenergic effects, but this risk needs to be balanced with the need for relief of airway obstruction.

Discussion: Angioedema is the result of increased capillary permeability with fluid loss into the surrounding tissue (edema). This ranges from peripheral edema (as in the present patient) to internal edema involving the gastrointestinal tract (on occasion causing obstruction). The concern is that the edema may involve the patient's airway, an obviously life-threatening event. The term *anaphylactic shock* refers to hypotension in the setting of the above. Whereas angioedema has many possible causes (discussed below), true anaphylaxis is an IgE-mediated process and in many patients has precedent in previous similar episodes.

Patients experiencing an allergic reaction may be able to identify a trigger, such as foods (seafood, peanuts), hymenoptera envenomations (bee stings), medications (penicillin) and environmental or topical agents (soaps, perfumes). It is important to ask whether patients have been treated for the same in the past, and whether they have ever required endotracheal intubation or a stay in an intensive care unit. If so, this places the patient in a higher risk category. Standard therapy for allergic reactions includes antihistamines (diphenhydramine), corticosteroids (methylprednisolone), and epinephrine (to increase adrenergic tone and vasoconstriction). Airway control is of paramount importance, and if the patient is not responding to therapy and the edema is progressive, endotracheal intubation is warrented for airway protection. Any delay in this measure may result in a difficult (or impossible) intubation once edema is severe. A cricothyroidotomy set should be available and ready to use if needed.

Angioedema has many other nonallergic causes. Patients with C1-esterase deficiency (an autosomal dominant trait resulting in deficient or defective C1-inhibitor affecting the compliment pathway) may present to the ED with the same clinical picture. This is historically referred to as *hereditary angioedema* as it was described in the 19th century. Although the mechanism of inhibition is unclear, many patients with known hereditary angioedema are prescribed androgens (e.g., danazol) for prophylaxis. Acute treament in the ED differs from that of the allergy-induced angioedema as this is *not* IgE-mediated. Ideally, replacement of C1-esterase should be instituted as soon as possible. However, in many institutions this product is unavailable. Instead, infusing fresh frozen plasma is an acceptable alternative for enzyme replacement.

In patients older than 65 years of age with a history of hypertension, angiotensin-converting enzymne (ACE) inhibitors should be considered the likely cause of angioedema. For more than a decade, this association has been well described. The drugs inhibit ACE by inactivating bradykinin and by inhibiting conversion of angiotenson I to angiotensin II. Both mechanisms result in vasodilation. The therapy for ACE-inhibitor induced angioedema is cessation of the drug. Any member of this class of drugs can cause angioedema, and a patient may have taken this particular medication (without problems) for quite some time prior to onset of these symptoms.

Clinical Pearls

1. Prior to any other action, establish a patent airway with effective breathing. If the patient is not responding to treatment, intubate early.

2. Not all facial edema represents an allergic response; remember heriditary angioedema and consider fresh frozen plasma administration as soon as possible.

3. After initial treatment, prolonged observation and hospitalization are necessary, as symptoms sometimes rebound.

4. If discharging the patient, establish follow-up with an allergist; write a prescription for an Epi-pen and instruct the patient on its usage.

REFERENCES

1. Grattan CE: Urticaria, angio-oedema and anaphylaxis. Clin Med JRCPL 2:20–23, 2002.
2. Kaplan AP: Chronic urticaria and angioedema. N Engl J Med 346:175–179, 2002.
3. Carugati A, Pappalardo E, et al: C1-inhibitor deficiency and angioedema. Molec Immunol 38:161–173, 2001.
4. Chiu AG, Burningham AR, et al: Angiotensin-converting enzyme inhibitor-induced angioedema: A multicenter review and an algorithm for airway management. Ann Otol Rhinol Laryngol 11:834–840, 2001.
5. Koury SI, Herfel LU: Anaphylaxis and acute allergic reactions. In Tintinalli JE, Kelen GD, Stapczynski JS: Emergency Medicine, 5th ed. New York, McGraw-Hill, 2000, pp 245–246.

PATIENT 68

A 34-year-old man with confusion, diaphoresis, and drooling

A 34-year-old man is brought to the emergency department via ambulance from the local farm where he works in the field. He was found on the ground by his coworkers, and they noted him to be agitated and confused.

Physical Examination: Vital signs: temperature 37.0°C; pulse 52; respiratory rate 28; blood pressure 110/62; room air pulse oximetry 93%. General appearance: awake, confused, and anxious with intermittent episodes of vomiting. Head: normal. Eyes: pin-point pupils. Mouth: drooling, breath with garlic odor. Lungs: diffuse wheezing, few coarse crackles. Cardiac: bradycardic without murmurs. Abdomen: nontender, active bowel sounds. Extremities: diffuse muscle fasciculations. Skin: diaphoretic. ECG: Sinus rhythm, QTc 550 msec.

Questions: What diagnosis can explain the patient's presentation? What is the mechanism of toxicity? What are the necessary therapeutic interventions?

Diagnosis: Organophosphate poisoning/cholinergic toxicity. Common insecticides such as diazinon and parathion are organophosphate compounds that act as powerful inhibitors of the enzyme acetylcholinesterase (ACHE) in the nervous system. This produces an excess of acetylcholine and overstimulation of its receptors. A cholinergic crisis is a clinical toxidrome involving the central, autonomic, and peripheral (neuromuscular junction) nervous systems with overstimulation of both nicotinic and muscarinic acetylcholine receptors.

Discussion: Poisoning is often secondary to accidental exposure in the home, during the production of the products, or in insect control workers. Absorption of the chemicals occurs by the inhalational, transdermal, transconjunctival, mucous membrane, and gastrointestinal routes. Metabolism occurs via hepatic enzyme degradation.

Clinical findings (see table) are caused by overstimulation of cholinergic receptors. The classic presentation is that of a patient who is unresponsive and has diaphoresis, muscle fasciculations, emesis, diarrhea, salivation, lacrimation, and urinary incontinence. The presentation can vary depending on the particular organophosphate and the amount and route of exposure. Most victims are symptomatic within 8 hours of a significant exposure. Acetylcholine stimulates both the sympathetic and the parasympathetic nervous systems, so the particular clinical effects depend on the predominant receptors affected. Significant nicotinic stimulation of the skeletal muscle leads to fasciculations, weakness, and eventually paralysis.

The diagnosis of organophosphate poisoning is based on several criteria: (1) A history suggestive of exposure to an insecticide, (2) findings suggestive of the toxidrome, and (3) laboratory acetylcholinesterase testing. A petroleum or garlic-like odor may be noted. The differential diagnosis for an organophosphate poisoning is large and includes all other causes of central nervous system alterations, seizures, pulmonary diseases with bronchospasm, and other toxic ingestions. Plasma and red blood cell cholinesterase assays may aid in following the course of treatment; however, they are unlikely to be available in the ED setting. Without treatment, the cholinesterase levels may take several months to return to baseline levels.

Treatment consists of decontamination, supportive care, prevention of further absorption, and the antidotes atropine and pralidoxime (2-PAM). Reversal of excessive muscarinic effects to prevent paralysis and cardiovascular effects is the primary goal of treatment. Decontamination includes removal of all clothing followed by complete external washing of the patient, including the scalp, hair, fingernails, skin, and conjunctivae, with soapy water. All hospital personnel should wear appropriate gloves, gowns, and protective gear. For large gastrointestinal ingestions, charcoal is indicated. There is no indication for removal of toxin via hemodialysis.

The patient should be supported with 100% oxygen, cardiac monitoring, and pulse oximetry. Seizures, profuse tracheal secretions, bronchospasm, or central nervous system depression are indications for early endotracheal intubation. To facilitate intubation, a nondepolarizing paralytic agent is recommended. Succinylcholine is contraindicated, as it is not metabolized in the setting of decreased serum cholinesterase activity and it can lead to prolonged paralysis.

Effects Seen in Cholinergic Toxicity

Sympathetic Effects	Parasympathetic Effects	Skeletal Muscle
Central nervous system	Central nervous system	
Confusion	Confusion	Fasciculations
Agitation	Hallucinations	Weakness
Hallucinations	Coma	Paralysis
Coma	Seizures	
Seizures	Miosis	
Mydriasis	Bronchorrhea	
Bronchodilation	Salivation, lacrimation	
Tachycardia	Bradycardia	
Hypertension	Urinary incontinence	
Hyperglycemia	Gastrointestinal distress, diarrhea, emesis	
Ketosis		
Urinary retention		

Therapy should not be withheld pending laboratory determination of ACHE level. For significant poisonings, atropine and pralidoxime are indicated. Atropine competitively antagonizes acetylcholine at muscarinic receptors, and it should be given immediately upon recognition of organophosphate poisoning. The dose is titrated to the effect of dried tracheobronchial secretions, which may require several hundred milligrams to reverse a massive overdose. The initial dose of atropine is 2 to 4 mg (adult) and 0.05 mg/kg (child). Failure to respond to a single test dose correlates well with organophosphate poisoning. The dose is doubled and given every 5 to 10 minutes until symptoms are relieved.

Pralidoxime is a compound that enhances the regeneration of ACHE. The ACHE enzyme is inactivated by the organophosphate compound, and then inactivation becomes permanent in a process called "aging" over 24 to 72 hours. If given early, pralidoxime aids in restoring acetylcholine and in reversing the muscarinic and nicotinic effects. However, pralidoxime is unable to restore acetylcholinesterase after aging has occurred. Initial pralidoxime dose is 1 to 2 g IV over 30 to 60 minutes followed by an infusion of 250 to 500 mg/hour titrated to the patient's symptoms.

Mild exposures may require 6 to 8 hours of ED observation after decontamination. Admission to an intensive care setting is required for any significant exposure. Most patients respond to 2-PAM within the first 48 hours. Death from organophosphates usually occurs in first 24 hours if untreated and is usually secondary to respiratory paralysis and central nervous system depression.

The present patient had a rapidly progressive worsening of his respiratory status, with the development of pulmonary edema and hypoxia. He improved slowly after the immediate administration of atropine and initiation of a pralidoxime infusion. He received a total of 25 mg of atropine. However, the emergency physician elected to intubate the patient using vecuronium. Activated charcoal was administered, and the patient was admitted to the intensive care unit. He remained on the ventilator for 48 hours and was successfully weaned and extubated. After 72 hours, his diarrhea and diaphoresis resolved. He was successfully weaned off the pralidoxime infusion. He was discharged from the hospital 5 days after his initial presentation.

Clinical Pearls

1. Muscarinic cholinergic symptoms can be remembered by the mnemonic SLUDGE: *s*alivation, *l*acrimation, *u*rination, *d*iarrhea, *g*astrointestinal distress, and *e*mesis.

2. Atropine treatment is titrated to dry the tracheal secretions and improve oxygenation; there is no universal correct dose, and massive overdoses often require hundreds of milligrams of atropine to control the tracheobronchial secretions.

3. The most common cause of treatment failure is inadequate atropinization.

4. Organophosphates such as sarin are the principal toxins found in many chemical warfare nerve gases.

REFERENCES
1. Robey W, Meggs W: Insecticides, herbicides, and rodenticides. In Tintinalli J (ed): Emergency Medicine: A Comprehensive Study Guide, 5th ed. New York, McGraw-Hill, 2000, pp 1174–1176.
2. Clark RF. Insecticides: Organic phosphorus compounds and carbamates. In Goldfrank L (ed): Toxicologic Emergencies, 6th ed. New York, McGraw- Hill, 1998, pp 1346–1357.

Joel Fein, MD

PATIENT 69

A 15-year-old boy with sudden-onset abdominal pain and vomiting

A 15-year-old boy presents to the emergency department reporting right-sided abdominal pain. He vomited twice in the past 2 hours but has not reported loose stools. The abdominal pain was sudden in onset, was sharp, and has waxed and waned since it started 2 hours ago.

Physical Examination: Temperature 37°C; pulse 105; respiratory rate 20; blood pressure 120/85. Chest: clear. Abdomen: slightly tender to deep palpation of right lower quadrant, right groin slightly tender. Genitalia: right side of scrotum swollen and red, tender right testicle (see figure).

Laboratory Findings: CBC: normal. Urinalysis: negative.

Questions: What are the major diagnostic considerations in this situation? What immediate interventions are needed?

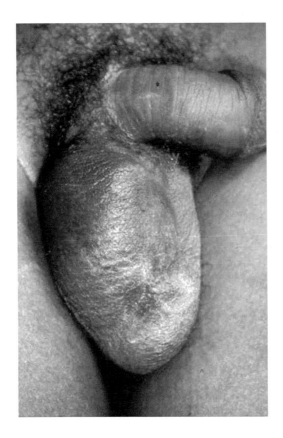

Diagnosis and Treatment: Right-sided testicular torsion. Initial management in high-suspicion cases should be manual detorsion, followed by operative detorsion and contralateral orchiopexy. In questionable cases, lack of blood flow to the testicle can be demonstrated by color Doppler ultrasonography.

Discussion: The most common causes of scrotal pain in older children and adolescents are testicular torsion, epididymitis, orchitis, and scrotal trauma. Other considerations include incarcerated inguinal hernia and torsion of the appendix testis. Pain of sudden onset suggests a vascular cause, possibly testicular torsion. Patients with testicular torsion invariably report nausea and/or vomiting. The absence of fever does not rule out epididymitis or orchitis. Pain due to traumatic injuries often resolves by the time that the patient gets to medical attention.

It is important to recognize that the child with scrotal pathology will often report lower abdominal or groin pain. A patient reporting abdominal pain should always have a genital examination performed. Conversely, it is important to examine the abdomen of all patients with scrotal pain to evaluate for peritoneal inflammation, intestinal obstruction, and abdominal masses.

Timing is crucial in the diagnosis and management of testicular torsion. In general, the prognosis is excellent if the testis is detorsed within 3 hours of symptom onset. After 8 hours, the salvage rate is below 25%, and salvage is rare after 24 hours of persistent ischemia.

Manual detorsion in the emergency setting can allow the testicle to remain viable until emergency surgery can be performed. When torsion occurs, the superior pole of the testicle frequently twists medially, toward the contralateral thigh. In the manual detorsion procedure, one holds the affected testicle between thumb and forefinger and untwists 360 degrees toward the ipsilateral thigh. If relief is noted, the testicle should be rotated another 360 degrees or more, since the usual twist is 720 degrees. Because testicles can rarely torse in the opposite direction, the direction can be reversed if more pain or swelling occurs after the initial maneuver. Sedation and analgesia may be warranted to facilitate the detorsion procedure. Surgical correction (bilateral orchiopexy) is still necessary after this maneuver, but the emergency detorsion procedure can help salvage the affected testicle.

Clinical Pearls

1. All patients with abdominal pain should undergo a thorough genital examination.
2. Testicular torsion is a surgical emergency, and laboratory and radiologic studies should not delay surgical management.
3. Manual detorsion in the emergency department may prevent testicular necrosis.

REFERENCES

1. Fein JA: Pathology in the privates: Acute scrotal swelling in children and adolescents. Pediatr Emerg Med Rep 2:47–56, 1997.
2. Lewis AG, Bukowski TP, Jarvis PD, et al: Evaluation of acute scrotum in the emergency department. J Pediatr Surg 30: 277–282, 1995.
3. Chamberlain RS, Greenberg LW: Scrotal involvement in Henoch-Schönlein purpura: A case report and review of the literature. Pediatr Emerg Care 8:213–215, 1992.
4. Gedalia A, Mordehai J, Mares AJ: Acute scrotal involvement in children with familial Mediterranean fever. Am J Dis Child 146:1419–1420, 1992.
5. Cattolica EV: Preoperative manual detorsion of the torsed spermatic cord. J Urol 133:803–805, 1985.
6. Knight PJ, Vassy LE: The diagnosis and treatment of the acute scrotum in children and adolescents. Ann Surg 200:664–673, 1984.
7. Cass AS: Testicular trauma. J Urol 129:299–300, 1983.

Kevin M. Takakuwa, MD
Jill M. Baren, MD, FACEP, FAAP

PATIENT 70

A 55-year-old man with unresponsiveness

A 55-year-old man with a history of congestive heart failure, alcohol abuse, and depression presents to the emergency department by 911 rescue after being found unresponsive by his daughter. He lives in a third floor apartment with closed windows and without fans or air conditioning. The rescue team estimates the apartment was 48.9° C, and his clothes were drenched in sweat, although he had no perspiration on his body.

Physical Examination: Vital signs: temperature 42.2° C; pulse 132; assisted respirations 16 by bag-valve with nasal intubation; blood pressure 80/44. Skin: dry. HEENT: pupils dilated and minimally responsive to light. Chest: clear to auscultation. Cardiac: regular tachycardia without gallops or murmurs. Abdomen: unremarkable. Extremities: no edema. Neuromuscular: unresponsive with Glasgow Coma Scale score of 3.

Laboratory Findings: CBC: unremarkable. Blood chemistries: Na 124, K 5.3, Cl 96, HCO_3 15, Bun 19, Cr 1.7, glucose 159. Urine dipstick: positive for blood, glucose, protein. ABG (after endotracheal tube intubation on 100% oxygen): pH 7.26, $PaCO_2$ 38, PaO_2 400. CK 1086, CK-MB 1.3, troponin 0.9. Coagulation studies: PT 13.8, INR 1.3, PTT 24.4. LFTs normal. ECG: wide complex sinus tachycardia, left bundle branch block. Chest radiograph: cardiomegaly. Unenhanced head CT: normal.

Questions: After immediate resuscitation and stabilization, what is the next most essential therapy for this patient? What is the cause of the urine abnormality? Why is creatine kinase level elevated?

Diagnosis and Treatment: Classic heat stroke. Rapid cooling must take place, as hyperthermia can permanently damage virtually any organ system.

Discussion: Heat stroke is defined as an elevated core body temperature to greater than 40°C accompanied by central nervous system (CNS) dysfunction. It usually includes anhydrosis, although the presence of sweating does not rule out the diagnosis. There are two forms: classic, or nonexertional, and exertional. Classic heat stroke results from exposure to high ambient environmental temperatures, usually in the setting of impaired heat regulatory mechanisms. Exertional heat stroke is due to prolonged exercise or activity in high temperatures in either acclimatized or unacclimatized individuals. The presenting characteristics of the two forms of heat illness are variable (see table). Hyperthermia occurs when the body's normal temperature homeostasis is interrupted by damage to the thermoregulatory center, allowing the body's temperature to rise unregulated. Denaturation and altered expression of heat shock proteins leads to cellular damage in multiple organ systems.

The CNS is the most profoundly affected of all organ systems. Symptoms range from fatigue, irritability, weakness, behavioral changes, and impaired judgment to stupor, delirium, paralysis, hallucinations, seizures, and coma. The renal, hepatic, cardiac, pulmonary, hematologic, and gastrointestinal systems are also sensitive to hyperthermic insult and can sustain permanent damage from direct cellular or functional injury. Damage throughout the body is related not only to the maximum core temperature but also to the length of exposure; prolongation of either increases the risks of morbidity and mortality.

Early response to hyperthermia includes tachycardia, the result of the body's attempt to circulate central blood to the periphery for dissipation via cutaneous vasodilation, and tachypnea, which manifests as respiratory alkalosis in classic heat stroke but can also be a compensatory mechanism for lactic acidosis in exertional heat stroke, in which patients are often dehydrated. Surprisingly, hypotension is reported only in one quarter of heat stroke patients, but its presence signifies poor prognosis.

Once the dyad of hyperthermia and CNS dysfunction are established, cooling should be immediately initiated. Many techniques have been suggested. Noninvasive cooling includes evaporation, immersion, and ice packing. Invasive methods include gastric, peritoneal, and even pericardial lavage with cool fluids. Experts recommend evaporative cooling to avoid shivering, normally a protective response that works against cooling. Patients should be fully undressed and sprayed with tepid water while the skin is electrically fanned. If shivering occurs, warmer air, warmer spray water, or skin massage should be used. Cooling should be discontinued when the core body temperature is lowered to 39°C, to avoid overcooling. Pharmacologic agents such as acetaminophen or dantrolene sodium do not speed the cooling process, as they can work only when the thermoregulatory mechanisms are operating normally.

The differential diagnosis of heat stroke must be broad, particularly if the CNS findings do not improve. Entities to consider include malignant hyperthermia, neuroleptic malignant syndrome, alcohol withdrawal syndrome, anticholinergic toxicity, stimulant toxicity, salicylate toxicity, meningitis, encephalitis, sepsis, brain abscess, cerebral falciparum malaria, status epilepticus, and thyroid storm.

Characteristics of Classic versus Exertional Heat Stroke

	CLASSIC	EXERTIONAL
Age	Elderly	Young
Health Status	Chronic illnesses, schizophrenia, alcoholism	Healthy
Activity Level	Sedentary	Strenuous activity
Time of Year	During heat waves	Variable
Renal Function	Oliguric	Acute renal failure with rhabdomyolysis
Coagulopathy	Mild	Disseminated intravascular coagulation common
Diaphoresis	May be absent	Usually present
Lactic Acidosis	Usually absent	Usually present

Clinical Pearls

1. Be particularly suspicious for heat-related illness in elderly patients, patients with comorbid diseases, or those with psychiatric disease, as they may lack the appropriate behavioral response to avoid high ambient temperatures.
2. Antipyretics are ineffective in cooling heat stroke patients
3. Ambient temperature does not need to be extreme to cause heat stroke. Patients with impaired metabolism or those who are intoxicated may lose normal heat dissipation mechanisms.

REFERENCES

1. Bouchama A, Knochel JP: Heat stroke. N Engl J Med 346:1978–1988, 2002.
2. Gaffin SL, Moran DS: Pathophysiology of heat-related illnesses. In Auerbach PS (ed): Wilderness Medicine, 4th ed. St. Louis, Mosby, 2001, pp 240–289.
3. Moran DS, Gaffin SL: Clinical management of heat-related illnesses. In Auerbach PS, ed: Wilderness Medicine, 4th ed. St. Louis, Mosby, 2001, pp 290–316.

Zachary F. Meisel, MD, MPH
John Pryor, MD

PATIENT 71

A 19-year-old man with a gunshot wound to the leg

A 19-year-old man with no significant past medical history presents to the emergency department after being shot in the left leg. A moderate amount of blood was noted at the scene. The police brought him to medical attention immediately.

Physical Examination: Temperature 36.7° C; pulse 105; respiratory rate 18; blood pressure 120/80. General: awake, anxious. Skin: warm, dry. HEENT: no signs of trauma. Neck: normal. Chest: clear and equal breath sounds. Cardiac: regular tachycardia, no gallop or murmurs. Abdomen: soft, nontender, nondistended, no wounds. Back and perineum: no wounds. Rectal: normal tone, negative for blood. Extremities: left lower extremity with 2 cm wound on posterior-lateral aspect of mid-calf with minimal gross blood and a small surrounding nonpulsating hematoma (see figure); no bruits, thrills, bony deformities, or other wounds. Dorsalis pedis and posterior tibialis pulses are palpable bilaterally. Neurologic: Glasgow Coma Scale (GCS) score of 15, moving all four extremities, strength normal, normal sensory examination.

Laboratory Findings: CBC: normal. Blood chemistries: normal. Anteroposterior and lateral radiographs of right tibia/fibula: no fractures; 2.0 cm × 1.5 cm nondeformed bullet in midline of lower leg 5 cm inferior to popliteal fossa, otherwise normal. Ankle brachial index (left leg:left arm): 0.7 (normal ≥ 0.9). Left lower extremity arteriogram: intimal irregularity of peroneal artery consistent with injury; no extravasation of contrast, no clot, no dissection, and strong distal arterial blood flow noted.

Questions: What can explain the patient's tachycardia? What are the delayed complications of this injury for which the patient is at risk?

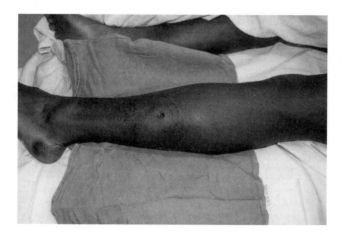

Diagnosis and Treatment: Peripheral vascular injury from penetrating trauma. Initial therapy includes intravenous crystalloid resuscitation, admission, and careful observation for development of ischemia and/or compartment syndrome. Tetanus immunization should also be given if the patient has not received a booster within the past 5 years.

Discussion: Gunshot wounds are a major source of morbidity and mortality in the United States. Transmission of large amounts of kinetic energy over a relatively small surface area from a firearm injury results in a particularly destructive pattern. All firearm injuries must be evaluated in a rapid and systematic fashion because undetected wounds to major blood vessels or organs can result in rapid hemodynamic collapse. Wounds may go undetected because the trajectory of a bullet is what determines tissue injury, and this trajectory is rarely obvious. Multiple gunshot wounds are frequent, and additional wounds are not always identified by prehospital personnel or even by patients themselves. Peripheral and seemingly superficial injuries can cause limb ischemia and/or compartment syndrome. Early detection and treatment of limb ischemia has been shown to directly correlate with limb salvage rates.

The standard trauma survey should be initiated for all gunshot wound victims upon arrival to the ED. In the present patient, the primary survey demonstrates palpable bilateral femoral and distal lower extremity pulses. However, the patient is also tachycardic, with a wound and surrounding hematoma in close proximity to a medium-size blood vessel. This should prompt closer secondary evaluation. The back, axillae, and perineum need to be fully exposed and examined. If this patient were actively bleeding, immediate digital compression would be applied.

Tachycardia in a trauma patient is always of concern. While anxiety and pain can explain a mild heart rate elevation, early shock must not be overlooked. Compensated hemorrhagic shock, often seen with a blood volume loss of 15% to 30% (750–1500 ml), may manifest as only mild tachycardia and normal blood pressure. Volume replacement through a large-bore peripheral intravenous line (14- to 16-gauge angiocatheter) with 1 to 2 L bolus of crystalloid fluid followed by rapid reassessment is appropriate.

The secondary survey for an isolated penetrating wound to the lower extremity involves identifying vascular, neurologic, and orthopedic injuries. Prompt plain radiography of the injured limb can identify the trajectory of the bullet as well as any fractures. Fractures from gun shot wounds, especially high-velocity firearms, are considered open fractures and may require antibiotics, operative irrigation, and débridement.

Examination of the injured extremity is primarily directed at identifying arterial injury. Physical signs of a major arterial injury are important to identify, since they indicate the need for immediate operative intervention. Physical findings are divided into clear signs of injury, "hard signs," and less clear signs, "soft signs" (see table). Management proceeds according to the following guidelines:

- If a patient has *any* hard signs of arterial injury, immediate surgical intervention for operative exploration and repair is warranted. Prompt revascularization (under 6 hrs) will optimize limb salvage. Angiography is reserved for only those patients with multiple areas of potential injury, such as shotgun wounds and multiple wounds to the extremities.
- If a patient has *no* hard *or* soft signs of arterial injury, significant arterial damage may be reliably excluded and further evaluation may not be warranted.
- Patients with soft signs of arterial injury often warrant further evaluation. Significant debate exists regarding the diagnosis and management of these potentially "occult" arterial injuries. Classically, angiography has been used to evaluate these injuries with nearly 100% sensitivity. More recently, the noninvasive ankle/brachial index has been used with success to screen patients for occult arterial injury in penetrating trauma (see table next page).

Rarely, significant hemorrhage can occur from a major venous injury without an associated arterial injury. If actively bleeding, injured veins may need to be surgically ligated, but often bleeding will become apparent only as the extremity is mobilized. For this reason, all patients with lower ex-

Physical Signs of Arterial Injury

HARD SIGNS	SOFT SIGNS
Pulsatile bleeding	Moderate/heavy bleeding at scene
Expanding or pulsating hematoma	Diminished palpable pulse
Palpable thrill or audible bruit	Injury/trajectory proximal to major artery
Pulselessness (distal to injury)	Peripheral nerve deficit

1. Apply cuff of sphygmomanometer distal to site of injury on affected leg.
2. Using a Doppler monitor, measure the systolic arterial pressure at the ankle (dorsalis pedis *and* posterior tibialis pulses).
3. Measure systolic arterial pressure at the brachial artery on the uninvolved upper extremity.
4. Calculate ratio of ankle arterial systolic pressure to brachial arterial systolic pressure.

tremity gun shot wounds should undergo a test of ambulation prior to discharge.

Vascular injury to a limb can result in ischemic tissue. Further injury can occur when the tissue is reperfused, generating the release of toxic cytokines. Compartment syndrome—a condition in which elevated tissue pressure within a limb fascial compartment compromises blood flow to the nerves and muscles within that compartment—is a common complication of such injuries. Patients with significant pain (out of proportion to injury) or edema may be manifesting signs of early compartment syndrome. Late signs of compartment syndrome include pallor, pulselessness, and paralysis. Compartment syndrome is a surgical emergency that requires urgent operative fasciotomy to release the compartment pressure. Patients with occult vascular injury require hospital admission to watch for signs of ischemia or compartment syndrome. Some patients with arterial injury may require prophylactic fasciotomy to prevent compartment syndrome.

If a major nerve injury is identified following penetrating trauma, nerve repair may be performed urgently or at a later date, depending on the clinical circumstances. Many patients with penetrating nerve injury need extensive physical and occupational therapy, which should be arranged prior to discharge.

Patients with penetrating injury to the distal lower extremity without evidence of vascular or orthopedic injuries can be safely discharged with close follow-up. Those with suspected vascular injuries require urgent vascular or trauma surgery consultation and hospital admission. The present patient was diagnosed with an occult peripheral arterial injury. He was admitted to the hospital for nonoperative management, including serial examinations for evaluation of ischemia and/or compartment syndrome. He was discharged from the hospital 48 hours later with intact strength, function, and sensation. Repeat angiogram performed on an outpatient basis 3 weeks post discharge revealed complete resolution of the injury.

Clinical Pearls

1. Be alert for hypovolemic shock in otherwise healthy trauma patients. Patients can lose up to 30% of their blood volume before manifesting vital sign abnormalities.

2. An initial abnormality found on examination of a penetrating extremity wound should not be discounted, even if it normalizes. All abnormal findings should be pursued to identify occult injury.

3. Fully expose all patients who have sustained gunshot wounds even if the wounds seem localized to the extremities. There may be additional torso, back, abdominal, or chest wounds that are not initially identified.

4. When discharging patients with penetrating injuries to the extremities, discuss potential signs and symptoms of occult vascular injury and late complications of peripheral vascular injury.

REFERENCES

1. Arrillaga A, Bynoe R, Frykberg E, et al: Practice management guidelines for penetrating trauma to the lower extremity. The EAST Practice Management Guidelines Work Group, 2002. www.east.org Accessed May 2003.
2. Modrall J, Weaver F, Yellin A: Diagnosis and management of penetrating vascular trauma and the injured extremity. Emerg Med Clin North Am 16:129–144, 1998.
3. Nassoura Z, Ivatury R, Simon R, et al: A reassessment of Doppler pressure indices in the detection of arterial lesions in proximity penetrating injuries of extremities: A prospective study. Am J Emerg Med 14:151–155, 1996.
4. Shackford S, Rich N: Peripheral vascular injury. In Feliciano D, Moore E, Mattox K (eds): Trauma, 3rd ed. Stamford, CT, Appleton & Lange, 1996, pp 819–851.
5. Fryberg E: Advances in the diagnosis and treatment of extremity vascular trauma. Surg Clin North Am 75:207–223, 1995.
6. Frykberg E, Dennis J, Bishop K, et al: The reliability of physical examination in the evaluation of penetrating extremity trauma for vascular injury: Results at one year. J Trauma 31:502–511, 1991.
7. Johansen K, Lynch K, Paun M, et al: Non-invasive vascular tests reliably exclude occult arterial trauma in injured extremities. J Trauma 31:515–522, 1991.

Vivian Hwang, MD
Philip R. Spandorfer, MD

PATIENT 72

An 18-year-old-man with polyuria, polydipsia, and lethargy

A previously healthy, 18-year-old-man is brought to the emergency department by his parents. His family reports that he had been outside in the hot sun most of the day and complained to them of feeling hot, dizzy, and weak. Furthermore, they relate a 2-day history of increased thirst associated with a decreased intake of solids and that he had to awaken multiple times during the previous night to urinate. On review of systems, they describe two episodes of nonbloody nonbilious emesis. They deny fever, diarrhea, or any other constitutional symptoms.

Physical Examination: Vital signs: temperature 37.6°C; pulse 140; respiratory rate 36; blood pressure 114/74; pulse oximetry 96% in room air. General: morbidly obese man who is sleepy but arousable. HEENT: eyes open to voice, PERRL, EOMI, dry mucous membranes, oropharynx clear, TMs clear bilaterally. Neck: supple. Chest: clear to auscultation bilaterally. Cardiac: tachycardiac, regular, no murmurs, gallops, or rubs. Abdomen: bowel sounds present, soft, obese, nondistended, diffuse tenderness, no peritoneal signs, no organomegaly. Extremities: no cyanosis/clubbing/edema, warm, less than 2-second capillary refill. Skin: no rashes. Neurologic: somnolent but arousable, follows commands appropriately, but remains fixated on intravenous line and the importance of not pulling it out; oriented to person and place; unsure of the date or the situation; remainder of neurologic examination is nonfocal.

Laboratory Findings: CBC: hemoglobin 17.0 g/dl, WBC 9700/μl, platelets 262,000/μl. Blood chemistries: sodium 135 mEq/L, potassium 5.9 mEq/L, chloride 85 mEq/L, bicarbonate 26 mEq/L, BUN 21 mg/dl, creatinine 1.7 mg/dl, glucose 1813 mg/dl, acetone <1:2. Arterial blood gas: pH 7.23, PCO_2 58 mmHg, PO_2 369 mmHg, base excess −5; serum osmolality 409 mOsm/kg (normal 275–295 mOsm/kg). Urinalysis: specific gravity 1.037, pH 5.5, >1000 mg/dl glucose, negative for ketones, nitrates, and leukocytes. Electrocardiogram: sinus tachycardia 140s, normal axis, normal intervals, nonspecific t wave changes.

Question: What disease entity can manifest with such profound hyperglycemia and yet have no ketosis present?

Diagnosis: Hyperglycemic hyperosmolar nonketotic syndrome

Discussion: Hyperglycemic hyperosmolar nonketotic syndrome (HHNK) is a life-threatening diabetic emergency characterized by hyperglycemia, hyperosmolarity, and dehydration. It is characteristic of non-insulin-dependent diabetes mellitus. Unlike diabetic ketoacidosis (DKA), patients typically lack severe ketosis and have only mild acidemia.

The elderly are at highest risk for developing HHNK. The average age of presentation is 60 years, but there is a wide age range that even includes pediatric patients. In up to two thirds of patients, HHNK is the first presentation of type II, non-insulin-dependent diabetes.

HHNK may be precipitated by a stress such as infection, myocardial infarction, stroke, or gastrointestinal bleeding. Other medical conditions known to precipitate HHNK include acute pancreatitis, subdural hematoma, pulmonary embolism, renal failure, heat stroke, severe burns, and endocrine disorders. Other factors include use of drugs that have a hyperglycemic effect such as glucocorticoids, use of drugs that cause dehydration such as thiazide diuretics, and noncompliance in the known diabetic.

Clinical manifestations in HHNK are a result of the profound dehydration that develops. The initiating event is hyperglycemia, which leads to an osmotic diuresis, causing loss of free water in addition to electrolytes such as sodium, potassium, magnesium, and phosphorus. As free water is lost in excess of electrolytes, a hyperosmolar hypovolemia develops. Patients may have a small ketosis, but in general, it is not to the same degree as in DKA. Although controversy exists, it is believed that patients with HHNK have sufficient insulin activity to inhibit the release of free fatty acid from adipose tissue but not enough to promote glucose uptake by cells. In addition, hyperosmolarity itself suppresses ketone formation by inhibiting lipolysis, which results in lower levels of free fatty acids to serve as substrate for ketogenesis.

Patients who develop HHNK have insidious onset of symptoms, including polydipsia, polyuria, fatigue, blurred vision, and weight loss. Medical attention is sought when the patient develops altered mental status. In fact, as many as 25% of patients present with coma. Interestingly, the severity of mental status changes has been found to correlate with the degree of hyperosmolarity and the rate at which it develops. It is important to recognize that if the osmolality is less than 345 to 350 mOsm/kg, coma is most likely not secondary to HHNK and another diagnosis should be investigated. Other neurologic findings related to HHNK include positive Babinski reflexes, nystagmus, visual loss, visual hallucinations, muscle fasciculations, unilateral or bilateral focal deficits, severe dysphagia, acute urinary retention, acute quadriplegia, and seizures. Gastrointestinal symptoms do not occur as often as in DKA.

Initial laboratory evaluation when HHNK is suspected includes serum electrolytes, complete blood cell count (CBC), arterial blood gases (ABG), urinalysis (UA), and electrocardiography (ECG). A search for underlying illness is warranted in these patients, and other studies such as a chest x-ray, urine culture, blood culture, amylase, lipase, liver function studies, and cardiac enzymes should be performed

Classically, patients with HHNK have a serum glucose >600 mg/dL, osmolality >320 mOsm/kg, pH >7.3, and bicarbonate >15 mEq/L. The measured serum sodium is factitiously low; the true value can be calculated by increasing the sodium by 1.6 mEq for every 100 mg/dl increase in glucose concentration over 200. Serum levels of potassium, magnesium, and phosphorus are typically normal or elevated upon initial presentation. However, as therapy for HHNK is instituted, these electrolytes will shift back from the extracellular to the intracellular compartments, causing serum levels to decrease.

Intravenous fluids are the mainstay in treatment of HHNK. Patients typically have a total body water deficit of about 20% to 25% representing approximately 9 L for an adult. Normal saline is the fluid of choice in the initial management of HHNK. If the patient is hypotensive, 2 L of normal saline should be rapidly infused. When the patient's blood pressure and urine output are acceptable, consider switching to 1/2 normal saline. Usually, patients require 3 to 4 L of fluid during the first 4 hours of therapy. In general, 50% of the calculated fluid deficit is replaced within the first 12 hours of therapy, with the rest replaced more slowly over the remaining 24 to 36 hours.

Fluid administration alone decreases the glucose concentration secondary to a dilution effect, and insulin therapy may not be necessary. However, patients with HHNK do respond well to insulin, and it is acceptable to start low-dose insulin intravenously at a rate of 0.05 to 0.1 U/kg/hr. When the glucose level falls below 250 mg/dl, it is important to add 5% dextrose to intravenous fluids and decrease the insulin drip by 50%.

Replacement of potassium is another important aspect of therapy. Plasma levels will fall during treatment of HHNK, so once urine output is established, potassium chloride can be administered at an infusion rate of 10 to 40 mEq/hour, depending on the initial potassium level. In general, it is not necessary to replace phosphate during the initial treatment of HHNK, unless there is severe hypophosphatemia. In addition, there is no indication for the use of bicarbonate, unless pH is less than 7.0.

Complications of HHNK and its treatment include large-vessel thromboembolism, disseminated intravascular coagulation, rhabdomyolysis, and cerebral edema. Dehydration may predispose patients to vascular occlusive disease and coagulation abnormalities. Nontraumatic rhabdomyolysis can occur in patients with decompensated diabetes and is characterized by creatine kinase levels greater than 1000 IU/L. Patients at highest risk for developing this complication are those with a markedly elevated serum osmolality and/or a high creatinine level. Cerebral edema is an extremely rare complication in adult patients with HHNK as compared to the pediatric population, in whom cerebral edema is the major cause of mortality. In adults, the mortality rate of HHNK, which is estimated to be between 10% and 17%, is mostly due to comorbid illnesses such as myocardial infarction. There has been no study showing that slow correction of hyperglycemic hyperosmolarity is advantageous, and rapid correction to a serum osmolality of less than 320 mOsm/L and plasma glucose to 250 to 300 mg/dl should be the goal of therapy.

The present patient received 4 L of normal saline within 3 hours while in the emergency department. Low-dose intravenous insulin therapy was started at 0.05 U/kg/hr. The patient was admitted to the intensive care unit for further management and was discharged with normal mental status 5 days later.

Clinical Pearls

1. HHNK is a potentially life-threatening diabetic complication characterized by hyperglycemia, hyperosmolarity, and dehydration. It is seen in patients with non-insulin-dependent diabetes.

2. HHNK is often precipitated by a stress, and it is important to search for a concomitant medical condition such as infection, myocardial infarction, or stroke.

3. Management of HHNK includes aggressive intravenous fluid administration, low-dose intravenous insulin therapy, and replacement of electrolytes.

4. Complications of HHNK and its treatment include large-vessel thromboembolism, disseminated intravascular coagulation, rhabdomyolysis, and cerebral edema.

REFERENCES

1. Magee MF, Bhatt BA: Management of decompensated diabetes: Diabetic ketoacidosis and hyperglycemic hyperosmolar syndrome. Crit Care Clin 17:75–106, 2001.
2. Gottschalk ME, Ros SP, Zeller P: The emergency management of hyperglycemic-hyperosmolar nonketotic coma in the pediatric patient. Pediatr Emerg Care 12:48–51, 1996.
3. Pope DW, Zun LS: Hyperosmolar hyperglycemic nonketotic coma. In Harwood-Nuss AL, Linden CH, Luten RC, et al (eds): The Clinical Practice of Emergency Medicine, 2nd ed. Philadelphia, Lippincott-Raven, 1996, pp 723–725.
4. Wang LM, Tsai ST, Ho LT, et al: Rhabdomyolysis in diabetic emergencies. Diabetes Res Clin Pract 26:209–214, 1994.
5. Fulop M, Rosenblatt A, Kreitzer SM, Gerstenhaber B: Hyperosmolar nature of diabetic coma. Diabetes 24:594–599, 1975.

PATIENT 73

A 79-year-old man with sudden loss of consciousness

A previously healthy, 79-year-old man suddenly lost consciousness while sitting in the local library. Witnesses noted no seizure activity. He spontaneously regained consciousness prior to the arrival of rescue personnel. In the emergency department, he was completely asymptomatic. He denied antecedent chest pain, shortness of breath, or palpitations.

Physical Examination: Vital signs: temperature 36.3°C; heart rate 83; respiratory rate 18; blood pressure 157/83. Skin: warm and dry. HEENT: normal. Neck: supple with +2 carotids; no audible bruit. Chest: clear bilateral breath sounds. Cardiac: no heave or thrill on palpation; nondisplaced point of maximal impact; regular rate; no murmur, rub, or gallop. Abdomen: soft and nontender; no rebound or guarding; rectal: heme negative. Extremities: normal. Neurologic: awake, alert, and oriented to person, place, and date. Cranial nerves 2–12 intact bilaterally; motor: normal bulk, tone, and strength; sensory: intact to all sensory modalities; cerebellum: normal; gait: normal.

Laboratory Findings: CBC: normal. Blood chemistries: normal. Electrocardiogram: normal sinus rhythm, normal intervals, no acute ischemia pattern.

Questions: What is the cause of this man's loss of consciousness? In the absence of a visible cause, is it safe for him to be discharged home? What are the indications for admission and further evaluation?

Diagnosis and treatment: Syncope; unknown cause. Based on an increased risk for possible cardiac origin, management should include admission to the hospital for inpatient cardiac monitoring and further evaluation.

The sudden loss of consciousness associated with the inability to maintain postural tone is the definition of syncope. The causes of syncope are myriad, ranging from simple to life threatening (see table). The challenge facing the clinician rests with the task of discerning benign from potentially fatal causes. Cardiac causes of syncope are often occult in presentation and carry a significant 1-year mortality rate of 18% to 33%.

Accurately diagnosing the cause of syncope can be challenging. A discernable cause is identified only 50% to 70% of the time. The cornerstone of the syncope evaluation remains a detailed history and thorough physical examination. Of the identifiable causes of syncope, history and physical examination alone may provide a diagnosis 50% to 80% of the time. Ancillary tests such as complete blood cell count (CBC) or serum electrolytes are useful only if indicated by the clinical scenario. For example, a CBC in the setting of an acute gastrointestinal bleed or serum glucose in the setting of an altered mental status of a diabetic patient may have higher yield than random

screening. Similarly, head computed tomography and electroencephalography are indicated only in the setting of abnormal neurologic findings or in the setting of possible seizure activity. A 12-lead electrocardiogram should always be included as an initial screening test in the evaluation of syncope, although it leads to definitive diagnosis in only a small portion of patients.

When a cause is identified, management is straightforward. Benign processes such as dehydration can be corrected in the ED. Acute life-threatening processes require admission and further therapy. For individuals in whom a cause has not been reliably identified, the dilemma is whether to admit the patient for further testing or discharge for outpatient evaluation. Given the high incidence of morbidity from cardiac causes of syncope, the physician must attempt to stratify the patient's risk for an occult cardiac process. Four separate criteria have been established to identify the patient at increased risk for cardiac syncope (see table). These risk factors cumulatively increase the potential risk for underlying occult cardiac causes of syncope; however, even just one risk factor is sufficient to raise concern for cardiac disease. A patient presenting with any of these variables in the setting of unexplained syncope should be admitted to a monitored bed for further evaluation.

The present patient was admitted to a monitored bed, as he did not demonstrate an overt cause of syncope by history and physical examination. Approximately 2 hours later he had a cardiopulmonary arrest. He was resuscitated and stabilized with a transvenous pacemaker and emergently taken to the cardiac catheterization laboratory for placement of a permanent pacemaker.

Causes of Syncope

Vasomotor/vascular
   Vasovagal
   Situational
   Carotid sinus syndrome
Orthostatic hypotension
   Hypovolemia
   Hemorrhage
Neurologic
   Transient ischemic attack
   Subclavian steal
   Migraines
   Subarachnoid hemorrhage
   Seizure
Medications
Psychiatric
Cardiac
   Structural/valvular
   Myocardial ischemia/infarction
   Dysrhythmias

Risk Factors for Cardiac Syncope

Age >45 years
History of ventricular dysrhythmia
History of congestive heart failure
Abnormal electrocardiogram (excluding
   nonspecific ST-T wave segment changes)

Clinical Pearls

1. Most patients with syncope look well by the time they arrive in the ED and no longer have symptoms; this should not dissuade the ED physician from a work-up and possible admission.

2. Expensive and comprehensive testing in the ED does not usually provide the diagnosis if history and examination do not.

3. Risk stratification helps to identify patients with potential cardiac cause of syncope.

REFERENCES

1. Panciolo AM, McNeil PM: Syncope. In Bosker, ed. Textbook of Adult and Pediatric Emergency Medicine. Atlanta GA, American Health Consultants, 2000.
2. Kapoor WN: Evaluation and management of the patient with syncope. JAMA 268:2553, 1992.
3. Linze M, Yang EH, Estes NA et al: Diagnosing syncope. Part 1. Value of history, physical examination and electrocardiography. The Clinical Efficacy Project of the American College of Emergency Physicians. Ann Inter Med 126:989, 1997.
4. Martin TP, Hanusa, Kapoor WN: Risk stratification of patients with syncope. Ann Emerg Med 29:4, 1997.

Amy L. Puchalski, MD
Kathy N. Shaw, MD, MSCE

PATIENT 74

An 18-month-old girl with vomiting, intermittent shaking, and refusal to walk

A previously healthy 18-month-old girl presents to the emergency department with non-bloody, non-bilious emesis intermittently over the past month. The episodes of vomiting are becoming progressively more frequent. For the past week, when her mother puts her down on the ground, she stands but refuses to walk. She has been intermittently irritable but can be consoled by her mother. For the past week, she seems to preferentially keep her eyes closed, but her mother noticed her eyes seem to "wiggle back and forth" whenever she opens them. She lost 2 pounds in the last 3 months and has no history of fever or trauma.

Physical Examination: Vital signs: temperature 37.6°C; pulse 130; respiratory rate 22; blood pressure 116/72. General appearance: cries intermittently but is consolable by mother. HEENT: no external signs of trauma, eyes are usually closed but when open, conjugate horizontal movements are noted; pupils symmetric and reactive. Neck: head held tilted to the left, no meningismus. Abdomen: soft, nondistended, no masses palpated, no hepatosplenomegaly. Neurologic: left 6th nerve palsy, normal strength in all extremities, 2+ deep tendon reflexes, no clonus, no truncal ataxia, refuses to walk.

Laboratory Findings: CBC: WBC 8600/μl, hemoglobin 10.9 g/dl, platelets 384,000/μl. Brain MRI: subtle meningeal enhancement around the brainstem, but no mass lesion or hydrocephalus. CSF: WBC 1, RBC 60, protein <10 mg/dl, glucose 50 mg/dl.

Questions: What further diagnostic tests would you pursue? What is the likely diagnosis?

Diagnosis: On further evaluation, the chest radiograph shows a retrocardiac density, and a subsequent chest computed tomography (CT) scan reveals a calcified left paraspinal mass extending to the level of the adrenal glands (see figures). The patient has opsoclonus-myoclonus secondary to neuroblastoma.

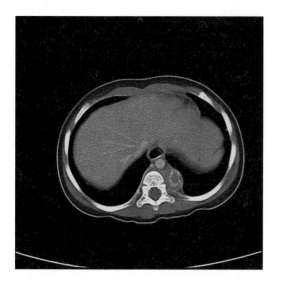 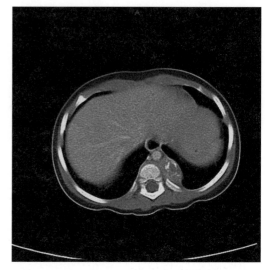

Discussion: Opsoclonus-myoclonus (OM), also known as "dancing eyes, dancing feet" syndrome, is characterized by rapid, repetitive, involuntary, conjugate eye movements in all directions. It can be associated with myoclonus of the extremities as well as cerebellar ataxia. In children, it is associated primarily with either viral encephalitis or neuroblastoma, in which case, it is considered a paraneoplastic syndrome. Neuroblastoma is the most common tumor of infancy and the most common extracranial malignancy of childhood, accounting for 8% to 10% of all pediatric malignancies. Sixty to 75% of patients have metastatic disease at presentation, and patients with lower stage neuroblastoma have a 90% survival. OM is found in 2% to 4% of all children with neuroblastoma, but primarily among those with favorable tumor histologic type, low-stage disease, and a paraspinal primary lesion and those who lack *N-myc* gene amplification.

The etiology of OM in patients with neuroblastoma is believed to be immune-mediated. It is hypothesized that the tumor expresses antigens similar to those on neurons, and the resultant immune response against the malignancy also damages the patient's nervous system. This theory is supported in a study by Antunes et al. examining the sera of 64 children with neuroblastoma. Antineuronal IgG was detected in 81% of the children with neuroblastoma-associated OM, but only 25% of those with OM alone. Similarly, a smaller study by Connolly et al, of nine patients with OM due to neuroblastoma, showed that all had IgM or IgG to Purkinje cells, whereas no control patients had similar antibodies. In addition, the current therapy for OM consists of immunosuppressive medication, further supporting an immune-mediated mechanism for OM.

The typical clinical course of OM usually progresses over several weeks to months, at times occurring before the tumor can even be detected. Children may first demonstrate behavioral changes such as irritability. They go on to develop an abnormal gait, which can progress to frank ataxia as well as manifesting the characteristic eye movements. Even after the tumor is resected, patients have persistent symptoms of OM. Although most children with OM associated with neuroblastoma survive the treatment of the tumor, they unfortunately suffer significant neurodevelopment impairment as a result of the OM. In one retrospective study of 29 children with OM due to neuroblastoma, 62% eventually had resolution of their OM symptoms, but 69% had persistent neurologic deficits (Russo et al). A study of 17 patients by Mitchell et al showed that all had delayed or abnormal neurocognitive development, including impairments in expressive language or fine and gross motor skills, oppositional behavior, and sleep problems. A similar study assessing neurologic outcomes showed that there is no relationship between the duration of symptoms prior to initiation of OM therapy and the degree of impairment (Hayward et al).

As mentioned previously, the treatment for OM consists of immunosuppression with prednisone, adrenocorticotropic hormone; intravenous immunoglobulin, cytoxan, and occasionally plasmapheresis. There are few data to evaluate which therapy is most effective in relieving the symptoms of OM. It is also unclear whether treatment of the OM symptoms diminishes the degree of eventual neurologic impairment. The present patient underwent surgical resection of her mass, and staging work-up revealed no evidence of metastatic disease. Her OM symptoms persisted after surgery for the tumor, and she was started on cytoxan and prednisone. At the time of discharge, her eye symptoms were improving and her irritability resolved.

Clinical Pearls

1. Children presenting with opsoclonus-myoclonus should be evaluated for neuroblastoma with imaging studies of the chest and abdomen as well as urine collection for vanillylmandelic acid/homovanillic acid.

2. Neuroblastomas associated with opsoclonus-myoclonus are usually low stage with good prognosis.

3. Patients with opsoclonus-myoclonus are frequently left with significant neurodevelopmental deficits.

REFERENCES

1. Mitchell WG, Davalos-Gonzalez Y, Brumm VL, et al: Opsoclonus-ataxia caused by childhood neuroblastoma: Developmental and neurologic sequelae. Pediatrics 109:86–98, 2002.
2. Hayward K, Jeremy RJ, Jenkins S, et al: Long-term neurobehavioral outcomes in children with neuroblastoma and opsoclonus-myoclonus-ataxia syndrome: Relationship to MRI finding and anit-neuronal antibodies. J Pediatr 139:552–9, 2001.
3. Antunes NL, Khakoo Y, Matthay KK, et al: Antineuronal antibodies in patients with neuroblastoma and paraneoplastic opsoclonus-myoclonus. J Pediatr Hematol Oncol 22:315–320, 2000.
4. Wheeler DS, Starr SR: Case 2: Neuroblastoma as a cause of opsoclonus. Pediatr Rev 19:281–283, 1998.
5. Connolly AM, Pestronk A, Mehta S, et al: Serum autoantibodies in childhood opsoclonus-myoclonus syndrome: Analysis of antigenic targets in neural tissues. J Pediatr 130:878–884, 1997.
6. Russo C, Cohn SL, Petruzzi MJ, Alarcon PA: Long-term neurologic outcome in children with opsoclonus-myoclonus associated with neuroblastoma: A report from the pediatric oncology group. Med Pediatr Oncol 28:284–288, 1997.
7. Hammer MS, Larsen MB, Stack CV: Outcome of children with opsoclonus-myoclonus regardless of etiology. Pediatr Neurol 13:21–24, 1995.

Iris Reyes, MD, FACEP

PATIENT 75

A 74-year-old man with chest pain

A 74-year-old non-English-speaking Chinese man is brought to the emergency room by his family. His granddaughter has limited English proficiency and explains that he has had chest pain for the past 2 days. It is difficult to understand her but the granddaughter is able to relate that he has had "heart problems."

Physical Examination: Vital signs: temperature: 37°C; pulse 80; respiratory rate 18; blood pressure 174/96. Skin: warm and slightly diaphoretic, multiple linear bruises on the upper back and chest (see figure, which shows similar bruises on a child). HEENT: normal. Neck: supple, no jugular vein distension. Chest: clear to auscultation. Cardiac: irregularly irregular, no murmurs or rubs. Abdomen: soft, nontender, normal. Extremities: trace bilateral pedal edema. Neuromuscular: normal.

Laboratory Findings: ECG: atrial fibrillation, normal axis, no ST-T wave abnormalities. CBC: normal. Blood chemistries: normal except elevated creatinine of 1.7; Cardiac isoenzymes: CK 580, relative index 4; troponin 2.0. Chest x-ray: normal.

Questions: Should you rely on the granddaughter to act as a translator when both she and the patient have limited English proficiency? What resources can you use to improve communication between you and your patient? Should you report the family to the authorities for elder abuse?

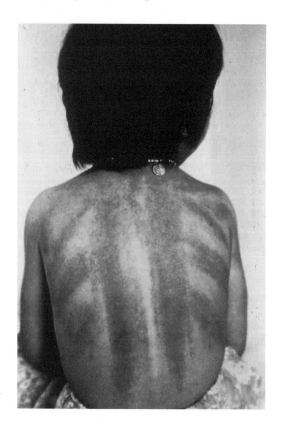

Diagnosis: Myocardial infarction. Cultural beliefs about illness have possibly contributed to a delay in seeking medical treatment. Limited English proficiency also is likely to play a role in the delivery of prompt and appropriate health care. Folk medicine practices may lead to misinterpretation of physical findings.

Discussion: Medical providers are facing significant challenges in providing care for patients from many cultures who speak many different languages and have diverse beliefs about illness causation and treatment. Census 2000 data revealed significant increases in minority and foreign-born populations in the United States. Many of these patients are cared for daily in emergency departments.

In March of 2002, the Institute of Medicine published a report highlighting significant racial and ethnic disparities in health care in the United States. In some cases, these disparities are associated with worse health outcomes. Examples of such disparities include the lower referral rates for cardiac catheterization for African Americans and inadequate use of analgesia in Hispanic patients with fractures compared to their white counterparts. Stereotyping, prejudice, and clinical uncertainty on the part of the provider can all contribute to disparate health care practices. Included in the Institutes of Medicine report is a recommendation to enhance patient-provider communication to reduce barriers to care in culturally diverse populations.

In March of 2001, the Office of Minority Health of the U.S. Department of Health and Human Services published a report defining the national standards for providing culturally and linguistically appropriate health care services. This report provides recommendations, guidelines, and mandates to which federally funded hospitals and other agencies must adhere. For example, these health care organizations must offer and provide language assistance services at no cost to each patient with limited English proficiency. This includes bilingual staff and interpreter services. Translation services must be provided at all points of contact in a timely manner, to optimize the outcome for each individual.

Cultural competency in health care includes addressing the numerous dimensions of the patient's culture, including health and illness beliefs, healing traditions, their decision-making style, locus of control, and the patient's social status within the family. In the present patient's case, the numerous bruises on his body are not the result of a physical assault. They are due to the Southeast Asian tradition of coining—the process of rubbing the body with a coin in an attempt to draw illness to the surface—which produces red raised areas or bruises. This alternative health practice is commonly seen in children and can easily be mistaken for child abuse. Familiarization with the patient's belief system and a careful, accurate history are essential for appropriate interpretation of illness and effective health care delivery.

Clinical Pearls

1. Use a culturally trained translator at the bedside or by phone in all situations in which limited English proficiency exists to optimize the patient's clinical outcome.

2. Recognize that patients have belief systems and alternative healing traditions that may be different from your own.

3. Avoid generalizations about all patients that identify with a particular racial, ethnic, or religious background; members of groups often do not share the same thoughts and beliefs with regard to health care.

REFERENCES

1. Smedley BD, Steta AY, Nelson AR, eds: Unequal Treatment: Confronting Racial and Ethnic Disparities in Health Care. Washington, DC, National Academy Press, 2003.
2. U.S. Department of Health and Human Services, Office of Minority Health: A practical guide for implementing the recommended national standards for culturally and linguistically appropriate services in health care. 2001. http://www.omhc.gov/clas/guide/.
3. Brach C, Fraser I: Can cultural competency reduce racial and ethnic disparities? A review and conceptual model. Med Care Res Rev 57:181–217, 2000.
4. Carrillo JE, Green AR, Betancourt JR: Cross-cultural primary care: A patient-based approach. Ann Intern Med 130:829–834, 1999.

PATIENT 76

A 5-day-old boy with bilious emesis

A 5-day-old boy presents to the emergency department 2 hours after a single episode of "green vomitus" and inconsolable crying. Prenatal course was uneventful. He was delivered vaginally without complications and stayed in the hospital for 48 hours after delivery. The mother reports some difficulty with breast-feeding and frequent spitting-up.

Physical Examination: Vital signs: temperature 37.4°C rectally; pulse 148; respiratory rate 52; blood pressure 68/44. General appearance: irritable and difficult to console. HEENT: moist mucous membranes; open, flat anterior fontanelle. Chest: clear. Cardiac: regular rate, rhythm; soft systolic murmur. Abdomen: soft, diffusely tender; absent bowel sounds; umbilical stump unremarkable. Genitalia: circumcised penis; descended, nontender testicles; no palpable hernia. Rectal: Yellow-green stool without occult blood. Extremities: normal. Skin: no lesions

Laboratory Findings: CBC: WBC 15,200/μl with 72% segmented neutrophils, 8% bands. Blood chemistry: electrolytes, blood urea nitrogen, creatinine normal. Abdominal x-ray with multiple air/fluid levels, no free air, minimally dilated loops of bowel.

Questions: How should you proceed with the evaluation of this patient? What specific diagnoses need to be excluded in a vomiting, irritable infant?

Diagnosis and Treatment: Intestinal malrotation. Bilious emesis in neonates can be a sign of significant abdominal pathology. Immediate surgical consultation is warranted while preparations are made for an upper gastrointestinal contrast study.

Discussion: Intestinal obstruction is found in 31% to 38% of neonates with bilious emesis. The differential diagnosis of vomiting with bilious emesis includes several anatomic entities (see table). This finding should prompt aggressive evaluation. Results of laboratory testing are usually normal or nonspecific. Plain abdominal radiographs are helpful if they reveal classic findings such as the presence of the "double bubble" sign (dilatation of the stomach and proximal duodenum) of duodenal atresia. However, neonates with significant gastrointestinal pathology may have subtly abnormal or normal plain radiographs. Therefore, the radiographic study of choice in patients with bilious emesis is an upper gastrointestinal series with oral contrast. Although the plain radiograph in this patient was not specific, the sudden onset of bilious emesis and abdominal tenderness was worrisome for intestinal malrotation.

Intestinal malrotation occurs as a result of failure of proper embryonic rotation of the tubular primitive gut. In the first trimester of development, the midgut rotates counterclockwise along the axis of the superior mesenteric artery and is fixed primarily at the cecum and the ligament of Treitz. The term *malrotation* is frequently used to encompass incomplete rotation, nonrotation of the midgut loop, and other variations of rotational abnormalities.

It is likely that many patients with malrotation remain asymptomatic throughout their lifetime. Some patients with malrotation are diagnosed in later childhood and adulthood during the course of the evaluation of complaints such as chronic abdominal pain or failure to thrive. However, the majority of patients who become symptomatic from malrotation present in the first year of life and most frequently in the first month after birth.

Causes of Bilious Emesis

Atresia of the duodenum, jejunum, or ileum

Hirschsprung's disease

Idiopathic

Malrotation with volvulus

Meconium ileus

Meconium plug

Symptoms arise via one of the following mechanisms: (1) compression of the duodenum distal to the insertion of the common bile duct by peritoneal bands, resulting in the characteristic bilious vomiting; (2) midgut volvulus (torsion of a loop of intestine), typically distal to the insertion of the common bile duct, also resulting in bilious emesis; and (3) torsion of the vascular pedicle, resulting in ischemia of the intestinal mucosa, which in turn results in severe abdominal pain and accompanying irritability.

Physical examination findings can range from normal (in patients with malrotation without intestinal obstruction or mesenteric ischemia) to significant abdominal distension and tenderness. When ischemia is prolonged, necrosis ensues, with passage of bloody, sloughed intestinal mucosa, peritonitis, metabolic acidosis, and subsequent systemic collapse. Significant bowel necrosis can occur as rapidly as a few hours. Small amounts of necrotic intestine can be resected, but this frequently leads to the short-gut syndrome, which requires long-term parenteral nutrition. The presence of larger amounts of infarcted intestine is often lethal. This underscores the need for emergency evaluation of patient with suspected malrotation, and neonates with bilious emesis should be presumed to have intestinal malrotation until proven otherwise.

Although the plain abdominal radiograph can be suggestive of malrotation, the imaging study of choice is an upper gastrointestinal series with contrast. However, as with many surgical emergencies, a toxic-appearing patient with worrisome history and examination findings may be taken directly to the operating room for exploratory laparotomy without any further diagnostic testing. Treatment for confirmed (or strongly suspected) malrotation is operative repair. While awaiting surgery, patients should undergo aggressive fluid resuscitation and nasogastric decompression as well as broad-spectrum antibiotic coverage.

The present patient had malrotation with volvulus confirmed by the upper gastrointestinal series, and he was taken emergently to the operating room. Perfusion to the small intestine was restored after correction of the malrotation, and there was no evidence of infarction. The patient had an uneventful postoperative course, and he was discharged to home without any significant sequelae.

Clinical Pearls

1. Neonates with bilious emesis need to be evaluated expeditiously since bowel necrosis can occur within hours.

2. Bilious emesis in neonates must be clearly differentiated from "spitting-up." The latter is extremely common and usually represents a far more benign cause such as gastrointestinal reflux.

3. Irritability and other nonspecific signs and symptoms must be taken seriously in a neonate. Sepsis, metabolic disorders, and congenital anatomic disorders should all be considered as potential causes.

REFERENCES

1. Godbole P, Stringer MD: Bilious emesis in the newborn: How often it is pathologic? J Pediatr Surg 37:909–911, 2002.
2. Clark LA, Oldham KT: Malrotation. In Ashcraft KW, Murphy JP (eds): Pediatric surgery. Philadelphia, WB Saunders, 2000, pp 425–434.
3. Lilien LD, Srinivasan G, Pyati SP, et al: Green vomiting in the first 72 hours in normal infants. Am J Dis Med 140:662–664, 1986.

Sandra Schwab, MD
Elizabeth R. Alpern, MD, MSCE

PATIENT 77

A 6-year-old boy with multiple injuries after a firecracker explosion

A previously healthy 6-year-old boy arrives via helicopter following the explosion of an M-80 firecracker in his hand. His mother found the boy after he ignited the firecracker in their home. The Trauma and Critical Care teams were notified prior to arrival of the patient and are present in the emergency department during the resuscitation. Upon arrival, the patient reports severe right hand and arm pain and is screaming that he cannot hear or see.

Physical Examination: Vital signs: temperature 37.2°C rectally; pulse 144; respiratory rate 21; blood pressure 144/56.

Primary Survey: Airway: patent. Breathing: spontaneous respirations and clear, equal breath sounds bilaterally. Circulation: heart regular rate and rhythm, no murmur. Strong distal radial and femoral pulses bilaterally. Brisk capillary refill. Disability: alert, responsive to all commands. Moving all extremities spontaneously.

Secondary Survey: General: crying child in distress. Head: multiple superficial shrapnel wounds over face with punctuate burns to bilateral eyelids. Right eye: pupil round and reactive, cornea and conjunctiva clear, no foreign body noted. Left eye: pupil irregular and poorly reactive, linear corneal abrasion (see figure). Ears: normal auricles, canals, and tympanic membranes. Chest: multiple superficial punctuate burns. Abdomen: soft, nontender. Extremities: right hand with partially avulsed first, second, and third digits; degloving of the skin of third, fourth, and fifth digits and palmer surface of hand (see figure); left arm/hand normal. Strong radial pulses bilaterally. Genital: penile meatus without blood. Rectal: normal tone, no gross blood. Back: nontender, no shrapnel wounds.

Laboratory Findings: CBC: normal. Hand x-ray: amputation of first digit distal phalanx with fracture of proximal phalanx. Amputation of the second digit through the proximal phalanx and fracture through the metacarpal shaft. Amputation through the third digit proximal phalanx with fracture of the metacarpal shaft. Forth and fifth digits intact. Chest x-ray: normal.

Questions: In addition to the loss of digits on the right hand, what is this child's other significant injury? What is the immediate course of action for this injury in the emergency department?

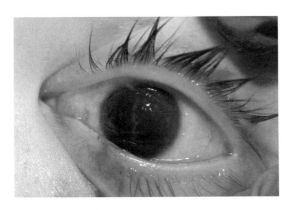 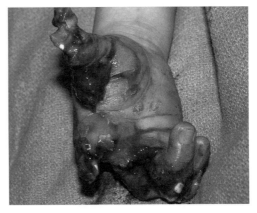

Images courtesy of Scott Goldstein, MD, Division of Ophthalmology, Hospital of the University of Pennsylvania, Philadelphia

Diagnosis: A left ocular global injury, which should be treated with a protective shield, pain control, and sedation to minimize intraocular pressure elevations, and emergency ophthalmology consultation.

Discussion: The present patient presents with multiple injuries that require immediate attention, including the avulsed digits and ocular global injury. In the face of multiple trauma, it is important to systematically approach the patient, conducting a primary and secondary survey, to properly diagnose and treat all existing injuries.

Each year, the U.S. Consumer Product Safety Commission tracks injuries and deaths caused by fireworks using the National Electronic Injury Surveillance System. An estimated 9500 patients were treated in emergency departments for firework injuries in 2001. Approximately 50% of these injuries occurred to children younger than 15 years of age. Children aged 5 to 14 years accounted for 35% of the total injuries. Injuries to males out-numbered those to females 3:1. Firecrackers, sparklers, and bottle rockets were the source of the majority of injuries. Contrary to the belief that parental supervision reduces injuries caused by fireworks, 54% of injured children are under direct supervision of an adult at the time of the accident.

The hands and eyes are most commonly affected in firework accidents and are associated with the highest morbidity. Up to one third of eye injuries result in permanent vision loss. Approximately 29% of children involved in a firework accident have primary ocular trauma.

Traumatic eye injuries can be categorized into closed globe or open globe. Closed globe injuries are those in which the eye wall remains intact. Open globe injuries are simply defined as a full-thickness wound to the eye wall. More specifically, a ruptured globe results from a blunt impact, subsequent increase in intraocular pressure, and finally rupture of the eyeball (and inside-out mechanism). In this case, the child had a blast injury and laceration of one eye wall, defined as a penetrating injury, another type of open globe injury. Laceration in which both an entrance and an exit wound can be identified in the eye is classified as a perforating injury. A retained foreign body is another example of open globe injury.

An open globe injury should be suspected with any evidence of ocular trauma. Corneal and scleral lacerations, irregular pupils, and hyphema are findings that are of concern for an open globe. The patient may present with pain and decreased visual acuity initially.

If a global injury is suspected, ophthalmologic examination should be stopped immediately. The eye should be covered with a shield that extends over the bony orbital structures. It is important to not introduce substances such as eye drops and antibiotics to the eye because these can be toxic to the inner eye contents. Consultation with an ophthalmologist should occur at this time.

In addition, it is important to keep the child from doing things that will raise intraocular pressure, as this may cause extrusion of the intraocular contents. This includes calming the child and controlling pain to prevent crying. The physician should also avoid any unnecessary interventions or uncomfortable examinations if possible.

The present patient immediately had a protective shield placed over the left eye. He was given morphine and midazolam for pain control and sedation. The right hand was dressed with saline gauze. The shrapnel wounds on chest were irrigated and covered. Orthopedics and Ophthalmology were consulted and the patient was taken to the operating room immediately for complete ophthalmologic examination in addition to hand débridment and completion amputation. The eye examination under general anesthesia revealed a left corneal laceration and traumatic hyphema. In addition, there was a puncture wound through the iris. Additional studies, including an ocular ultrasonogram and computed tomography scan, verified the absence of an intraocular foreign body or retinal detachment. The patient eventually developed a post-traumatic cataract that required further surgical intervention and did suffer vision loss. In addition, he required complete amputation of his first, second, and third digits to the metacarpals. He returned to the operating room multiple times for wound débridement and skin graft placement.

Clinical Pearls

1. All patients with multiple trauma require a primary and secondary survey to identify life-and-limb threatening as well as any additional injuries.

2. Children account for approximately 50% of firework injuries, with the hands and eyes being the most common body parts injured.

3. An open globe injury should be suspected in a blast injury, especially if findings such as corneal lacerations, irregular pupils, and hyphema are found.

4. If an open globe injury is suspected, the eye examination should be stopped immediately. The eye should be protected with a large shield and Ophthalmology should be consulted at that time. Every effort should be made to avoid rises in intraocular pressure.

REFERENCES

1. Green M, Race P: 2001 Fireworks Annual Report: Fireworks-Related Deaths, Emergency Department Treated Injuries and Enforcement Activities During 2001. US Consumer Product Safety Commission, 2002.
2. American Academy of Pediatrics, Committee on Injury and Poison Prevention, 2000–2001: Fireworks-related injuries to children. Pediatrics 108:90–191, 2001.
3. Rychwalski PJ, O'Halloran HS, Cooper HM, et al: Evaluation and classification of pediatric ocular trauma. Pediatr Emerg Care 15:277–279, 1999.
4. Smith GA, Knapp JF, Barnett TM, Shields BJ: The rockets' red glare, the bombs bursting in air: Fireworks-related injuries to children. Pediatrics 98:1–9, 1996.

Lauren Daly, MD
Joseph Zorc, MD

PATIENT 78

A 12-month-old girl with altered mental status

A previously healthy 12-month-old girl presents with a 3-day history of sleepiness, vomiting, and decreased oral intake. Her mother reports irritability over the past 2 weeks. The emesis is nonbloody and nonbilious, with multiple episodes each day. Her mother denies history of fever, diarrhea, cough, rhinorrhea, rash, ingestions, trauma, or movements suggestive of seizure.

Physical Examination: Vital signs: temperature 37.3°C; pulse 100; respiratory rate 22; blood pressure 92/56; pulse oximetry 98% in room air. General appearance: awakens only to painful stimuli. HEENT: normocephalic atraumatic, fontanelle closed; pupils equal, round, but sluggishly reactive 4 mm to 3mm; mucous membranes dry. Neck: supple. Cardiac: RRR, no murmurs. Respiratory: normal. Abdomen: soft, normoactive bowel sounds, possible mass in RUQ. Rectal: guaiac negative. Skin: no rashes, capillary refill 4 seconds. Neurologic: Glasgow Coma Scale score 9 (opens eyes to pain, cries to pain, withdraws to pain), decreased tone throughout musculature, DTR 2+ symmetrically.

Laboratory Findings: CBC: normal. Blood chemistries: Na 140, K 4.2, Cl 102, CO_2 20, BUN 10, Cr 0.3, glucose 135. Liver function tests: normal. Serum/urine toxicology screens: pending. Blood culture: pending.

Question: What emergency interventions should be pursued?

Treatment: Attention to airway, breathing, and circulation are foremost in the care of this patient. This patient has evidence of currently protecting her airway with adequate respiratory effort; however, she has signs of dehydration not associated with elevated heart rate. Cardiorespiratory monitoring and intravenous access should be immediately obtained.

Discussion: A multitude of pediatric diagnoses can manifest with altered mental status. These diagnoses range in their severity and the degree of intervention needed. As such, an organized and efficient approach to patient stabilization and differential diagnosis is required. Stabilization efforts should immediately address the airway, breathing, and circulation (the ABCs) of an obtunded patient. The decision to intubate a child because of altered mental status should be individualized based on the suspected cause and the work-up that is planned. For example, a child with a known seizure disorder who is postictal is likely to improve with minimal supportive care, such as blow-by oxygen, and close observation. The condition of a child with acute head trauma, however, is likely to worsen, and aggressive airway management is indicated. A Glasgow Coma Scale score should be documented, to follow changes in the patient's neurologic status over time and to evaluate the need for increasing airway support. Initial management of children with altered mental status also includes assessing the "Ds" of dextrose and disability. Therefore, an immediate measurement of blood glucose is indicated. Hypoglycemia is a common cause of altered mental status in children, most commonly due to ketotic hypoglycemia in an otherwise healthy child with a prolonged fasting state.

Empiric therapy for altered mental status includes administration of naloxone to reverse a potential opioid ingestion. Naloxone can be given safely in a full reversal dose (0.1 mg/kg up to 2 mg), as withdrawal is generally not a concern in children. In contrast, flumazenil, a benzodiazepine reversal agent, should not be given empirically for altered mental status because it may precipitate seizures and interact with other unsuspected toxins such as cyclic antidepressants. Thiamine replacement is generally not indicated in children because deficiency requires long-standing poor nutrition, such as is seen in adult alcoholics.

Once the patient is stable, the clinician's task shifts to differentiating the cause of the mental status change. A useful mnemonic that includes the most common causes of mental status change in pediatrics is "VITAMINS" (see table).

With the differential diagnosis in mind, the clinician should perform a directed history and physical examination. Key elements of the history include access to medications and other toxins and recent changes in the home environment, such

Mnemonic for Altered Mental Status:
VITAMINS

Vascular	Infarct, intraparenchymal/subarachnoid hemorrhage, arteriovenous malformation, sinus venous thrombosis
Infections	Meningitis, encephalitis, sepsis, brain abscess, toxin-producing (e.g., Shigella)
Trauma	Subdural/epidural hemorrhage, postconcussive, "shaken baby" or other nonaccidental trauma
A lot of toxins	Medications (e.g., benzodiazepenes, barbiturates, opioids, cyclic antidepressants), alcohol, carbon monoxide
Metabolic	Hypoglycemia, diabetic ketoacidosis, posthypoxic encephalopathy, hypoxemia, acidosis, hyponatremia, dehydration, uremia, inborn errors of metabolism
Intussusception	
Neoplasms	Brain tumor, obstructive hydrocephalus
Seizure	Postictal state, clinical/subclinical status, absence seizure

as a new caretaker, a situation that may be associated with occult head trauma and abuse. A head-to-toe physical examination is needed, with a particular focus on vital signs, cranial nerves and neurologic examination, and abdominal examination. Intussusception as a cause of altered mental status is unique to pediatrics and may manifest with episodes of recurrent pain, vomiting, bloody stools, or abdominal mass. If intussusception is suspected, a barium enema is indicated, as clinical examination or plain radiographs are insufficient to rule out the diagnosis.

Further studies should be individualized based on the history and physical examination. Electrolytes, renal and liver function tests, an ammonia level, and a venous blood gas measurement can detect many of the metabolic causes of altered mental status, although inborn errors of metabolism may require further studies. Lumbar puncture should be deferred in obtunded patients until imaging has been performed, usually by noncontrast head computed tomography(CT). Patients with intracranial mass lesions can present with depressed mental status in the absence of focal neurologic findings.

In the present patient, a suspicion of an abdominal mass in the context of vomiting made intussusception a consideration. A barium enema was obtained and resutls were negative. On reexamination and x-rays, this mass was consistent with palpable fecal material. On further review, the patient had progression of signs of increased intracranial pressure, including persistent vomiting, low heart rate despite signs of dehydration, and minimally reactive pupils. A head CT scan led to the final diagnosis of brain tumor with obstructive hydrocephaly that was treated by emergency placement of a ventriculoperitoneal shunt followed by chemotherapy and radiation.

Clinical Pearls

1. Use a structured differential diagnosis, such as the VITAMINS mnemonic, to guide the history and physical examination in a patient with altered mental status.
2. Flumazenil is not used as empiric therapy in patients with altered mental status, as it may precipitate seizure or interact with other toxins.
3. Lumbar puncture is contraindicated in patients with altered mental status until imaging confirms absence of an intracranial mass.

REFERENCES

1. Hasbun R, Abrahams J, Jekel J, et al: Computed tomography of the head before lumbar puncture in adults with suspected meningitis. N Engl J Med 345:1727–1733, 2001.
2. Zorc J J: A lethargic infant: Ingestion or deception? Pediatr Ann 29:104–107, 2000.
3. Pershad J, Monroe K, Atchison J: Childhood hypoglycemia in an urban emergency department: Epidemiology and a diagnostic approach to the problem. Pediatr Emerg Care 14:268–271, 1998.
4. Hoffman RS, Goldfrank LR: The poisoned patient with altered consciousness: Controversies in the use of a 'coma cocktail'. JAMA 247:562–569, 1995.

PATIENT 79

A 20-year-old man with a gunshot wound to the left buttock

A 20 year old man ambulates into the emergency department escorted by police. He has been shot in his left buttock while sitting in his car, apparently the victim of an attempted car-jacking. He reports pain in the area of the wound and numbness in his left foot. He has no significant past medical, surgical, or family history. He has no drug allergies and denies the use of tobacco, alcohol, or illicit drugs.

Physical Examination: Vital signs: temperature 37.6°C; pulse 120; respiratory rate 16; blood pressure 106/58; room air oxygen saturation 99%. General appearance: well developed, no acute distress. HEENT: normal. Lungs: normal. Heart: tachycardiac with occasional irregular beats, grade II/VI systolic murmur, no rub or gallop. Abdomen: normal. Genitourinary: normal. Rectum: normal. Extremities: 2-cm wound left posterior thigh/buttock, tender around wound and along anterior aspect of thigh; peripheral pulses intact. Pelvis: stable. Neurologic: deep tendon reflexes 2+ bilateral ankles and knees, down-going planter reflexes; decreased sensation to pinprick and light touch in L4/5 distribution of left leg. Left foot strength: 3/5 for flexion/extension, 0/5 for inversion/eversion, otherwise normal. Ankle-brachial indices: left dorsalis pedis (DP) 1.17, left posterior tibialis (PT) 0.96, right DP 0.83, right PT 0.87.

Laboratory Findings: CBC, Chemistries: normal. ECG: see figure. Portable abdominal and pelvic radiograph: foreign body visualized in soft tissue near left hip (see figure on next page). Chest x-ray: see figure on next page. Emergency Medicine Bedside Ultrasonogram/FAST scan: no free fluid in abdomen, foreign body in right ventricle, no fluid in pericardial sac. CT scan abdomen/pelvis: large distorted bullet fragment near left hip with evidence of damage to left femoral vessels, no other pathologic lesions.

Question: What *one* diagnosis would explain all these findings (i.e., atrial flutter, bullet fragment in the right ventricle, no apparent myocardial injury, bullet fragment near the hip)?

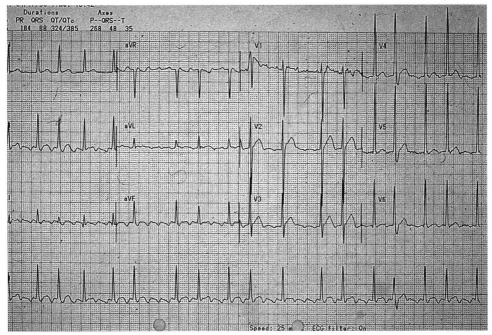

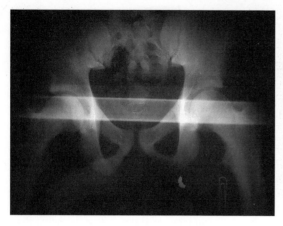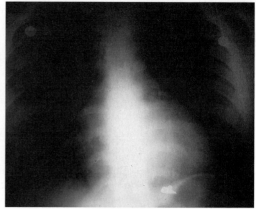

Diagnosis: Bullet embolism. This is the only diagnosis that can explain *all* the findings.

Discussion: The evidence for this diagnosis is as follows:

1. The patient was shot only once, and no exit wound is visualized.

2. The bullet appears deformed on the pelvic x-ray. It struck bone and a fragment entered the femoral vein; hence the damaged vessels seen on computed tomography scan.

3. The foreign body seen on the chest x-ray has a motion artifact.

4. There is no damage to the myocardium on ultrasonogram. The bullet floated into the right ventricle from the pelvic veins and caused the patient's rhythm disturbance.

Bullet embolism was first discussed in the medical literature in 1834. Since then, there have been at least 180 reported cases, with recent increase in frequency due to the increased numbers of civilian gun owners and subsequent gun shot injuries. Since many of these guns are low-caliber weapons (<0.22), this has also increased the number of bullet emboli, since bullets that are smaller in diameter and lighter in weight have a better chance of floating into a blood vessel.

Factors that determine whether damage will be done and where a bullet will lodge include the bullet's kinetic energy, mass and shape, and site of origin, and the patient's position and blood pressure. Suspect the possibility of bullet embolism under the following circumstances:

1. No exit wound found

2. No bullet seen on radiographs

3. Bullet in a strange or new location

4. A "disappearing" bullet

5. Foreign body with motion artifact overlying cardiac silhouette on radiograph

6. Loss of peripheral pulses

Bullets that have landed in the heart need not always be removed; these are often benign. Adverse effects associated with cardiac foreign body include pericardial effusion, valvular disease, thrombus formation, dysrhythmias, embolism out of the heart, and cardiac neurosis/psychosis. Most experts agree however, that bullets that are free in a cavity, sharp in nature, larger than 5 mm, or are located in the left heart should be removed. Traditionally, the only surgical option was a midline sternotomy with or without cardiopulmonary bypass. More recently, percutaneous transvenous retrievals have been performed with success.

The bullet in the present patient was removed using a snare catheter that was inserted via a right internal jugular cutdown (see figures on next page). The patient was cardioverted at 100 J into sinus rhythm and discharged 24 hours after his initial presentation.

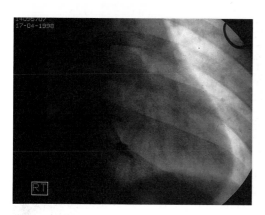 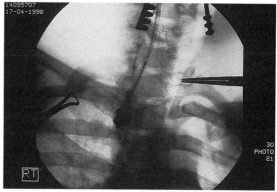

Clinical Pearls

1. Maintain a high level of suspicion for bullet embolism or the diagnosis will certainly be missed.

2. If no bullet is seen where it is expected, search the patient as well as ancillary radiographs.

3. Unusual symptoms remote from the site of entry should prompt a search for bullet embolism.

REFERENCES

1. Berkan O, Gunay L: An unusual case of birdshot embolism. Circulation 66:707–708, 2002.
2. Kalimi R: Bullet embolization from the left internal iliac vein to the right ventricle. J Trauma 52:772–774, 2002.
3. Wales L: Delayed presentation of right ventricular bullet embolus. Ann Thorac Surg 72:619–620, 2001.
4. Obermeyer RJ: Embolization of bullet to the right ventricle. Am J Surg 179:189, 2000.
5. Roberts JR, Hedges JR, eds: Clinical Procedures in Emergency Medicine, 3rd ed. Philadelphia, WB Saunders, 1998.
6. Rajmani K, Fisher M: Bullet embolism. N Engl J Med 339:812, 1998.
7. Headrick JR Jr, Mugosa M, Carr MG: Venous bullet embolism: Controversies in management. Tenn Med 90:103–105, 1997.
8. O Neill PJ, Feldman DR, Vugic I, Byrne TK: Trans-jugular extraction of bullet embolus to the heart. Military Med 161:360–361, 1996.
9. Mattox KL, Beall AC Jr, Ennix CL, Debakey ME: Intravascular migratory bullets. Am J Surg 137:192, 1979.

Aaron Donoghue, MD

PATIENT 80

An 8-month-old boy with hypocalcemic seizures

An 8-month-old boy is brought to the emergency department with a chief symptom of twitching movements of his arms. His mother reports that she observed a 2- to 3-minute period of twitching movements of both arms; she also states that the baby was "breathing funny" but denied cyanosis. She denies fever, vomiting, diarrhea, respiratory symptoms, history of trauma, or any chance of ingestion. She has brought the child to an emergency department twice in the past 10 days following similar brief episodes; she states that no specific work-up has been done.

Physical Examination: Vital signs: temperature 37.1°C.; pulse 148; respiratory rate 28; blood pressure 97/71. General appearance: alert, no distress. HEENT: mucous membranes moist. Chest: clear to auscultation bilaterally. Cardiovascular: normal S1 and S2, no murmur. Abdomen: soft, nontender, no organomegaly. Genitourinary: normal male genitalia. Extremities: warm, pulses normal; left wrist slightly deformed appearing; baby cries when left arm is moved. Skin: warm and dry; no rash. Neurologic: cranial nerves intact, strength 5/5 in all groups, DTRs 2+.

Laboratory Findings: Blood chemistries: Na 137, K 5.3, Cl 107, CO_2 20, BUN 3, Cr 0.2, glucose 86; calcium 4.7 mg/dl (normal range 9–11 mg/dl), phosphorus 5.5 mg/dl (normal range 2.5–4.5 mg/dl), magnesium 1.6 mEq/L (normal range 1.3–2.0 mEq/L), alkaline phosphatase 663 U/L (normal range 150–420 U/L), ionized calcium 0.65 mmol/L (normal range 0.95–1.35 mmol/L). Wrist radiograph: see figure. Electrocardiogram: see figure.

Question: How would you manage this patient?

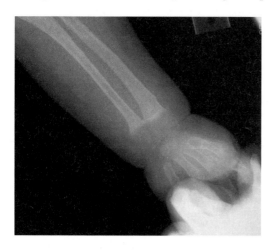
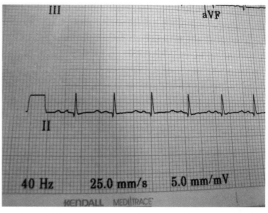

Treatment: Admission to inpatient telemetry unit (due to evidence of prolonged QT interval on ECG), intavenous and oral calcium supplementation, and treatment with ergocalciferol.

Discussion: The present patient was diagnosed with rickets; the relevant features are hypocalcemia, elevated alkaline phosphatase, and typical radiographic changes with splaying and cupping of long bone metaphyses. The present patient also suffered a pathologic fracture of his ulna and radius, as shown in the figure.

The term *rickets* signifies a failure of mineralization of osteoid tissue in growing bone, most often due to a deficiency or abnormality in the vitamin D pathway. Earlier in the 20th century, this was almost uniformly due to lack of nutritional intake of vitamin D. Currently, in industrialized countries, because of supplementation of vitamin D in foods, nutritional rickets is less common, but it can still occur in patients who have insufficient intake of appropriate foods or lack of exposure to sunlight. The active form of vitamin D in the body, 1,25-dihydroxyvitamin D, represents the end point of a synthetic pathway involving both dietary intake of vitamin D and photochemical conversion of vitamin D_3 (naturally present in human skin) to 1,25-hydroxyvitamin D in the liver followed by further hydroxylation in the kidney to 1,25-dehydroxyvitamin D. This active form facilitates intestinal absorption of calcium as well as deposition of calcium in developing bone. It is deficiencies within this vitamin D pathway, rather than calcium deficiency alone, that lead to rickets.

Children with darkly pigmented skin are more susceptible to rickets, and in seasonal climates, the clinical presentation of a young child with rickets is believed to occur more commonly in the winter when sun exposure is decreased. Other chronic conditions that can lead to rachitic changes include renal conditions causing excessive phosphaturia, renal tubular acidosis, hepatic disease, and several rare genetic deficiencies of enzymes and receptors within the vitamin D pathway. One case-control study of children in Nigeria showed no significant difference in dietary calcium intake, but found that patients with rickets had a greater proportion of first-degree relatives with rickets and a shorter mean duration of breast feeding.

Children presenting with rickets can vary greatly in their symptoms, among them skeletal deformity or injury, failure to thrive, abnormal radiographic findings, or symptoms related to hypocalcemia such as seizures or tetany. Case reports exist of infants presenting with stridor and laryngospasm and dilated cardiomyopathy secondary to severe hypocalcemia caused by nutritional rickets. The clinical findings of rickets are most pronounced in the skeletal system, with the site of the abnormality relating to the child's age and the region of greatest skeletal growth. In newborns with congenital rickets, the skull may be most affected (craniotabes); in infants, the ribs (rachitic rosary) and the long bones of the arms may be most abnormal; leg bone changes and bowing are unlikely to be noticeable until a child is ambulatory. Radiographic changes are the most reliable diagnostic tool, with widening and irregularity of the epiphyses and metaphyseal cupping along with osteopenia. Laboratory findings are inconsistent, and frank hypocalemia is not common. The alkaline phosphatase level is typically moderate elevated and slowly normalizes with proper treatment. It is important to bear in mind the wide variability of historical, laboratory, and radiographic data that can be present in patients with rickets. One case series of 21 adolescents diagnosed with rickets, by Narchi et al, found that 19 of 21 had serum hypocalcemia, but only 8 of 18 patients (44%) who underwent radiographic evaluation had changes consistent with rickets. In children with significant hypocalcemia, it is important to rule out significant cardiac effects as evidenced by prolongation of the QT interval; if present, telemetry monitoring should be instituted.

Treatment of rickets depends on the underlying cause but in most cases involves supplementation with both calcium and vitamin D analogues. Hospitalization should be reserved for patients with symptomatic hypocalcemia at presentation. Failure to respond to vitamin D therapy should prompt an endocrine evaluation for a cause of vitamin D resistant rickets. Most children with rickets respond to therapy with healing of bony changes within 2 to 4 weeks, and the overall prognosis is excellent for complete recovery.

With regard to the present patient, further history yielded that the baby was exclusively breastfed and that his mother maintained a strict vegan diet. He was given oral calcium carbonate, intravenous calcium gluconate, and daily doses of ergocalciferol; he was admitted to a telemetry unit for his hospital stay but had no significant cardiac events. A complete skeletal survey yielded evidence of pathologic fractures of both wrists and marked rachitic changes in both femurs and tibias. He underwent casting of both fractured wrists. He was gradually weaned off intravenous calcium as his laboratory values normalized, and he was discharged home on hospital day 7 on an oral regimen of calcium carbonate and supplemental vitamin D.

Clinical Pearls

1. Rickets occurs in children at all social and economic levels.
2. Life-threatening complications of hypocalcemia include laryngospasm, QT interval prolongation, and seizures.
3. Correction of severe hypocalcemia should occur on an inpatient basis.

REFERENCES

1. Narchi H, El Jamil M, Kulayat N: Symptomatic rickets in adolescence. Arch Dis Child 84:501–503, 2001.
2. Hale DE: Endocrine emergencies. In Fleisher G, Ludwig S, eds: Textbook of Pediatric Emergency Medicine. Philadelphia, Lippincott Williams & Wilkins, 2000.
3. Thacher TD, Fisher PR, Pettifor JM, et al: Case-control study of factors associated with nutritional rickets in Nigerian children. J Pediatr 137:367–373, 2000.
4. Abdullah M, Bigras JL, McCrindle BW, Mustafa A: Dilated cardiomyopathy as a first sign of nutritional vitamin D deficiency rickets in infancy. Can J Cardiol 15:699–701, 1999.
5. Halterman JS, Smith SA: Hypocalcemia and stridor: An unusual presentation of vitamin D-deficient rickets. J Emerg Med 16:41–43, 1998.
6. Barness LA, Curran JS: Nutrition. In Behrman RE, Kliegman RM, Arvin Am (eds): Nelson Textbook of Pediatrics. Philadelphia, WB Saunders, 1996.

Lauren Daly, MD
Elizabeth R. Alpern, MD, MSCE

PATIENT 81

A 7-year-old girl with abdominal and back pain after a motor vehicle collision

A 7-year-old girl presents to the emergency department after being involved in a motor vehicle collision. She was a passenger in a car that struck a parked trailer. She was in the back seat restrained with a lap belt only. There was a question of loss of consciousness at the scene, but she is now alert and reports abdominal and lower back pain.

Physical Examination: Vital signs: temperature 37.2°C orally; pulse 106; respiratory rate 24; blood pressure 100/59; pulse oximetry 98% on room air. General appearance: alert but uncomfortable. HEENT: active epistaxis, no lacerations or deformities of head, PERRLA, EOMi, no oral trauma. Neck: immobilized in cervical-spine collar. Cardiac and respiratory: normal. Back: slight tenderness to palpation over L1-L5. Abdomen: soft but tender bilateral lower quadrants with rebound and slight guarding; erythematous abrasion across lower quadrants (see figure). Extremities: atraumatic. Neurologic: GCS 15, 5/5 strength all extremities.

Laboratory Findings: CBC: normal. Electrolytes and liver function tests: normal. Chest, abdomen, pelvis radiographs: normal.

Questions: What injury syndrome does this patient's constellation of symptoms likely represent? What further diagnostics are indicated? How could these injuries have been prevented?

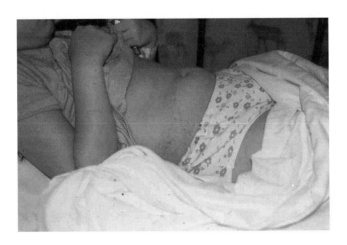

Answers: Seat belt syndrome; abdominal computed tomography(CT) and radiographic imaging of the lumbar spine; by following guidelines for age-and size-appropriate child restraint devices.

Discussion: The "seat belt syndrome" is an injury pattern seen in children restrained with lap belts only or lap-shoulder belts in motor vehicle crashes when the device fits them improperly. Originally described in adults, case reports of this syndrome in children have become more frequent, and the prevalence is estimated between 0.2% of all restrained children in motor vehicle collisions (MVCs) and 1.5% of all restrained children who present to emergency departments after being involved in a crash. The characteristic injury pattern is a triad of abrasions/bruising to the lower abdomen/pelvis area (the "seatbelt sign"), intra-abdominal injuries, and injuries to the lumbar spine. Although a variety of intra-abdominal injuries can occur, there is a significant incidence of gastrointestinal tract perforation (usually small bowel).

GI tract perforation may be difficult to detect on initial examination. Because a small disruption of the intestinal lumen may cause a slow leak, free air or fluid may not be appreciated on initial radiograph or abdominal CT scan. Even a contrast study may be compromised, since the material may not have traversed the length of injured bowel by the time the images are taken. This fact, and recent literature citing a significantly increased risk of intra-abdominal injury with the presence of an abdominal wall hematoma, has led to the recommendation of admission for serial abdominal examinations even in the face of normal initial radiographic studies. Our patient was diagnosed with a duodenal hematoma and ischemic injury to her jejunum, along with a rectus sheath hematoma by abdominal CT.

Seat belts are designed for adult body proportions and so, due to this fact and because children tend to move forward on the seats of cars for comfort reasons, seat belts tend to ride high on the abdomen of children, rather than low over the pelvis. The poorly positioned seat belt exerts a vector of force on a child in a crash that allows severe flex-ion of the lumbar spine and entrapment of bowel between the belt and the spinal column, creating a mechanism for bowel hematoma or perforation. The extreme flexion of the spine may also lead to either compression fractures or Chance fractures of the lumbar vertebrae. The present patient ultimately underwent a magnetic resonance imaging (MRI) scan of the lumbar spine due to persistent pain and was found to have a contusion of L3 and L4.

The appropriate restraint devise for children is determined by age and weight factors. An infant should be placed in a rear-facing infant or convertible safety seat until at least 1 year of age and 20 pounds. A rear-facing infant seat should never be placed in the front seat of a vehicle with an airbag. The safest place for all children is in the rear seat. After the child is 1 year of age and greater than 20 pounds, she may be transitioned to a forward-facing child safety seat until the maximum height and weight allowed by the seat. Once the height and weight limits of the child safety seat have been reached, the child should be transitioned to a belt-positioning booster seat (usually appropriate for children 40–80 pounds). A belt-positioning booster seat should be used until the vehicle safety belt fits properly. This is achieved when the lap-shoulder belt of the car can be comfortable positioned across the chest with the lap component low and snug across the thighs. The child should be tall enough to sit with his back against the seat back and his legs comfortably bent at the knees.

More recent literature alerts the clinician to a fourfold higher incidence of head injuries in children inappropriately restrained with lap or lap-shoulder belts rather than booster/child seats, thought to be due to the children displacing the shoulder belt behind the back for comfort. Consistent with these data, the present patient suffered a nasal fracture as well.

Clinical Pearls

1. In children with history of lap belt use in motor vehicle crashes, abdominal and lumbar spine injuries must be ruled out.

2. Even if initial radiographic findings are normal, admission for serial abdominal examinations is recommended for children with the "seat belt sign."

3. Children inappropriately restrained in lap belts have a significantly higher risk of head injury than if restrained in age-and size-appropriate devices.

REFERENCES

1. American Academy of Pediatrics Committee on Injury and Poison Prevention: Selecting and using the most appropriate car safety seats for growing children: Guidelines for counseling parents. Pediatrics 109:550–553, 2002.
2. Durbin D, Arbogast K, Moll E: Seat belt syndrome in children: A case report and review of the literature. Pediat Emerg Care 17:474–477, 2001.
3. Chandler CF, Lane JS, Waxman KS: Seatbelt sign following blunt trauma is associated with increased incidence of abdominal injury. Am Surg 63:885–888, 1997.
4. Albanese CT, Meza MP, Gerdner MJ, et al: Is computed tomography a useful adjunct to the clinical examination for the diagnosis of pediatric gastrointestinal perforation from blunt abdominal trauma in children? J Trauma 40:417–421, 1996.
5. Hardacre JM, West KW, Rescorla FR, et al: Delayed onset of intestinal obstruction in children after unrecognized seat belt injury. J Pediat Surg 25:967–969, 1990.

PATIENT 82

A 33-year-old man refusing ambulance transport after a seizure

Emergency services are activated for a 33-year-old man who has just had a seizure in front of his house. When the paramedics arrive, the patient is postictal. The patient's wife states that he has a known seizure disorder, but today's seizure seemed longer than usual, prompting her to call for an ambulance. The patient's mental status improves during the course of his evaluation. He states that he takes phenytoin for seizures but that he may have missed a "few" doses. He admits to drinking "two beers" earlier in the day.

Physical Examination: Vital signs: pulse 96; respiratory rate 16; blood pressure 144/88; the ambulance does not carry a thermometer so temperature is not recorded. Skin: no lesions. HEENT: slight smell of ethanol on the breath; no evidence of trauma. Chest: clear to auscultation. Cardiac: regular rate without murmurs or gallops. Abdomen: nontender. Extremities: no signs of trauma. Neuromuscular: the patient cooperates with the paramedics and is oriented to person, place, time, and circumstances. No gross motor deficit is appreciated. As the paramedics complete their assessment, the patient stands up abruptly and yells "I'm not going to the hospital, and you can't make me!"

Laboratory Findings: Prehospital data are limited. The patient's blood sugar is 112 mg/dl, and room-air oxygen saturation by pulse oximetry is 99%.

Questions: If the paramedics were to contact you for online medical command, how would you advise them to manage this situation? What are the risks of leaving the patient at the scene versus directing the paramedics to transport him against his expressed wishes?

Management: Management involves a careful assessment of the patient's mental capacity to refuse care. The patient's refusal is then honored, or the patient is treated against his wishes.

Discussion: The management of patients who refuse medical care can be challenging under the best of circumstances. In the relatively isolated environment in which emergency medical services (EMS) providers often operate, these scenarios may be even more difficult. EMS personnel may lack immediate law enforcement back-up in the event that the patient becomes confrontational or violent, and consultation with an online medical command physician for guidance may not be an option. Encounters in which a patient refuses care or transport to the hospital may be associated with an adverse outcome for the patient as well as liability for the EMS system. A patient who is not transported may deteriorate and even die, resulting in a lawsuit for patient abandonment or wrongful death. At the same time, a patient who is transported against his or her expressed wishes may charge the EMS system with battery or false imprisonment.

Most patients who refuse prehospital care have a favorable outcome. However, the fact that a patient refuses care does not mean that his or her condition is not serious or potentially life-threatening. Studies of the outcome of patients who refuse transport by EMS demonstrate that a small percentage re-contact EMS for recurrence of the same problem in the next few days. Many of these patients are transported to an emergency department for treatment. Some are admitted to the hospital, and a few die. Therefore, EMS systems should develop written policies and procedures addressing patient refusal of care, often after consultation with legal counsel and local law-enforcement agencies. This will ensure that these situations can be handled in a way that ensures the patient's safety and minimizes liability.

Just as patients have the right to consent to treatment, they also have the right to refuse treatment, even if that decision is in conflict with a health care provider's professional opinion. For a patient to be considered to have the mental capacity to refuse treatment, he or she must (1) be alert and oriented to person, place, time, and circumstances; (2) be able to express an understanding of the seriousness of the medical condition; (3) understand the treatment being offered, its benefits, and the risks associated with refusing that treatment, including the possibility of permanent disability or death; and (4) be informed of alternative treatment options. A patient's mental capacity may be affected by the underlying medical emergency, severe pain, use of intoxicants such as ethanol, and baseline intelligence and level of education.

Assessing a patient's capacity for medical decision making is an imperfect process that must take into account the gravity of the medical emergency, associated physical findings of the condition, and other factors. An elderly patient with chest pain, hypotension, and diaphoresis, who is refusing care, has a much greater risk of an adverse outcome than does a patient with a small abrasion on the hand. It is far more important that health care providers convince a patient with a serious medical condition to accept care and transport than a patient with a minor problem. Analogously, health care providers must be far more rigorous in establishing a patient's capacity when the medical condition is serious as opposed to minor. A patient with a sprained thumb and mild alcohol intoxication who is refusing transport may, under most circumstances, be safely left at the scene with appropriate instructions and documentation. While it could be argued that his capacity is impaired by ethanol, the consequences of his refusal are minor. Furthermore, the hazards associated with transporting him against his will may outweigh the benefits. In contrast, an individual with a gun shot wound to the chest, who is oriented, hemodynamically stable, but refusing care, may, in most cases, be transported against his will. While it could be argued that he has a normal mental status, his expressed wish is so unreasonable and so inconsistent with what most people would request under the circumstances that his capacity to refuse may be questioned.

All cases of patient refusal of care must be carefully documented. This should include the circumstances, vital signs and physical findings, a detailed description of the patient's capacity, and the presence of intoxicating agents or painful injuries. The health care provider should also document that the benefits of therapy and the risks of refusing therapy were explained to the patient, as were any available alternative therapies. Finally, if the patient is believed to have the capacity to refuse, he or she should sign an against-medical-advice form, be encouraged to seek follow-up care, and re-contact EMS if the condition recurs or deteriorates. Before releasing the patient, it is also advisable to involve a medical command physician in the decision-making process. Studies have demonstrated that when physicians speak to patients who are refusing care, in many cases the patients will change their mind. Physician involvement should be documented in the medical record.

In the present patient's case, the paramedics contacted a medical command physician to discuss their options. They all believed that the patient had the mental capacity to refuse transport. In accordance with their written protocol covering this situation, the paramedics advised the patient of the risks associated with his refusal of transport and had him sign an against-medical-advice form. The patient was instructed to follow up with his primary care physician. The wife was advised to re-contact EMS if the patient's condition deteriorated.

Clinical Pearls

1. Patients who are able to demonstrate the capacity to make decisions have the right to refuse medical care, even if health care providers disagree with this decision.

2. The principles outlined for refusal of care in the prehospital setting can also be applied in the ED setting.

3. Family members or friends should be considered allies to health care providers when patients refuse transport. Often patients can be encouraged to seek treatment through these individuals.

4. All patient encounters involving refusal of care should be documented in detail.

REFERENCES

1. Mechem CC, Barger J, Shofer FS, Dickinson ET: Short-term outcome of seizure patients who refuse transport after out-of-hospital evaluation. Acad Emerg Med 8:231–236, 2001.
2. Weaver J, Brinsfield K, Dalphond D: Prehospital refusal of transport policies: Adequate legal protection? Prehosp Emerg Care 4:53–56, 2000.
3. Cohn BM, Azzara AJ: Medical treatment: Consent and refusal. In Legal Aspects of Emergency Medical Services. Philadelphia, WB Saunders, 1998, pp 33–50.
4. Moss ST, Chan TC, Buchanan J, et al: Outcome study of prehospital patients signed out against medical advice by field paramedics. Ann Emerg Med 31:247–250, 1998.
5. Schmidt TA, Mann C, Federiuk CS, et al: Do patients refusing transport remember descriptions of risks after initial advanced life support assessment? Acad Emerg Med 5:796–801, 1998.
6. Alicandro J, Hollander JE, Henry MC, et al: Impact of interventions for patients refusing emergency medical services transport. Acad Emerg Med 2:480–485, 1995.
7. Zachariah BS, Bryan D, Pepe PE, Griffin M: Follow-up and outcome of patients who decline or are denied transport by EMS. Prehosp Disaster Med 7:359–364, 1992.
8. Holroyd B, Shalit M, Kallsen G, et al: Prehospital patients refusing care. Ann Emerg Med 17:957–963, 1988.

Angela M. Mills, MD
Jill M. Baren, MD, FACEP, FAAP

PATIENT 83

A 75-year-old man status post fall onto right hip

A 75-year-old man who lives in a nursing home lost his balance and fell onto his right hip. He reports only right hip pain and denies any other symptoms.

Physical Examination: Vital signs: temperature 36.3°C; pulse 85; respiratory rate 18; blood pressure 125/70. Skin: no lesions. HEENT: normal: Chest: clear to auscultation. Cardiac: regular rate without gallops or murmurs. Abdomen: normal. Extremities: right leg shortened and outwardly rotated with tenderness to palpation over greater trochanter and proximal femur. Knee: nontender. Neurovascular: dorsalis pedis pulses equal bilaterally and sensation intact.

Radiographic Findings: Right hip radiograph: see figure.

Questions: How does one evaluate hip pain after trauma? How are hip fractures classified and managed?

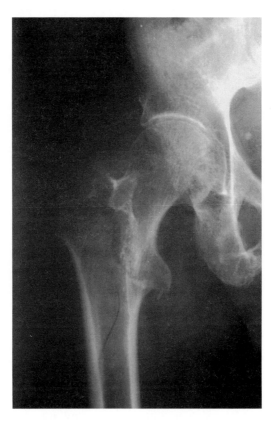

Diagnosis: Right intertrochanteric hip fracture

Discussion: In young healthy adults, major trauma (motor vehicle crashes and falls from significant height) is responsible for most hip fractures. Elderly individuals may sustain hip fractures from relatively minor trauma due to pre-existing bone disease such as osteoporosis.

Evaluation of the patient with traumatic hip pain consists of a detailed history, a complete examination, and appropriate radiography. Examination of the hip should include observation for deformities, bruises, or lacerations; palpation for irregularities or tenderness; active and passive range of motion; and a thorough neurovascular assessment. The inability to bear weight or ambulate due to hip pain requires further evaluation. Standard radiography of the hip includes anteroposterior (AP) and lateral views. The physician must also determine the need for radiography of the pelvis, femur, and knee when evaluating hip pain after trauma. The inability to ambulate may heighten suspicion for an occult fracture, and if plain radiographs do not reveal a fracture, further evaluation with magnetic resonance imaging (MRI) or nuclear bone scan is required.

Hip fractures can be divided into femoral head and neck fractures (intracapsular) and trochanteric, intertrochanteric, and subtrochanteric fractures (extracapsular). Femoral neck fractures most commonly occur in older adults with osteoporosis and can lead to significant complications, including avascular necrosis, nonunion, deep infection (osteomyelitis or septic arthritis), and pulmonary embolism. Intertrochanteric fractures are more common in elderly women with osteoporosis, result in an externally rotated and shortened extremity, and may be associated with hemodynamic instability from substantial blood loss. Subtrochanteric fractures are usually caused by direct blunt trauma with a fall and occur in both elderly and young patients. These fractures are also associated with hemodynamic instability, nonunion, and fat embolism. The majority of hip fractures require surgical management, and orthopedic consultation should occur early.

The radiograph shows a comminuted right intertrochanteric fracture extending into the femur. Intertrochanteric fractures extend between the greater and lesser trochanters of the femur, where there is an excellent blood supply. On examination, there may be swelling, bruising, and pain with range of motion or weight bearing. The majority of these fractures require operative management with internal fixation allowing for faster recovery of mobilization and decreased mortality. The mortality rate is 10% to 30% in the first year following surgery. Long-term complications include infection, mechanical failure, and implant migration.

The present patient was admitted to the orthopedic surgery service and underwent an open reduction and internal fixation of his right intertrochanteric hip fracture. He recovered quickly and was discharged home on regular physical therapy.

Clinical Pearls

1. The patient with hip pain following trauma with no fracture on radiograph but unable to bear weight or ambulate must have further evaluation for occult fracture.

2. Major trauma victims with hip or pelvic fracture or dislocation must have other injuries excluded (intra-abdominal, retroperitoneal, and genitourinary).

3. Hemodynamic instability in the setting of hip fracture suggests an associated vascular injury, which must be aggressively treated.

REFERENCES
1. Gurr DE, Gibbs MA: Femur and hip. In Marx JA, Hockberger RS, Walls RM, et al, eds: Rosen's Emergency Medicine, 5th ed, vol 1. St. Louis, Mosby, 2002.
2. DeLee JC: Fractures and dislocations of the hip. In Rockwood JC Jr, Green DP, Bucholz RW, eds: Rockwood and Green's Fractures in Adults, 4th ed, vol 2. Philadelphia, JB Lippincott, 1996.
3. Koval KJ, Zuckerman JD: Hip fractures II: Evaluation and treatment of intertrochanteric fractures. J Am Acad Orthop Surg 2:150–156, 1994.

Philip R. Spandorfer, MD

PATIENT 84

A 20-month-old girl with fever, vomiting, and diarrhea

A previously healthy 20-month-old girl presents to the emergency department with a 1-day history of illness. Her parents relate that she has had five episodes of vomiting. Although there was no blood in the vomitus, they think that the last episode was green tinged. Furthermore, she has had nine episodes of nonbloody, loose, watery diarrhea. Her mother states that every time the child drinks the bottle, she vomits the entire amount. The patient began to feel warm to the touch about 1-hour prior to presentation. Her parents are unable to comment on her urine output because every diaper they change has a diarrheal stool. She is in day care, but the parents are unaware of any ill contacts. She does not have a history of recent travel or new food exposures.

Physical Examination:　Vital signs: temperature 38.2°C rectally; pulse 161; respiratory rate 28; blood pressure 95/54; weight 16.2 kg. General appearance: tired and worn-out appearing, not toxic (see figure). HEENT: tears present, eyes are not sunken; mucous membranes dry; no meningismus. Lungs: clear to auscultation bilaterally. Cardiac: tachycardiac, but otherwise regular rhythm without murmurs appreciated. Abdomen: bowel sounds present, abdomen soft and nontender, no hepatosplenomegaly detected. Extremities: capillary refill at 1.5 seconds. Neurologic: somnolent, otherwise normal.

Laboratory Findings:　Electrolytes within normal limits, glucose 68, urinalysis normal.

Questions:　What is the most likely diagnosis? How dehydrated is this patient, and what is the most appropriate treatment?

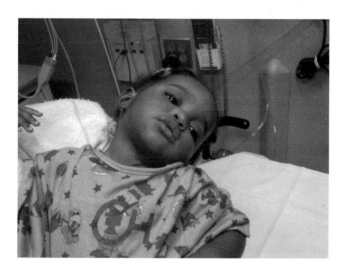

Diagnosis: Acute gastroenteritis. She is moderately dehydrated, and oral rehydration therapy should be instituted.

Discussion: Gastroenteritis is one of the leading causes of dehydration in pediatric patients. The diagnosis of acute gastroenteritis is typically a clinical diagnosis based on the history of diarrhea with or without vomiting. It is tempting to diagnosis a patient who presents with vomiting alone as having gastroenteritis; however, since diarrhea has not developed, there is no enteritis. There are numerous diagnoses that frequently manifest with vomiting alone and risk being misdiagnosed as gastroenteritis. A few of the many important diagnoses not to overlook are brain tumors, head trauma, or any cause of increased intracranial pressure, lower lobe pneumonias, appendicitis, pancreatitis, hepatitis, hernias, urinary tract infection/pyelonephritis, or testicular/ovarian torsion. The importance of avoiding diagnosing vomiting alone as gastroenteritis is to prevent the significant morbidity that may be involved if the diagnosis is incorrect.

Once gastroenteritis is correctly diagnosed, the challenge of accurately predicting the degree of dehydration remains. Several classification systems have been developed by organizations such as the World Health Organization (WHO) and the American Academy of Pediatrics (AAP). These systems categorize patients as mildly (1–4%), moderately (5–9%), or severely dehydrated (≥ 10%). Although these systems have been extensively used, they have not been studied in a prospective manner and assessed for validity and reliability. There may be considerable overlap for an individual patient, with some features consistent with mild dehydration and other features consistent with either moderate or severe dehydration.

Gorelick et al conducted a prospective study of the commonly assessed features of a dehydrated patient and developed a classification system that addressed these issues. This scoring system has been determined to be reliable and valid to predict the degree of dehydration. Patients are assessed for 10 clinical features and given a point for each feature that is present (see table). If the patient scores 0 points, he or she is not dehydrated, 1 to 2 points is mildly dehydrated, 3 to 6 points is moderately dehydrated, and 7 to 10 points is severely dehydrated. Although this scoring system is helpful, it is difficult to remember all 10 features accurately during the clinical evaluation of a patient. A model based on 4 of the 10 features was found to have the same diagnostic accuracy as the full model. These four features include ill appearance, absence of tears, dry mucous membranes, and capillary refill greater than 2 seconds. If none of the four features are present, then the patient is not dehydrated; if one is present, then the patient is classified as mildly dehydrated; two signifies moderate dehydration; and the presence of three or four features represents severe dehydration.

The appropriate treatment to be instituted first in a mild or moderately dehydrated patient is oral rehydration therapy (ORT). Numerous organizations, including the WHO, AAP, Centers for Disease Control and Prevention, and Canadian Pediatric Society, endorse the benefits of ORT for children who are mild to moderately dehydrated.

The 10-Point Dehydration Score, Listed by Descending Positive Predictive Value

CLINICAL FINDING	SENSITIVITY (95% CI)	SPECIFICITY (95% CI)	PPV	NPV
Decreased skin elasticity	0.35 (0.23–0.49)	0.97 (0.92–0.99)	0.57	0.93
Capillary refill >2 sec	0.48 (0.35–0.61)	0.96 (0.90–0.99)	0.57	0.94
Ill appearance	0.59 (0.46–0.71)	0.91 (0.84–0.95)	0.42	0.95
Absent tears	0.67 (0.53–0.78)	0.89 (0.82–0.94)	0.40	0.96
Abnormal respirations	0.43 (0.30–0.56)	0.86 (0.78–0.91)	0.37	0.94
Dry mucous membranes	0.80 (0.67–0.89)	0.78 (0.70–0.85)	0.29	0.99
Sunken eyes	0.60 (0.47–0.72)	0.84 (0.76–0.90)	0.29	0.95
Abnormal radial pulse	0.43 (0.30–0.56)	0.86 (0.78–0.91)	0.25	0.93
Tachycardia (>150)	0.46 (0.32–0.61)	0.79 (0.72–0.87)	0.20	0.93
Decreased urine output (parental report)	0.85 (0.73–0.93)	0.53 (0.44–0.62)	0.17	0.97

PPV, positive predictive value; NPV, negative predictive value.

From Gorelick MH, Shaw KN, Murphy KO: Validity and reliability of clinical signs in the diagnosis of dehydration in children. Pediatrics 99:e6, 1997; with permission.

ORT is defined as the process of calculating a specific volume of fluid to be administered to a patient over a given time interval and administering the fluid orally in small, frequent aliquots. Appropriate oral rehydration solution (ORS) should be used. For most patients, 50 to 100 ml/kg corrects the fluid deficit from acute gastroenteritis. The exact mechanics of the time interval is variable, depending on the patient's response to hydration. Administering ORS over a 4-hour time interval in aliquots every 5 minutes is one alternative. Other options include 5 ml of ORS every minute for 1 to 2 hours. Patients may be syringe-fed or may be allowed to drink the aliquot from a bottle or cup. If the patient refuses to drink, then syringe administration is the preferred method.

ORT utilizes the sodium glucose cotransport mechanism in the intestine to promote water, electrolyte, and glucose absorption. This cotransport mechanism works with an optimal stoichiometric ratio of 1 molecule of sodium to 1 molecule of glucose. Appropriate ORS have sodium to glucose ratios in the 1:1 (WHO ORS) to 1:3 (Pedialyte) range.

If ORT were unsuccessful due to the patient's refusal or inability to stay ahead of the vomiting or diarrhea output, then intravenous fluids would be the appropriate next step. Advantages of ORT over intravenous fluids include the simplicity of ORT, the painless nature of the therapy, the ability of ORT to be used outside of a medical environment as well as for future episodes of dehydration, the speed with which patients recover, and the ability to provide glucose as a substrate during the rehydration phase on a routine basis. This last point should be emphasized, since approximately one third of moderate to severely dehydrated children also have documented hypoglycemia.

The present patient was thought to have viral gastroenteritis. Using the dehydration score discussed previously, the patient is moderately dehydrated (dehydration score 4/10 or 2/4). Her parents were taught how to administer ORT using 10 ml of Pedialyte every 5 minutes. Although the first few aliquots were a little challenging to administer, the patient soon realized that she felt better with the slow syringe feeds. After 2 hours of ORT, the child was markedly improved. Her vomiting had resolved and she had produced urine. Her parents were able to continue the treatment at home. On follow-up, the patient continued to have diarrhea for approximately 4 days and her parents had to intermittently use ORT techniques when she refused to drink oral fluids. She improved over the next several days and had returned to baseline activity by 1 week.

Clinical Pearls

1. Vomiting alone should not be diagnosed as gastroenteritis. To diagnosis gastroenteritis, the acute onset of diarrhea needs to be present with or without vomiting.

2. Oral rehydration therapy (ORT) is defined as the process of measuring out a specific volume of fluid to be administered, typically with an oral syringe, over a given time frame.

3. ORT is a fast and simple way to institute therapy in a dehydrated patient.

4. ORT provides glucose as a substrate to dehydrated patients early in the treatment phase.

REFERENCES

1. Atherly-John YC, Cunningham SJ, Crain EF: A randomized trial of oral vs intravenous rehydration in a pediatric emergency department. Arch Pediatr Adoles Med 156:1240–1243, 2002.
2. Gorelick MH, Shaw KN, Murphy KO: Validity and reliability of clinical signs in the diagnosis of dehydration in children. Pediatrics 99:e6, 1997.
3. American Academy of Pediatrics, Provisional Committee on Quality Improvement, Subcommittee on Acute Gastroenteritis: Practice parameter: The management of acute gastroenteritis in young children. Pediatrics 97:424–436, 1996.
4. World Health Organization: The Treatment of Diarrhea: A Manual for Physicians and Other Senior Health Workers. WHO/CDD/SER/80.2 Rev.3. Geneva, World Health Organization, 1995.
5. Hirschhorn N, Lindenbaum J, Greenough WB III, Alam SM: Hypoglycemia in children with acute diarrhea. Lancet 2: 128–132, 1966.

Worth Everett, MD

PATIENT 85

A 64-year-old woman with bloody stools

A 64-year-old woman with a history of hypertension and rheumatoid arthritis presents to the emergency department for evaluation of massive bleeding per rectum. She had large grossly bloody bowel movements at home, on the way to the ED, and in the ED. She denied any other symptoms. She takes naproxen for pain control.

Physical Examination: Vital signs: temperature 37.5°C; pulse 110; respiratory rate 18; blood pressure 170/100. General appearance: appears comfortable. Skin: warm, pink, no diaphoresis. HEENT: conjunctiva pink, moist mucous membranes. Cardiac: regular tachycardia without murmurs or gallops. Chest: clear to auscultation bilaterally. Abdomen: normoactive bowel sounds, no tenderness, no guarding, no masses. Extremities: no edema or cyanosis, 2+ symmetric radial and femoral pulses. Digital rectal examination: grossly bloody, dark clots, slowly oozing. Neurologic: awake, alert, normal.

Laboratory Findings: CBC: hemoglobin 10 g/dl, platelets 346,000/mm^3. Blood chemistries: normal. Coagulation profile: normal. ECG: sinus tachycardia without ischemia or infarction. Nasogastric lavage: clear without blood or coffee-ground material. Anoscopy: no masses, polyps, or fissures visualized; copious dark blood clots. Bleeding scan (see figure): active bleeding lesion identified in the sigmoid colon.

Questions: What is the most likely cause of this patient's lower gastrointestinal bleeding? What therapy should be initiated? What diagnostic tests should be considered?

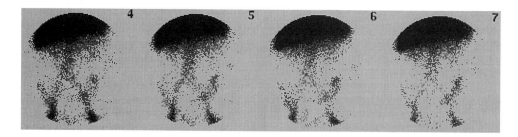

Diagnosis and Treatment: Lower gastrointestinal bleed from a sigmoid diverticular vessel. Priority is initial hemodynamic stabilization. Diagnostic options include anoscopy, colonoscopy, bleeding scan, and angiography.

Discussion: Gastrointestinal bleeding that originates from a source distal to the ligament of Trietz defines a lower gastrointestinal bleed. Although less common than upper gastrointestinal bleeding, lower gastrointenstinal bleeding is increasingly common because of its association with advancing age in conjunction with an aging population. The colon is the most common site of bleeding, although severe epistaxis, oropharyngeal, esophageal, and brisk upper gastric/duodenal bleeds also can manifest with grossly bloody stools due to the cathartic effects of large volumes of blood. Although diverticular bleeding vessels and arteriovenous malformations make up the majority of identifiable anatomic sources, there are other causes to consider (see table).

Bloody stool, either hematochezia (maroon or bright red stool) or melena (black tarry stool), is the cardinal physical finding or patient complaint. A history of stool frequency and color can be informative about the severity of the current episode. Frequent bright red stools suggest either a distal source or a brisk upper tract source, whereas black stools indicate blood from a proximal source with slower gastrointestinal transit time. Prior gastrointestinal medical and surgical problems and current medications are important to consider. Other patient-solicited historical factors have been shown to be of limited clinical usefulness.

The majority of lower gastrointestinal sources bleed intermittently and resolve spontaneously more than 80% of the time. This does not preclude a complete physical examination and diagnostic evaluation. Hemodynamic support and stabilization should occur simultaneously with the evaluation. Two large-bore intravenous lines and crystalloid fluid (normal saline or lactated Ringer's solution) should be started. Blood should be sent for type and cross-match if emergency or urgent blood transfusion is anticipated. Other routine blood tests should include complete blood cell count (CBC) and coagulation profiles. Elderly patients and those with a history of coronary disease, symptoms suggesting ischemia, and shock should undergo an electrocardiogram (ECG) to evaluate ischemia/infarction as a secondary complication. Orthostatic vital signs are commonly requested but add little clinical significance to serial monitoring of hemodynamics and CBC. Anoscopy is a fast and simple procedure that can identify extreme distal bleeding sources such as internal hemorrhoids, rectal muscosal tears, and rectal polyps/masses. Nasogastric lavage is important to expeditiously evaluate gastric bleeding sources.

Consultation with a gastroenterologist should occur early to coordinate diagnostic evaluation and definitive therapy. Colonoscopy is the study of choice for lower gastrointestinal bleeding events that have stopped. In addition to identifying the likely origin of bleeding, direct visualization of the entire large bowel permits evaluation of suspicious masses and lesions. The procedure can be both diagnostic and therapeutic. However, profuse bleeding and the need for bowel preparation often make emergency use prohibitive. For ongoing bleeding, angiography is indicated. Angiography is also both diagnostic and therapeutic, because embolization is an option when a bleeding lesion is identified. The study is invasive and has its own risk of morbidity.

A reasonable alternative for a stable patient is the technetium bleeding scan, a nuclear study that uses radiolabeled red blood cells or sulfur colloid to identify suspected sources of bleeding that exceed 0.1 ml/minute. After intravenous injection of the tracer, continuous phase imaging over the abdomen and pelvis is performed. Delayed static scans can be acquired for up to 24 hours if needed. Definitions of what constitutes a "positive" scan vary. For active bleeds, early tracer activity (termed "blush") identified in the abdominal/pelvic region, but outside of normal vascular distributions and normal organ activity, is considered positive. Results of a bleeding scan can then be used to guide angiographic embolization or colonoscopy.

Diagnostic yield of all procedures widely varies from 40% to 95%. Profuse bleeding and hemodynamic instability are indications for surgical consultation. Abdominal computed tomography(CT) has no role in the setting of acute gastrointestinal bleeding.

*Causes of Lower Gastrointestinal
Bleeding in Adults*

Diverticular disease
Angiodysplasia
Neoplasms/polyps
Inflammatory bowel disease
Medication induced (anticoagulants,
nonsteroidal anti-inflammatory drugs)
Infection (bacterial, viral, parasitic)
Massive upper gastrointestinal sources

The present patient passed several additional large maroon stools in the ED but remained hemodynamically stable. Gastroenterology was consulted and a bleeding scan was performed. An actively bleeding lesion was identified in the sigmoid region of the colon (see figure: extravasation of tracer at left iliac vessel just distal to the aortic bifurcation). The patient underwent a successful angiography-guided embolization of the bleeding vessel but required transfusion of 2 units of red blood cells. She was admitted to the ICU and discharged 2 days later with an uneventful hospital course. Follow-up colonoscopy revealed diverticular disease.

Clinical Pearls

1. Lower gastrointestinal bleeding resolves spontaneously in more than 80% of cases. However, most patients experience intermittent bleeding and therefore require a diagnostic evaluation.

2. In female patients, it is important to distinguish and confirm the site of bleeding as vaginal versus rectal.

3. Consider colonoscopy, a bleeding scan, or angiography for diagnostic evaluation in conjunction with gastroenterology consultation. Diagnostic yields of these studies vary from 40% to 95%.

4. Bleeding scans are noninvasive and appropriate for stable patients, and findings help guide therapeutic angiography or colonoscopy.

REFERENCES

1 Peter DJ, Dougherty JM: Evaluation of the patient with gastrointestinal bleeding: An evidence based approach. Emerg Med Clin North Am 17:239–261, 1999.

2. Bono MJ: Gastrointestinal emergencies: Lower gastrointestinal tract bleeding. Emerg Med Clin North Am 14:547–556, 1996.

3. Emslie JT, Zarnegan K, Siegel ME, Beart RW: Technetium-99m-labeled red blood cell scans in the investigation of gastrointestinal bleeding. Dis Colon Rectum 39:750–754, 1996.

Anthony W. Rekito, MD
William H. Shoff, MD, DTM&H

PATIENT 86

A 23-year-old man with shoulder pain after a fall

A 23-year old man with a negative past medical history presents to the emergency department complaining of right shoulder pain after a fall from his bicycle. He reports landing awkwardly on his right hand and arm after losing control and crashing. He denies loss of consciousness, head trauma, or any other complaints.

Physical Examination: Vital signs: pulse 105; blood pressure 118/66; respiratory rate 18; room air oxygen saturation 100%. General appearance: in distress secondary to pain in right shoulder; supporting right arm. Neck: nontender, with full range of motion. Chest: clear, nontender. Cardiac: heart rate regular without murmur or gallop. Abdomen: nontender; bowel sounds active. Back: nontender. Extremities: right shoulder with abnormal contour; supporting right forearm with left hand; resists any movement of left or right shoulder; unable to touch right palm to left shoulder. Neurologic: no focal deficit. Skin: minor abrasions bilaterally on knees and elbows.

Laboratory Findings: Anteroposterior (AP) and scapular Y radiographs (pre-and post-reduction) of the injured right shoulder: see figures (radiographs courtesy of AJ Dean, MD, Hospital of the University of the Pennsylvania).

Questions: What injury has this man sustained? What can be done to make him more comfortable? What other injuries should be considered?

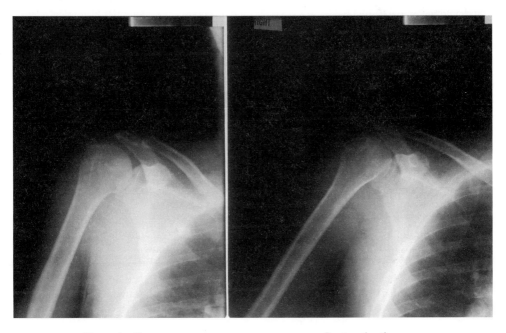

Pre-reduction   Post-reduction

AP VIEWS

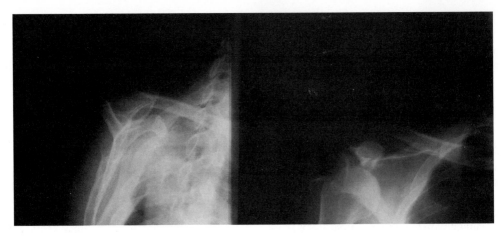

Pre-reduction   Post-reduction

SCAPULAR Y VIEWS

Diagnosis and Treatment: Anterior dislocation of the right shoulder with a greater tuberosity fracture. Treated by closed reduction and immobilization.

Discussion: Anterior shoulder dislocation is the most common joint dislocation encountered in the ED. Reduction is accomplished by a number of methods; however, care must be taken to avoid a number of complications. The glenohumeral joint is frequently dislocated because of its size and configuration. It is a weak joint capsule with a relatively high incidence of injury. Anterior dislocations account for more than 95% of all shoulder dislocations, whereas posterior dislocations account for 1.5% to 4% and inferior dislocations for less than 1%. The distribution of shoulder dislocations is bimodal, with peak incidences at age 20 to 30 in men and age 60 to 80 in women.

Patients with anterior shoulder dislocations, usually present with the injured arm held in slight abduction and internal rotation. The mechanism of injury is typically a combination of abduction, extension, and external rotation such as is produced by a fall on an outstretched hand. Rarely, a direct blow to the posterior shoulder can produce this injury. On physical examination, the shoulder is "squared off," with loss of the normal rounded deltoid contour. The humeral head may be palpable anteriorly beneath the clavicle (subcoracoid dislocation). There is resistance to abduction and internal rotation with consequent inability to touch the opposite shoulder.

A careful evaluation is necessary to rule out associated injuries. Potential injury to the axillary artery, although rare, is assessed by comparing radial pulses. Sensation over the lateral aspect of the upper arm must be tested to discern injury to the axillary nerve (4–12%). The motor component of the axillary nerve supplies the deltoid muscle, which should be tested after reduction. Neurovascular deficit is not a contraindication to closed reduction. Rotator cuff injuries occur in 10% to 15% of cases, particularly in primary dislocations in patients older than 40 years of age.

Radiographic studies prior to attempts at reduction document the type of dislocation and evaluate for associated fractures. The typical shoulder series consists of an AP view and an axillary or scapular Y view. The typical anterior dislocation is characterized by subcoracoid position AP view. It may be more obvious in the Y view. Humeral head and neck fractures should be ruled out, since significant displacement may be a contraindication to closed reduction. When certain of the diagnosis (recurrent dislocation with minimal trauma), some emergency physicians may skip prereduction radiography, because it does not alter management. Other osseous injuries that may occur are acromion fracture, coracoid fracture, glenoid rim fracture (bony Bankart lesions), greater tuberosity avulsion (10–15%), and posterolateral humeral head compression (Hill-Sachs lesion, 11–50%).

Several methods of closed reduction have proven safe and effective. Operator familiarity and patient comfort should guide selection of method. Conscious sedation should be utilized because it maximizes patient relaxation and analgesia. The Stimson technique involves a prone patient on the edge of the stretcher with the affected arm hanging toward the floor. Five to 15 pounds of weight are suspended from the wrist or arm, allowing for slow steady traction. This technique may require 20 to 30 minutes and slight rotation of the humerus to achieve reduction. The scapular manipulation technique also requires a prone patient with the affected arm hanging perpendicular to the floor. Once traction is applied and the patient is relaxed, the superior aspect of the scapula is stabilized with one hand while the inferior tip of the scapula is pushed medially toward the spine. The external rotation method involves the patient lying supine with the affected arm fully adducted and flexed 90 degrees at the elbow. One applies slow external rotation, pausing for pain, until the shoulder is reduced. In the traction-countertraction technique, the patient is supine with a sheet wrapped around the upper chest and under the axilla of the affected shoulder, by which an assistant provides countertraction. Axial traction is then applied to the affected arm with a sheet wrapped around the forearm and the elbow bent 90 degrees. Successful reduction by any technique is recognized by a slight lengthening of the affected arm and an audible and palpable "clunk" at the instant of reduction.

Postreduction care involves radiographs to document reduction and to identify fractures not evident on prereduction images. A repeat neurovascular and range of motion examination should be completed and documented. The shoulder is immobilized, using a shoulder immobilizer or a sling-and-swathe, until orthopedic follow-up. Appropriate oral analgesics should also be provided prior to discharge from the ED.

Posterior shoulder dislocations are much less common, and greater than 50% are missed on initial presentation because the radiograph may appear normal. The injury occurs as a result of excess force applied to an adducted, internally rotated, flexed humerus. The precipitating events include seizures, electrical shocks, and falls. On physical examination, the anterior shoulder is flat with a prominent coracoid. The humeral head may even be palpable beneath the acromion on the posterior shoulder. Neurovascular injuries are uncommon. On AP radiographs, the findings are subtle. Look for a distance of greater than 6 mm between the anterior glenoid labrum and the humeral head, giving it a "rifle barrel" appearance. It is more easily diagnosed by posterior displacement of the humeral head on the axillary view. Orthopedic consult is warranted because of the rarity of this injury. When missed, the posterior dislocation becomes locked for weeks to months, usually necessitating surgical intervention.

The extremely rare inferior shoulder dislocation (luxatio erecta) results from a hyperabduction injury levering the humerus against the acromion. The patient presents with the arm locked overhead in 110 to 160 degrees abduction, the elbow flexed, and the hand placed on or behind the head. Orthopedic consultation is required for management. Complications of this dislocation include severe soft-tissue injury, proximal humerus fractures, and detachment of the rotator cuff.

Clinical Pearls

1. More than 90% of shoulder dislocations are anterior, specifically subcoracoid.
2. Prereduction radiographs may not be necessary under appropriate clinical circumstances.
3. Always test for sensation in the distribution of the axillary nerve.

REFERENCES

1. Daya MR: Shoulder trauma. In Ferrera PC, Colucciello SA, Marx JA, et al, eds: Trauma Management: An Emergency Medicine Approach. St. Louis, Mosby, 2001.
2. Shuster M, Abu-Laban RB, Boyd J: Prereduction radiographs in clinically evident anterior shoulder dislocation. Am J Emerg Med 17:653–658, 1999.
3. Wen DY: Current concepts in the treatment of anterior shoulder dislocations. Am J Emerg Med 17:401–407, 1999.
4. McNamara R: Management of common dislocations. In Roberts JR, Hedges JR, eds: Clinical Procedures in Emergency Medicine, 3rd ed. Philadelphia, W.B. Saunders, 1998.

PATIENT 87

A 2-year-old boy with diffuse red rash for 2 days

A 2-year-old boy presents with abrupt onset of a red rash 2 days ago. It initially started on the face and then spread to the hands, feet, trunk, and extremities. The first lesions were round but now they have a variety of shapes. The child also has a mild upper respiratory illness associated with fever and sores on the lips and oral mucosa. There is no difficulty breathing and no ill contacts in the family.

Physical Examination: General appearance: alert toddler who is slightly irritable but well hydrated and comfortable. Skin: diffuse erythematous maculopapular rash on hands, feet, face (see figure), trunk, and extremities. Lesions are polymorphous, mostly round, and some have a "target" appearance (see figure). HEENT: shallow ulcerations on the tongue, buccal mucosa, and lips but no oral vesicles. The ulcerations on the lips and around the mouth have a slight vesicular and honey-crusted appearance.

Questions: What is the most likely diagnosis? What infectious cause is not likely associated with this condition?

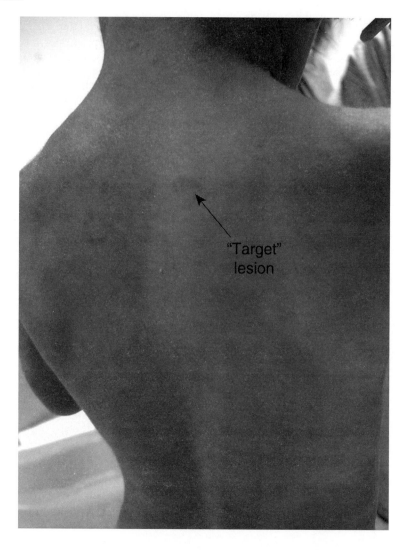

"Target" lesion

Diagnosis: Erythema multiforme minor with herpes simplex infection

Discussion: Erythema multiforme (EM) is a rash commonly seen in the ED. The rash is thought to be an immune-mediated acute hypersensitivity reaction from exposure to a sensitizing antigen. Precipitants of EM are myriad, but no cause is identified in up to 50% of cases. The most common drugs associated with EM are trimethoprim-sulfamethoxazole, cefaclor, phenytoin, and penicillins. Foods such as nuts and shellfish and infections with many agents (viral, bacterial, protozoal, and fungal) have also been implicated. Several infections that deserve special mention are herpes, streptocoocal, and mycoplasma infections, as these are some of the most commonly associated with EM.

Patients may initially report a prodrome of itching, burning, and malaise. The rash develops symmetrically and can begin on any part of the body. It has a predilection for the hands and feet and may be present on the palms and soles. Lesions may at first be solitary but often become confluent. Lesions are also of mixed type, and although they are most commonly erythematous and maculopapular, they may also be vesicular, bullous, or urticarial. The hallmark lesion is an erythematous macule with central clearing, referred to as a "target lesion," and these often establish the diagnosis.

Two forms of EM have been described: EM minor, in which there is cutaneous involvement alone or with slight mucous membrane involvement on one surface such as the mouth and limited systemic symptoms, and EM major, which is more extensive with skin and mucosal involvement and systemic symptoms such as fever, chills, or malaise. With significant mucosal involvement, the rash is often characterized instead as Stevens-Johnson syndrome and must be recognized as a true emergency requiring close monitoring and fluid support.

Treatment for EM consists of support and reassurance for the patients and family as well as discontinuation of any identified precipitants. Treatment should also be directed at underlying infections. Antihistamines, both oral and topical, can be used to control pruritus. For more severe cases, patients may require hospitalization for intravenous fluids and pain control.

Herpes simplex infection was considered the most likely precipitant in the present patient with EM minor. Treatment with acyclovir and antipruritics was initiated in the ED, and the patient was discharged home. The lesions persisted for approximately 3 weeks, and at follow-up they were noted to be nonpruritic, mostly macular, and slightly hyperpigmented. Within 4 weeks, the patient experienced complete resolution of the rash.

Clinical Pearls

1. The most common infectious causes of EM are herpes, mycoplasma, and streptococcal infections.

2. EM with extensive mucous membrane involvement (Stevens-Johnson syndrome) can be very severe and often necessitates hospitalization.

3. Treatment for EM is predominantly supportive but is also aimed at elimination of the precipitating agent.

REFERENCES

1. Gruskin K: Rash—maculopapular. In Fleisher GR, Ludwig S (eds): Textbook of Pediatric Emergency Medicine, 4th ed. Philadelphia, Lippincott Williams & Wilkins, 2001, pp 507–508.
2. Hurwitz S: Clinical Pediatric Dermatology: A Textbook of Skin Disorders of Childhood and Adolescence. Philadelphia, WB Saunders, 1993.

INDEX

B

Back pain
  seat belt syndrome-related, 237
  upper, aortic dissection-related, 38–40
Bacterial diseases. *See also* specific bacteria
  invasive, 83
Barium contrast enema, as intussusception treatment, 17
Benzocaine, as methemoglobinemia cause, 47
Beta-agonists, as asthma exacerbation treatment, 96
Beta-blockers
  as acute myocardial infarction treatment, 14
  as alcohol withdrawal treatment, 63
  as hypoglycemia cause, 32
  as thyroid storm treatment, 192, 193
Biliary obstruction, acute pancreatitis-related, 138–140
Blast injuries, firecracker accident-related, 225–227
Bleeding scans, for lower gastrointestinal bleeding evaluation, 249, 250
β-blockers. *See* Beta-blockers
Blood pressure. *See also* Hypertension; Hypotension
  systolic, in elderly patients, 116
Blood transfusions, in ruptured ectopic pregnancy patients, 72
Blunt trauma, 76–78, 128–130
Bordetella pertussis, as pertussis ("whopping cough") cause, 101
Borrelia burgdorferi, as Lyme disease cause, 35
Botulism, in infants, 145–147
Botulism immune globulin, as infant botulism treatment, 146, 147
Boyle's Law, 69
Bradycardia, anorexia nervosa-related, 54–56
Brain, child abuse-related atrophy of, 74, 75
Brainstem, intracerebral hemorrhage-related dysfunction of, 121
Brain tumors
  as altered mental status cause, 228–230
  as headache cause, 136
Bronchoscopy, rigid, use in pediatric patients, 92, 93
Bruises
  child abuse-related, 75
  coining-related, 220–221
Bulimia nervosa, 55
Bullets. *See also* Gunshot wounds
  as embolism cause, 231–233
Buttocks, gunshot wound to, 231–233

C

Cadioversion, as supraventricular tachycardia treatment, 5, 6
Calcium, as hyperkalemia treatment, 164
Calcium carbonate, as rickets treatment, 235
Calcium channel blockers, as subarachnoid hemorrhage treatment, 89, 90
Calcium gluconate, as hyperkalemia treatment, 163
Campylobacter jejuni
  as Guillain-Barré syndrome cause, 25
  as methemoglobinemia cause, 47

Cancer. *See also* specific types of cancer
  neutropenic fever associated with, 106–108
  Salmonella arizonae infection associated with, 118
Candidiasis, mucocutaneous, Addison disease-related, 175
Carboxyhemoglobin levels, in carbon monoxide poisoning, 113
Cardiac arrest
  methemoglobinemia-related, 47
  pit viper envenomation-related, 156
Cardiac output, in dilated cardiomyopathy, 110
Cardiomyopathy, dilated, 109–111
Cardiovascular disease, *Salmonella arizonae* infections associated with, 118
Carotid sinus syndrome, as syncope cause, 215
Cataracts, post-traumatic, 226
Catecholamines, in diabetic ketoacidosis, 50
Cavitary lesions, pulmonary, tuberculosis-related, 141–144
CD4 count, use in tuberculosis diagnosis, 142
Cefaclor, as erythema multiforme cause, 255
Cefotaxime, 2–3
  as bacterial meningitis treatment, 127
  as meningococcal disease treatment, 196
  as neonatal conjunctivitis treatment, 28
  as pneumococcal meningitis treatment, 83
Cefotetan, as pelvic inflammatory disease treatment, 133
Cefoxitin, as clenched-fist injury/human bite wounds treatment, 152
Ceftriaxone
  as bacterial meningitis treatment, 127
  as Lyme disease treatment, 35, 36
  as meningococcal disease prophylaxis, 195
  as neonatal conjunctivitis treatment, 28
  as pelvic inflammatory disease treatment, 133
  as pneumococcal meningitis treatment, 83
Central nervous system disorders, hyperthermia-related, 206
Central nervous system infections, as headache cause, 136
Cephalosporins, as bacterial meningitis treatment, 127
Cerebral perfusion pressure (CPP)
  in stroke patients, 86, 87
  in subarachnoid hemorrhage patients, 89
Cerebrospinal fluid analysis, in bacterial meningitis diagnosis, 126, 127
Cerebrospinal fluid pressure, elevated, 181–182
Cervical spine injuries, mandible fracture-associated, 172
Cesarean sections, emergency, 20, 21
Charcot's triad, 139
Chest
  blunt traumatic injuries to, 128–130
  pain in. *See* Pain, in chest
Child abuse
  as altered mental status cause, 229
  coining misdiagnosed as, 221

Corynebacterium, as human bite wound-related infection cause, 152

Cough
    mediastinal mass-related, 53
    nocturnal, asthma-related, 95
    of pertussis ("whooping cough"), 100, 101

Cranial nerve palsy/dysfunction
    intracerebral hemorrhage-related, 121
    Lyme disease-related, 35
    pit viper venom-related, 156

C-reactive protein
    as Kawasaki disease indicator, 166–167
    in pediatric invasive bacterial infection indicator, 83
    as pelvic inflammatory disease indicator, 132–133

Creatine kinase
    as rhabdomyolysis indicator, 213
    as rhabdomyolysis marker, 185, 186, 187

Crotaline antivenom, 155, 157

Crying, in infants
    as child abuse precipitating factor, 74
    excessive, 10, 11, 12
    intussusception-related, 17

Cryotherapy, contraindication as crotaline snakebite treatment, 156, 157

Cullen's sign, 139

Cultural competency, in health care, 220–221

Cushing-Kocher response, 121

Cyanosis
    as apparent life-threatening event (ALTE) component, 188, 189
    methemoglobinemia-related, 46, 47, 48
    pertussis ("whooping cough")-related, 101, 102

Cyst, ruptured ovarian, 179

Cytoxan, as opsoclonus-myoclonus treatment, 218–219

D

Dalton's Law, 69

"Dancing eyes, dancing feet," 218

Decontamination, of organophosphate poisoning patients, 201, 202

Dehydration
    altered mental status-related, 229
    anorexia nervosa-related, 55
    gastroenteritis-related, 245–247
    hyperglycemic hyperosmolar nonketotic syndrome-related, 212, 213
    as methemoglobinemia risk factor, 47, 48
    severity classification of, 246

1,25-Dehydroxyvitamin D, 235

Delirium tremens, 63

Depression, anorexia nervosa-related, 55, 56

Dermatitis, irritant, differentiated from lichen sclerosis et atrophicus, 58

Dexamethasone, as thyroid storm treatment, 192

Dextrose
    as hyperglycemic hyperosmolar nonketotic syndrome treatment, 212
    as hyperkalemia treatment, 164

Diabetes mellitus
    ketoacidosis associated with, 49–51
        as appendicitis mimic, 66
        as hyperkalemia cause, 163
        pediatric Addison disease-related, 175

Dialysis. *See also* Hemodialysis
    as thyroid storm treatment, 192

Diaphoresis, organophosphate poisoning-related, 200, 202

Diarrhea
    diabetic ketoacidosis-related, 50
    gastroenteritis-related, 245, 246, 247
    meningococcal infection-related, 194
    as methemoglobinemia risk factor, 46, 47, 48
    organophosphate poisoning-related, 200, 202

Diazepam, as alcohol withdrawal treatment, 63, 64

Diffuse axonal injuries, shaken baby syndrome-related, 74

Digits, hair-thread tourniquet-related strangulation of, 10–12

Digoxin, as hyperkalemia cause, 163, 164

Diplopia, idiopathic intracranial hypertension-related, 181, 182

Disopyramide, as hypoglycemia cause, 32

Disseminated intravascular coagulation
    hyperglycemic hyperosmolar nonketotic syndrome-related, 213
    pancreatitis-related, 139
    rhabdomyolysis-related, 186

Diuretics, potassium-sparing, as hyperkalemia cause, 163

Domestic violence
    injuries caused by, 43–44
    toward pregnant patients, 21

Doxycycline
    as Lyme disease treatment, 36
    as pelvic inflammatory disease treatment, 133
    as rickettsial disease treatment, 83

Drugs. *See also* specific drugs
    as hypoglycemia cause, 31–33
    as rhabdomyolysis cause, 186

Dysmetria, intracerebral hemorrhage-related, 121

Dyspepsia, gallstones-related, 104

Dyspnea
    acute hypercapneic respiratory failure-related, 148, 149
    blunt chest trauma-related, 128
    latex allergy-related, 168, 169
    mediastinal mass-related, 52, 53
    thyroid storm-related, 191
    tuberculosis-related, 142

E

Echocardiography, of dilated cardiomyopathy, 110

Edema
    cerebral
        diabetic ketoacidosis-related, 51
        hyperglycemic hyperosmolar nonketotic syndrome-related, 213
        shaken baby syndrome-related, 74

Edema (*Cont.*)
  facial, 197–199
  Kawasaki disease-related, 166
  pulmonary
    as acute respiratory failure cause, 149
    pit viper venom-related, 156
Ehrlichia infections, 83
Eikenella corrodens, as human bite wound-related infection cause, 152, 153
Elderly patients
  abdominal aortic aneurysm in, 97–99
  acute abdomen in, 115–116
  acute hypercapneic respiratory failure in, 148–150
  acute inferior wall myocardial infarction in, 13–15
  angiotensin-converting enzyme inhibitor-related angioedema in, 198
  cholecystitis in, 116
  heat-related illness in, 205–207
  hip fractures in, 243–244
  medication-induced hypoglycemia in, 31–33
  myocardial infarction in, 220–221
  syncope in, 214–216
  vital signs in, 116
Electrocardiography
  of acute myocardial infarction, 13, 14, 15
  of dilated cardiomyopathy, 109, 110
  in hyperkalemia patients, 162–164
  rickets-related abnormalities on, 234, 235
  for syncope evaluation, 215
Electrolyte abnormalities, rhabdomyolysis-related, 186
Electromyography
  for Guillain-Barré syndrome diagnosis, 25
  for infant botulism diagnosis, 146, 147
Embolism
  bullet-related, 231–233
  dilated cardiomyopathy-related, 108
  pulmonary, as acute respiratory failure cause, 149
Encephalitis, as opsoclonus-myoclonus cause, 218
Encephalomalacia, cystic, 74
Encephalopathy
  hypertensive, 159–161
  pertussis ("whooping cough")-related, 101
Endocrinopathies, as dilated cardiomyopathy cause, 110
Endotracheal intubation
  in angioedema patients, 198
  in asthmatic patients, 96
  as emergency respiratory support, 149
  in latex allergy patients, 169
  in mediastinal mass patients, 53
  noninvasive ventilation prior to, 149, 150
  in organophosphate poisoning patients, 201, 202
Enterobacter, as neutropenic fever cause, 107
Enterovirus infections, 83
Epididymitis, 204
Epiglottitis, meningococcal infection-related, 195
Epinephrine
  as anaphylaxis treatment, 169
  as angioedema treatment, 198

Epinephrine (*Cont.*)
  as cardiac ischemia cause, 198
  as severe asthma treatment, 96
Episcleritis, meningococcal disease-related, 196
Epistaxis, pertussis ("whooping cough")-related, 101
Epstein-Barr virus infections, 83
Errors, in medication administration, 31–33
Erythema
  clenched-fist injury/human bite wound-related, 152
  oropharyngeal, Kawasaki disease-related, 166
Erythema migrans, Lyme disease-related, 34, 35, 36
Erythema multiforme minor, herpes simplex infection-related, 254–255
Erythrocyte sedimentation rate
  in Kawasaki disease, 166–167
  in pelvic inflammatory disease, 132–133
Erythromycin, as pertussis ("whooping cough") prophylaxis and treatment, 101
Erythromycin ointment, as neonatal conjunctivitis treatment, 28
Escherichia coli
  as fever and petechiae cause, 83
  as meningitis cause, 127
  as methemoglobinemia cause, 47
  as neutropenic fever cause, 107
  as spontaneous bacterial peritonitis cause, 2, 3
Estrogen cream, as urethral prolapse treatment, 23
Ethambutol, as tuberculosis treatment, 143
Ethanol withdrawal syndrome, 62–64
Etomidate, use in asthmatic patients, 96
Exercise, as rhabdomyolysis cause, 186
Exercise tolerance, asthma-related decrease in, 95
Eye discharge, neonatal conjunctivitis-related, 27, 28, 30

F
Face
  edema of, 197–199
  traumatic injuries to, 171–173
Falls, as facial fracture cause, 171–173
FAST examination, in trauma patients, 77
Fatty-acid oxidation defects, as dilated cardiomyopathy cause, 110
Femur, osteomyelitis of, 118
Fenoldopam, as hypertensive emergency treatment, 161
Fetal distress, maternal trauma-related, 19–21
Fetus, effect of maternal trauma on, 19–21
Fever
  bacterial meningitis-related, 127
  clenched-fist injury/human bite wound-related, 152
  gallstones-related, 103
  Kawasaki disease-related, 165–167
  Neisseria meningitides infection-related, 82–84
  neutropenic, 106–108
  osteomyelitis-related, 117
  petechiae associated with, 82–84
  as supraventricular tachycardia cause, 4, 5, 7
  tuberculosis-related, 141, 142

Fibrinolytic therapy
  adverse effects of, 14
  contraindications to, 14
  for myocardial infarction, 14, 15
Firecracker accident injuries, 225–227
Fitz-Hughes-Curtis syndrome, 132
Floppiness, in infants, differential diagnosis of, 146
Fluid therapy, for hyperglycemic hyperosmolar non-
    ketotic syndrome, 212, 213
Flu-like symptoms, carbon monoxide poisoning-re-
    lated, 112
Flumazenil, contraindication in obtunded patients,
    229, 230
Fluoroquinolone, as clenched-fist injury/human bite
    wound treatment, 152
Folate supplementation, in alcoholics, 64
Folk medicine practices, 220–221
Food
  aspiration of, 92
  Salmonella arizonae transmission in, 118, 119
Foreign bodies
  aspiration of, 91–93
  cardiac, 231–233
  clenched-fist injury/human bite wound-related, 152
Formication, 63
Fractures
  bowing, 184
  buckle (torus), 183–184
  in children, 183–184
  clenched-fist injury/human bite wound-related, 152
  greenstick, 184
  gunshot wounds-related, 209
  of the hip, 243–244
  mandibular, 171–173
  pelvic, implication for patient transport, 70
  physeal (growth plate), 184
  rickets-related, 234, 235
  of skull, in children, 74
Fresh frozen plasma, as hereditary angioedema treat-
    ment, 198
Furosemide
  as idiopathic intracranial hypertension treatment, 182
  patient noncompliance with, 1

G
Gallbladder, Kawasaki disease-related hydrops of,
    166
Gallstones, 103–105
  hemolytic anemia-related, 139, 140
  as pancreatitis cause, 139
Gastroenteritis
  acute, 245–247
  infectious, as appendicitis mimic, 66
  Salmonella arizonae infection-related, 118
Gastroesophageal reflux, in neonates and infants, 189,
    224
Gaze deviation, intracerebral hemorrhage-related, 121
Genital lesions, in children, 57–59
Gentamicin, as pelvic inflammatory disease treatment,
    133

Glasgow Coma Scale scores
  in intracerebral hemorrhage patients, 121, 122
  in pediatric patients, 229
Globe, traumatic injuries to, 225–227
Glucagon, in diabetic ketoacidosis, 50
Glucocorticoids, as thyroid storm treatment, 192, 193
Glucose, as dehydration treatment, 247
Glucose-6-phosphate dehydrogenase deficiency, 47,
    48
Glycoprotein IIb/IIIa receptor antagonists
  as acute coronary syndrome treatment, 61
  contraindication in intracerebral hemorrhage, 121
Grey-Turner sign, 139
Groin pain, slipped capital femoral epiphysis-related,
    124
Growth hormone, in diabetic ketoacidosis, 50
Guanethidine, as thyroid storm treatment, 192
Guillain-Barré syndrome, 24–26
Gunshot wounds
  to buttocks, 231–233
  as peripheral vascular injury cause, 208–210

H
Haemophilus influenzae
  as fever and petechiae cause, 83
  as meningitis cause, 127
  as neonatal conjunctivitis cause, 29
Hair-thread tourniquets, 10–12
Hallucinosis, alcohol withdrawal-related, 63
Hand
  clenched-fist injury/human bite wounds to, 151–153
  firecracker accident-related injuries to, 225–227
Headaches
  carbon monoxide poisoning-related, 112
  classification of, 136
  idiopathic intracranial hypertension-related, 181,
      182
  intracerebral hemorrhage-related, 121
  Lyme disease-related, 34, 35, 36
  meningococcal infection-related, 195
  methemoglobinemia-related, 47
  migraine, 135–137
    as syncope cause, 215
  subarachnoid hemorrhage-related, 88, 89, 90
Head injuries, child abuse-related, 73–75
Health care
  racial and ethnic disparities in, 221
  refusal of, 240–242
Hearing loss, meningococcal disease-related, 196
Heart
  bullets lodged in or near, 231–233
  traumatic rupture of, 129
Heart block, hyperkalemia-related, 163
Heartburn. *See also* Gastroesophageal reflux
  gallstones-related, 104
Heart rate
  in elderly patients, 115, 116
  during supraventricular tachycardia, 4, 5
Heat stroke, 205–207
Helicopter transport, of patients, 68

Pain (*Cont.*)
pelvic inflammatory disease-related, 131–134
in pregnant patients, 19–21
seat belt syndrome-related, 237, 238
testicular torsion-related, 203–204
in back
abdominal aortic aneurysm-related, 98, 99
seat belt syndrome-related, 237
in chest
acute coronary syndrome-related, 60–61
aortic dissection-related, 39, 40
blunt trauma-related, 128, 129
myocardial infarction-related, 13–15, 220–221
thyroid storm-related, 191
as unstable angina, 60–61
epigastic, aortic dissection-related, 40
in groin, slipped capital femoral epiphysis-related, 124
in hip, slipped capital femoral epiphysis-related, 124
in knee, 123–125
left flank, abdominal aortic aneurysm-related, 97, 98, 99
pelvic, ruptured ectopic pregnancy-related, 71–72
right upper quadrant
gallstone pancreatitis-related, 139
gallstones-related, 104
pelvic inflammatory disease-related, 132
scrotal, 203–204
in shoulder, septic arthritis-related, 7–9
in thigh, slipped capital femoral epiphysis-related, 124
Palpation, abdominal, for abdominal aortic aneurysm detection, 98
Pancreatitis, acute, 138–140
Papilledema, idiopathic intracranial hypertension-related, 182
Parainfluenza virus infections, 83
Paralysis, Guillain-Barré syndrome-related, 24–26
Peak expiratory flow, during asthma exacerbations, 95
Pelvic inflammatory disease, 131–134
Penetrating injuries
to the extremities, 208–210
ocular, 225–227
Penicillin
as erythema multiforme cause, 255
as Lyme disease treatment, 36
Penicillin allergy, in clenched-fist injury/human bite wound patients, 152, 153
Penis, squamous cell carcinoma of, 58
Pentamidine, as hypoglycemia cause, 32
Pericardial effusion, cardiac foreign body-related, 232
Pericarditis, meningococcal, 195
Perihepatitis, 132
Peritonitis, spontaneous bacterial, 1–3
Petechiae
fever associated with, 82–84
Neisseria meningitides infection-related, 82–84
Pharyngitis, streptococcal, 83
Phenobarbital, as alcohol withdrawal treatment, 64

Phentolamine, as hypertensive emergency treatment, 161
Phenytoin, as erythema multiforme cause, 255
Phimosis, lichen sclerosis et atrophicus-related, 58
Photophobia
meningococcal infection-related, 195
subarachnoid hemorrhage-related, 88, 89
Physical examination, of infants, 11, 12
Pit viper bites, 154–158
Placental abruption, motor vehicle accident-related, 20
Plasmapheresis, as opsoclonus-myoclonus treatment, 218–219
Pleural effusions, gallstone pancreatitis-related, 139
Pneumonia
as acute respiratory failure cause, 149
as diabetic ketoacidosis risk factor, 50, 51
lower-lobe, as appendicitis mimic, 66
meningococcal infection-related, 195
pertussis ("whooping cough")-related, 101
Pneumocystis carinii, 142
Salmonella arizonae infection-related, 118
Pneumothorax
blunt trauma-related, 128, 129, 130
implication for patient transport, 67, 68, 69
mediastinal mass treatment-related, 53
pertussis ("whooping cough")-related, 101
tension, blunt chest trauma-related, 129, 130
Poisoning, 79–81
Polydipsia, hyperglycemic hyperosmolar nonketotic syndrome-related, 211
Polymerase chain reaction, for pertussis ("whooping cough") diagnosis, 101
Polyuria, hyperglycemic hyperosmolar nonketotic syndrome-related, 211
Potassium chloride, as hyperglycemic hyperosmolar nonketotic syndrome treatment, 212–213
Pralodoxime, as organophosphate poisoning treatment, 201, 202
Prednisone
as asthma exacerbation treatment, 95
as opsoclonus-myoclonus treatment, 218–219
Pregnancy
as aortic dissection risk factor, 39
as diabetic ketoacidosis risk factor, 50
ectopic
pelvic inflammatory disease-related, 133, 134
ruptured, 71–72
traumatic injuries during, 19–21
Pro-opiomelanocortin, as hyperpigmentation cause, 175
Propofol, as alcohol withdrawal treatment, 64
Propranolol, as thyroid storm treatment, 192
Propylthiouracil, 192
Protective clothing, for hospital personnel
N-95 masks, 142, 143
in organophosphate poisoning treatment, 201
Pruritus, erythema multiforme-related, 255
Pseudomonas, as neonatal conjunctivitis cause, 29
Pseudomonas aeruginosa, as neutropenic fever cause, 107

Ticaracillin/clavulanate, as clenched-fist injury/human bite wounds treatment, 152
Ticks, as Lyme disease vectors, 35–36
Tinea versicolor, differentiated from lichen sclerosis et atrophicus, 58
Tinnitus, idiopathic intracranial hypertension-related, 181, 182
Tongue, "strawberry," Kawasaki disease-related, 166
Tourniquets
    contraindication as crotaline snakebite treatment, 156, 157
    hair-thread, as strangulated digit cause, 10–12
Tracheal shift, blunt chest trauma-related, 129, 130
Transient ischemic attacks, as syncope cause, 215
Translation services, for non-English speaking patients, 221
Transport
    patient's refusal of, 240–242
    of pediatric trauma patients, 67–70
Trauma
    blunt, 76–78, 128–30
    as headache cause, 136
    multiple
        firecracker accident-related, 225–227
        in gunshot injury patients, 209, 210
        as indication for patient transport, 67–70
    during pregnancy, 19–21
    as rhabdomyolysis cause, 185–187
    thoracic, 128–130
Trauma centers, transport of pediatric patients to, 67–70
Trichomonas, as pelvic inflammatory disease cause, 132
Trimethoprim sulfa/clindamycin, as clenched-fist injury/human bite wounds treatment, 152
Trimethoprim sulfa/metuoxazole, as erythema multiforme cause, 255
Tuberculin skin testing, in human immunodeficiency virus-positive patients, 142, 143
Tuberculosis
    in human immunodeficiency virus-positive patients, 141–144
    latent, 143
Tumor lysis syndrome, 53
Turner's syndrome, as aortic dissection risk factor, 39

U
Ultrasonography
    for appendicitis diagnosis, 66
    emergency medicine bedside, 104–105
        of abdominal aortic aneurysm, 98
        for acute pancreatitis evaluation, 138, 139, 140
        for syncope evaluation, 177, 178, 179, 180
    of gallstones, 103, 104, 140
    of intussusception, 17
    transabdominal, for gallstone detection, 140
    transvaginal, 71, 72
    in trauma victims, 77
Unresponsiveness, hypoglycemia-related, 31–33

Urethral prolapse, in children, 22–23
Urethritis, meningococcal, 195
Urinalysis, for rhabdomyolysis diagnosis, 185, 187
Urinary retention, hematocolpos-related, 41–42
Urticaria, anaphylaxis-related, 169

V
Vaginal bleeding
    pelvic inflammatory disease-related, 132
    ruptured ectopic pregnancy-related, 71–72
    urethral prolapse-related, 22–23
Vaginal discharge, pelvic inflammatory disease-related, 131, 132–133
Valproic acid, as hypoglycemia cause, 32
Valvular heart disease, cardiac foreign body-related, 232
Vancomycin
    as meningococcal disease treatment, 196
    as pneumococcal meningitis treatment, 83
Vascular injuries
    hip fracture-related, 244
    peripheral, gunshot wound-related, 208–210
Vasculitis
    Kawasaki disese-related, 166, 167
    meningococcal disease-related, 196
Vasospasm, subarachnoid hemorrhage-related, 89
Vegetarianism, maternal, as rickets risk factor, 235
Venous injuries, gunshot wound-related, 209–210
Ventricular fibrillation, hyperkalemia-related, 163
Verapamil, contraindication in children, 5
Vision loss
    firecracker accident-related, 226
    idiopathic intracranial hypertension-related, 182
Vital signs, in elderly patients, 116
Vitamin D, as rickets treatment, 235
Vitamin D deficiency, as rickets cause, 235
Vitiligo, differentiated from lichen sclerosis et atrophicus, 58
Volvulus, intestinal malrotation-associated, 223
Vomiting
    Addison disease-related, 174
    alcohol withdrawal-related, 63
    in altered mental status patients, 228, 230
    bacterial meningitis-related, 127
    bilious, in neonates, 222–224
    carbon monoxide poisoning-related, 112
    diabetic ketoacidosis-related, 49, 50
    gallstones-related, 104
    gastroenteritis-related, 245, 246, 247
    idiopathic intracranial hypertension-related, 181, 182
    induced, in bulimia nervosa patients, 55
    intracerebral hemorrhage-related, 121
    Kawasaki disease-related, 166
    meningococcal infection-related, 194, 195
    methemoglobinemia-related, 46
    opsoclonus-myoclonus-related, 217
    pertussis ("whooping cough")-related, 100, 101
    shaken baby syndrome-related, 73, 74
Vulvar carcinoma, lichen sclerosis et atrophicus-related, 58